# WE DID THE BEST WE COULD

## How To Create Healing Between The Generations

**Lorie Dwinell and Ruth Baetz**

With contributions by
Patsy Burnett Carter • Constance B. Huey • Chandra Smith

**Health Communications, Inc.**
**Deerfield Beach, Florida**

**Library of Congress Cataloging-in-Publication Data**

Dwinell, Lorie, 1939-
    We did the best we could/by Lorie Dwinell; with contributions by
    Ruth Baetz...[et al.].
        p.    cm.
    Inclues bibliographical references.
    ISBN 1-55874-269-7
    1. Parent and adult child.   I. Baetz, Ruth.   II. Title.
HQ755.86.D95 1993                                    93-24747
306.874—dc20                                              CIP

©1993 Lorie Dwinell
ISBN 1-55874-269-7

Publisher: Health Communications, Inc.
            3201 S.W. 15th Street
            Deerfield Beach, Florida 33442-8190

*Cover design by Barbara Bergman*

# DEDICATIONS

Lorie dedicates this book to
my beloved Aunt LaDean Jones, my clients
and my bungee-cord friends

Ruth dedicates this book to
Sandra Jo

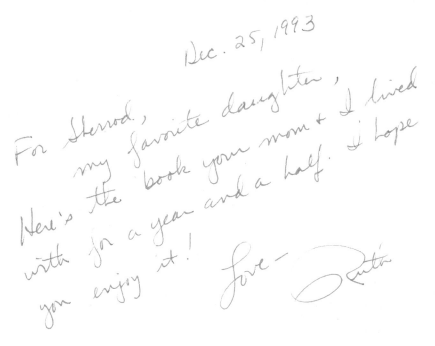

Dec. 25, 1993

For Sherrod, my favorite daughter, Here's the book your mom + I lived with for a year and a half. I hope you enjoy it! Love— Ruth

# CONTENTS

## SECTION 1: OUR PARENTAL TOOLBOX

## SECTION II: THE BIG PICTURE

## SECTION III: OUR HEALING JOURNEY

# ACKNOWLEDGMENTS

In September 1990, I decided to take a one-year sabbatical to rest, reflect and complete the book I had been developing during the prior three years. But nothing is ever as simple as we hope it will be. Within a month, crises hit my life, and the sabbatical for my writing had to be shared with grief work.

It was at this point I discovered that although I felt as though I were in a 15,000-foot free fall, I was not without support. I had "bungee-cord" friends who surrounded me with loving care.

I worked on this book as I was able to. I asked three colleagues, Constance B. Huey, Patsy Burnett Carter and Chandra Smith, for help.

First, I asked them to help me test out the viability of my model in a series of Parents of Adult Children workshops. Second, I asked them to write chapters based on the sections of the workshops they led.

Because each of us was in trauma in her own life, our planning meetings became a combination of personal growth, support and workshop brainstorming. The love and support we gave each other during our planning sessions freed us to be more effective both personally and professionally.

By the beginning of 1992, I had gone through a year of grief recovery and was thoroughly stalled on the book again. Connie and Patsy, who had already completed their chapters, began to function as my pitchforks-in-the-rump. They were excited about the model's potential for helping parents and about their chapters.

They each had asked Ruth Baetz, a gifted psychotherapist, writer and editor, to edit their chapters. Ruth was like magic.

As a psychotherapist, she was excited by the book and deeply committed to the ideas it represented. She was passionate about the book's completion and had been essential to the fine work that Connie and Patsy had completed.

She joined me as co-author of the book and took on the job of shepherding the entire project — cajoling, suggesting, coordinating and editing. I owe Ruth a tremendous debt of gratitude.

We have a book! This book could not have been completed without Connie, Patsy, Chandra, Ruth and my secretary, Alice Mezias. It also could not have been completed without all of my bungee-cord friends who have loved and supported me throughout the course of this project. Please bear with me as I thank each person who has contributed to my life and to this project.

First, I would like to thank Alice Mezias. Alice not only typed the entire manuscript from beginning to end but, as a parent of children entering adulthood, gave me essential feedback. I have been loved and supported by Alice from the very beginning of our relationship many years ago, and I anticipate that Alice and I will grow old together, forever good friends.

I would like to thank Sandy Ruvelson for her loving patience and her "Atta-girl" encouragement. Sandy read each chapter (or listened while I read it to her over the phone) and tested out the exercises both from the perspective of a parent and from the perspective of an adult child. Her feedback and support have been invaluable.

I would also like to thank Barbara Nichols, my editor at Health Communications, Inc., for her belief in this project and her patience with the realities of my life over the past two years. Thanks also to editors Patricia Reese Boyd and William Heyward for fine-tuning the manuscript.

I extend my gratitude to Peter Vegso and Gary Seidler of both Health Communications, Inc. and U.S. Journal Training, Inc. and to Dan Barmettler of the Institute for Integral Development. Without the work offered by each of these men, I would have lacked the financial resources to complete this book. Their belief in this project has helped it come to fruition.

My closest friends have literally loved me back to health over the past two years. They not only supported me in the writing of this book but also, more important, supported me in what has been the most difficult and, oddly enough, the most exciting and rewarding time in my life. I feel especially the deepest gratitude to my friends: Claudia Black, Jack Fahey, Bill Ferguson, Mike Berni, Doug Haldeman, Dawn Baker, Bill and Nancy Thorn, Elaine DuCharme, Marcia Parish, Pat McCullough, Jane Terry, Marilyn Mason, JoAnn Krestan, Claudia Bepko, Roxy Lerner, Stephanie Covington, Rebecca Brown, Annette Chaudet, Greg and Cathy Bates, Sarah and Don Lowell, Carol Allen and Pat Dunn, Matalie Wham, Nancy Archer, Judy Nottrott, Marian Greher, Kay D'Angelo, Sally Graves, Nan Whitaker-Emrich, Susan Grout, Sybil Vaughn, Craig Bader, Elaine Tyrie, John and Carol Halleran, Carla and Stu Clark, Sue Flood, Pat Walker, David Dickman, Jan McKamy, Julie Holladay, Jim and Jean Northrup, Ken and Mary Fox, Del and Jean Fogelquist, A. Carol McDaniel, Mary LeLoo, Caren Monastersky, Susan Rush, Judy Kimmell and Barbara Mack.

I would also like to thank the many wonderful clients I have had the privilege of working with over the past several years: Thank you for trusting me and for entrusting yourselves and your work to me.

Last, but not least, I would like to thank my 74-year-old mother, my 86-year-old stepdad, both of my brothers, Bill and David Dwinell; my wonderful sisters-in-law Karen and Pat; and my nieces Kathy, Erica and Jeanine.

I deeply wish my beloved aunt, LaDean Jones, after whom I was named, were still alive to read this book: Aunt Dean, you were one of my "good-mother people." I hope you're sitting on the edge of a cloud in heaven reading a copy of this book right now. I hope you know how much I love you and how important you have been in my life.

# INTRODUCTION

## All Parents Do The Best They Can
## And Their Best Is Never Good Enough

It's true. All of us parents do the best we can, and our best is never good enough. Such is the nature of being human, limited and imperfect.

This book is intended to help us take a realistic and compassionate look at the young parents we once were. It is those young parents we are judging when we criticize or feel guilty about our imperfect parenting, and we must see them clearly before we can judge them with any justice. We may eventually need to own up to, or even apologize for, some mistakes we made as parents. But first we need to remove ourselves from the current climate of parent-bashing and put our parenting into its proper context.

This book is for all of us who wonder what effect our parenting has had on our children. It is for the wide variety of us — stepparents, co-parents, foster parents, grandparents who raised grandchildren and, of course, biological parents.

Some of us who have suffered from addiction have enough recovery to look at our children and our children's problems with feelings of shame and personal responsibility. Some of us are in the midst of our midlife crisis, evaluating the first half of our lives and wanting to clear up the messes of the past before we take on the second half. Some of us are feeling the pressures of being the sandwich generation — caught between the needs and expectations of our elderly parents, on the one hand, and our children and our grandchildren on the other.

We will look at the tools and attitudes we brought to parenting. What did we really know when we began parenting? We will look at the context in which we parented — at the events in our extended family and in the culture that influenced our parenting. We will work through our own feelings about our parenting so we are prepared, if we choose, to dialogue with our children and heal the pain between us.

This book is about hope and encouragement. It is also about a journey, and it is not a journey for sissies. It takes courage and commitment to face our fears, especially the feared condemnation by our children.

It is far easier, although in the long haul far more emotionally expensive, either to deny the reality of our remorse, shame and guilt or to avoid dealing with the issues between ourselves and our children altogether. If we fail to take this journey, we pay a price by having perfunctory, empty, guilt-tinged interactions with the children to whom we gave life and with whom we began this journey of parenting with such good intentions.

Parenting is difficult for everyone, but it has been especially difficult for those of us who have been recovering from any major life dysfunction — depression, substance abuse, mental problems, eating disorders and so forth. While I intend this book to help all parents who have undergone the arduous task of parenting in the past 60 years, it is most especially for parents in recovery.

Most parents who are in recovery know the history I'm about to recount. I tell it here because it's important for all of us — whether we are in recovery or not — to see how on earth we got into this situation with our children. It didn't happen overnight, and it didn't happen just to our individual family. It's part of a worldwide movement that's been going on for over 60 years. For whatever reason, it began with the treatment of alcoholism.

## Demon Rum

At the turn of the century the most widely recognized addictive disorder was alcohol addiction. The power attributed to it was evident in epithets like "evil spirits," "demon rum" and so on.

Individuals afflicted with alcohol addiction were not called alcoholics, but instead were called inebriates, drunkards and derelicts. They were characterized as weak-willed sinners who needed to see the error of their ways and repent or as wayward souls who needed to get right with God in order to recover.

As you can well imagine, the legitimate treater for such individuals was the church, a potential haven for sick souls. Alcohol addiction was seen as a manifestation of moral failing and lack of character. There was little or no recognition that these individuals had a disease or an addiction.

From the 1920s through the 1940s, alcohol addiction was redefined when Freudian and psychodynamic explanations of behavior hit the belief system of the larger culture. Individuals who were alcohol-addicted were no longer seen as sinners, but as people with deep-seated psychoneurotic disorders.

The church, therefore, was no longer the legitimate treater of these poor, wretched souls. Now medicine, particularly psychiatry, was The Way, The Truth and The Light. Through analysis, alcoholic drinking would disappear and the alcoholic would be able to drink normally. From the addictive drinker's perspective, this was like offering to redecorate the living room while the house was on fire.

## AA Is Born

It was within this social climate that Alcoholics Anonymous (AA), the self-help psychotherapy system that has become the model for all subsequent 12-Step programs, was founded in June 1935. With its inception, a new definitional system was developed. Alcohol addicts were now called alcoholics and seen as suffering from an addiction or illness. This meant they were burdened with both an allergy of the body and a compulsion of the mind, which, when taken together, made being a temperate, reasonable drinker impossible.

Alcoholics Anonymous has helped many addicted drinkers stop the downward spiral of self-destructive and other-destructive drinking. After its inception, it spread rapidly throughout North America and eventually took root in other countries as well. In

July 1990, Alcoholics Anonymous celebrated its 55th anniversary in Seattle, Washington, with 46,000 Alcoholics Anonymous and Al-Anon members from all over the world celebrating "55 Years, One Day at a Time."

Alcoholics Anonymous provided an antidote to the despair of the addicted drinker. Through the support of others similarly afflicted, it offered a chance of recovery from this illness. With its emphasis on the psychological as well as the spiritual aspects of addiction, it provided an opportunity to stop addictive drinking while gaining emotional and spiritual insight into one's behavior. Through the recommended 12-Step format, one could repair the damage done to one's relationship with self and others.

Anything that can be used can be abused. While Alcoholics Anonymous, under the best of circumstances, can provide an opportunity for sobriety and for emotional and spiritual growth, under the worst of circumstances it can be used to avoid looking at how one's early life contributed to developing an addiction and to avoid looking too closely at the effect one's alcoholism has had on others. This is not the intent of Alcoholics Anonymous, nor is there a suggestion that Alcoholics Anonymous be changed in any way. It is simply a descriptive statement of the misuse to which this self-help system can be put.

Alcoholics Anonymous encourages letting go of the past. At the Ninth Step, one makes amends to anyone who was harmed. Then one is encouraged to keep current one's personal inventory of harm done and one's amends, but not to look to the past for causes or more detailed damage done. It is feared that dwelling on the past will trigger alcoholic self-pity and an addiction relapse, as in "Poor me, poor me, pour me a drink."

## Al-Anon Is Born

Al-Anon is the self-help psychotherapy system for family members, friends and colleagues of individuals suffering from alcoholism. Al-Anon is now over 40 years old. It has the capacity to cool off the over-reactiveness of individuals who are relating to alcoholics.

Over the years, many terms have been applied to this over-reactive response to addiction: enabling, co-alcoholism, over-responsibility or co-dependency. But whatever term we choose to use, the process is the same: Al-Anon helps individuals detach with love from the consequences of someone else's addictive behavior and stop the over-responsible reactions that feed into the alcoholic's continued drinking.

One of the paradoxes of relating to an addicted person is that one cannot not respond. Even in not responding, one is responding. So Al-Anon helps friends and family members shift from inappropriate, unhealthy and disabling responses to healthier, more appropriate responses focused on the co-alcoholic's own self and needs.

By definition, co-dependency is the chronic abuse or neglect of self in favor of someone or something else. Al-Anon members learn that since they didn't cause, and hence can't cure or control, the alcoholic's drinking, they need to stop neglecting themselves and their own needs.

Again, anything that can be used can be abused, and Al-Anon is no exception. The detachment Al-Anon recommends, which is so essential to the co-dependent person's recovery, can move partners into a nonintimate, perfunctory, fixed-distance relationship. This helps them avoid the accumulation of hurt and anger generated during the active years of addiction.

It can also help partners avoid the inner guilt both feel about the effects alcoholism and co-dependency have had on family life. "Letting go of the past" can fend off an awareness of any real and imagined damage done to the children.

My statements are intended to be descriptive, not critical, of Al-Anon. I would not propose any changes in Al-Anon. As it now stands, it is an excellent example of a self-help psychotherapy system and meets a very vital need.

## The Capsule Of Transport

You will notice I have started to use *addiction* rather than just *alcoholism* or *alcohol addiction*. Let me explain this shift.

In the late 1960s in the United States, mental health problems, alcoholism and drug addiction were seen as separate issues both by the individuals recovering from these problems and by governmental agencies. It was important to alcoholics not to be seen as "dope fiends" or "mental cripples." Ironically, it was just as important to drug addicts not to be seen as "winos" or "crazies."

Then in the 1970s the drug treatment establishment began to recognize that addiction was addiction, that many drugs were cross-addicting with one another and that the addictive process was quite similar regardless of the specific actions of different drugs. Workers in the addiction field began to talk about substance abuse addictions. At first, *substances* just meant alcohol and other drugs; later food was included as well.

Next, the definition of addiction was expanded even more as it came to be recognized that any thing, substance or process that altered our experience of ourselves or of reality could constitute an addiction. As Milkman and Sunderwirth point out in *Craving For Ecstasy,* anything could serve as a "capsule for transport" — fame, power, sex, work, ideas, spending, earning, food, excitement, drugs, alcohol, relationships, even self-help books and groups — altering our experience of ourselves and our world in an addictive way.

## The Tender Turtle

Let me go back to the family's perspective. Family members of newly recovering addicts characteristically hold their breaths during the two to five years of early recovery when their newly abstinent family member is at high risk for relapse. This period is what I call the tender turtle time.

Any addiction is like the hard protective shell of a desert box turtle. The addiction/shell protects addicts from feeling the degree to which their lives are out of control, shame-filled and self- and other-destructive. Recovery is like sliding our hands under the turtles' thick protective shells of addiction and ripping them off. Then we put these bloody tender turtles back in their environments, minus the shell, and say, "Cope." You can see why the turtles have all they can do simply staying sober, and why the turtles are in no position to hear in much detail how their addiction has hurt family members.

Family members, full of pain themselves as a result of living with active addiction, are loath to rock the boat or discuss past hurts also. In fact, they will do anything in their power to prevent a relapse in the addict.

With the founding of Alcoholics Anonymous in 1935, I believe the entire culture began holding its breath, waiting to see if Alcoholics Anonymous and later Al-Anon could really help stop the cycles of destructive drinking and destructive co-dependency. As more individuals were helped by AA, by Al-Anon and by public and private treatment resources, the recovery movement was born. Subsequently it gathered tremendous momentum as recovering people carried the message that recovery was possible, both from substance abuse and from the mirror illness of co-dependency.

## Recovery Takes Time

Addiction recovery, whether substance or process addiction, is a time-dependent process. It takes many years for tender turtles, no matter what addiction made up their shells, to develop new, healthier coping responses and communication skills. It also takes many years — not months, but years — for them to work through their feelings about having been addicted and about the effects that their addiction had on their families.

One mother, at the five-year mark in her recovery, stated, "Thank God, my alcoholism has not affected my children." She said this in spite of evidence that her addiction, which had developed when her youngest son was 12 years old, had dramatically affected his life course.

When such a parent is in early recovery, the guilt she feels about how her addiction has affected her children is often temporarily lessened by a tremendous sense of relief. She has learned a name for the illness with which she is afflicted, and she has learned there is a way back to wholeness via recovery. She is in the honeymoon or pink-cloud period of early recovery.

Being in the honeymoon phase, this mother was unable to acknowledge that the age of 12 is a developmentally critical time for any child, but it is especially so for a young male trying to separate from an attractive, seductive mother with whom he is overly close. Her drunken, sexually inappropriate behavior toward her son and toward other men in her environment had both disgusted him and made him hesitant to separate from her for fear there would be no one else to protect her from harm. At the 11-year mark in her recovery, this same mother, no longer needing her turtle shell of denial, was able to mourn the influence of her addiction on her son's life.

Parents who are in any 12-Step program, such as Alcoholics Anonymous, Al-Anon, or Co-dependency Anonymous, often make amends to their children by using the Fourth, Fifth, Eighth and Ninth Steps.

Step 4. Made a searching and fearless moral inventory of ourselves.

Step 5. Admitted to God, to ourselves, and to another human being the exact nature of our wrongs.

Step 8. Made a list of all persons we had harmed and became willing to make amends to them all.

Step 9. Made direct amends to such people whenever possible, except when to do so would injure them or others.

The amends made are genuine and heartfelt, but can seem highly ritualized, nonemotional and robot-like because parents feel terror when they name aloud to their children the actions they regret. The parents' anguish during this process can be so great that an inadvertent "Don't-talk" message can be conveyed to the children. Their words may say, "I have a disease. I am not responsible for having a disease. My behavior was symptomatic of my disease. I have harmed you. I didn't mean to. I am sorry." Meanwhile, their tone and body language may say, "And this is the last time I want to talk about it. I've said I'm sorry and I'm not going to say it again or allow you to beat me up."

Rather than opening the door and creating dialogue, such an amends process can lead to an emotional cutoff. The parents and children can move into a fixed-distance, perfunctory relationship — each person carrying pain, unexpressed feelings and unspoken words. A powerful invisible barrier has been constructed between them that reads, "No Trespassing. Danger Zone. High Potential for Explosion. Keep Out."

## ACoA Is Born

It was not until about 1977 that children who had grown up in addicted families felt able to believe that there were enough culture-wide recovery resources on board for them to break their silence. With the ACoA (Adult Children of Alcoholics) movement, they could begin to work through the unmourned losses of their childhoods, which they had had to deny and delay processing until they could trust that recovery was a real possibility for the parental generation.

In a sense, over 40 years of successful substance abuse recovery in the culture functioned as an emotional safety net for these children of alcoholic parents. Finally they could break the conspiracy of silence that had told them all their childhoods, "There's nothing wrong here. Don't talk about it; don't trust; don't feel."

I believe, by the way, that the ACoA movement came into being in response to two things: First, the demonstrated track record of AA and Al-Anon; second, the growing recognition in the therapy and recovery fields that addiction attempts to cover emotional pain that has been rooted in our childhoods. ACoA uses the proven 12-Step methods of AA and Al-Anon to address psychic pain directly.

Just as the definition of addiction was eventually expanded to include substance and process addictions, so also the definitional system of the Children of Alcoholics movement has been expanded to become the Adult Children of Alcoholics/Dysfunctional Families movement. Individuals who include themselves in it are encouraged to look for the origins of their present pain in their childhood family experiences and in their interactions with their parents.

Whereas Alcoholics Anonymous sobers up the family system and Al-Anon cools it down, Adult Children of Alcoholics self-help groups tend to heat it up dramatically. ACoA speaks directly to the pain that these adult offspring of alcoholics have experienced as children.

The Adult Children of Alcoholics movement is basically a grief work movement. Under the best of circumstances, Adult Children of Alcoholics groups can provide a place to grieve over the losses of childhood, to identify hurts and to hold parents accountable for harm done, both real and imagined. Under the worst of circumstances, again remembering that anything that can be used can be abused, Adult Children of Alcoholics meetings can become a place to play the blame game, can become a chapter of "Whiners Anonymous" and can be a place to stay unforgiving and emotionally cut off from family members.

If we failed our children — if we did the best we could and feel or fear it wasn't good enough — we are accountable first and foremost to ourselves and then to our children. But the current atmosphere of parent-bashing and holding parents totally responsible for all of our children's adult problems is not an atmosphere that promotes dialogue between the generations.

---

### Reader's Note

This book is based on the work of well-known family therapist Lorie Dwinell. All first-person statements in the text, such as "I discovered," "my workshop," "my clients," and so forth, refer to Dwinell's work.

Ruth Baetz, a therapist herself, was the wordsmith for this book.

# CHAPTER

# 1

# Please Don't Shoot
# The Piano Player

W̲e live in odd times. Ours is the first generation of parents whom the younger generation feels it has the right to hold directly accountable for how our parenting has affected them in adulthood.

Most of us feel angry about this turn of events. Many of us, in fact, wonder from time to time, "Hey, when did they change the rules? How come, after I tried so hard to be responsible, to play fair and to do what I was told, I get judged by my children, using a set of rules that didn't even exist when I began playing the game?"

Most of us also feel emotions ranging from mild discomfort to debilitating shame and guilt. We look back with the wisdom and

1

maturity of the present on the job we did as parents and think, "If only I had known this . . . . If only I had (or hadn't) done that. . . ." Many of us live in a guilt- and shame-filled silence, sure that everyone can see how we failed. We judge ourselves unmercifully from within, and we wait in abject terror for what seems like the inevitable confrontation with our children.

Parenting is probably the most important job we will ever undertake in the course of a lifetime, and it's also the job for which we are the most ill prepared.

I remember seeing a billboard along a Seattle roadside several years ago that poignantly spoke to this issue. In the center of the billboard sat a baby with a tag attached to its diaper. The tag read, "A baby is the only complicated piece of machinery delivered without a set of instructions."

The only set of instructions most of us received for the job of parenting came from our own experience of having been parented, for better or for worse. We absorbed our parents' values and methods unconsciously, often completely unaware of what we had learned until we heard ourselves using a familiar tone of voice or familiar words with our own children.

Some of us never gave the parenting methods we learned a moment's thought. As a matter of fact, we never thought about whether we wanted to be parents at all. Our generation, now in its mid-40s and older, was not allowed the luxury of questioning whether or not children would be part of our lives. Getting married, having children and getting a job were rock-solid societal expectations. They were the rites of passage that said we were now grown-ups.

We did what we thought we were supposed to do, never or seldom questioning how it was to be done. Unconsciously we drew on the models of parenting we had experienced in our own childhoods. We unwittingly lived out the rule: You can't know what you don't know — and what you do know is usually what you yourself have experienced.

Another substantial group of us are the parents I call the 180-degree-pendulum-swing parents. We are the ones who actively and consciously rejected some or all of the parental modeling we experienced in our families as we grew up. We vowed to give our children a better childhood than we ourselves had had.

The problem was that knowing what we *didn't* want to do as parents didn't mean we knew what we *did* want to do. Many of us simply did the opposite of what our own parents had done and hoped for the best. If our parents had been rigid, we were permissive. If our parents had been chaotic, we were structured.

Then when "modern" concepts of parenting were made popular with the influence of child-rearing experts such as Benjamin Spock, those of us in the 180-degree-pendulum-swing group breathed a sigh of relief. We could now take on this most difficult of all tasks with some degree of assurance that modern experts would guide us. Now we wouldn't fail.

But, alas, the experts often didn't agree with one another, or they had maladjusted children themselves, in spite of their theories. About the time we had mastered one theory of parenting, along came a new expert who said we had been doing it all wrong. What a confusing enterprise!

We began showing up in therapy with anxiety neuroses we had developed while trying to be perfect and deliberate parents. Parenting in the newly emerging multiple-option society of the last half of this century was not only proving to be a difficult task, but seemed also to be creating almost as many problems as we modern parents had set out to solve.

This scenario was further complicated by being played out against a backdrop of constant cultural turmoil. The mythologist, Joseph Campbell, in *The Power of Myth*, says that the end product of 50 years of unprecedented social change in contemporary society has been a loss of the myths and rituals that inform our humanness.

We had lost all our familiar support systems and had little that was useful to put in their places. Although our contemporary society had made us "resource rich," our resources were secondary people — counselors, attorneys or teachers. Gone were the days when we could rely on the primary resource people of our extended family — parents, grandparents, aunts, uncles — and on long-time friends of our neighborhood or village. Now we lived hundreds of miles from the neighborhoods of our birth and paid secondary resource people to help us solve problems that once were discussed over a cup of coffee at the kitchen table. We "processed" our feelings with therapists rather than "telling our troubles" to family members and friends.

By the time our children were adults or almost adults, the Adult Children of Alcoholics (ACoA) movement had arrived on the scene. Within a few years the movement had expanded to include adult children from any kind of dysfunctional family, and across the nation we parents and our grown children began to look at our relationships.

Let me talk a bit about this movement because the filter through which we and our children now look at our relationships has been influenced to a great degree by it.

## Adult Children

The ACoA movement is basically a grief work movement. Unlike Alcoholics Anonymous and Al-Anon which say, "The past is the past; don't sit on the pity pot; deal with the reality of now," Adult Children of Alcoholics says, "The past is relevant; its fingerprints are affecting the present. Review the past; mourn the past. Open up the old wounds that had to be denied in childhood and feel the repressed feelings of then, now. Listen to your wounded inner child. Then let the pain go so that you can move on in your life."

The wounded inner child whom ACoA members talk about is the sad, hurt, empty, fearful, angry child in each of us whose developmental needs were not appropriately met.

Nancy Whitaker-Emrich, an addictionologist and family therapist in Portland, Oregon, states that each of us as adults has three child selves operative inside us at any given time:

1. The wounded child
2. The wonder child — the open-hearted, naive, loving, trusting child, who is the child we are at birth
3. The loyal child — the part of us that remains loyal to our family. (Though the loyal child in us can say anything it pleases about its family, woe be unto other people if they do.)

Addiction or any major family dysfunction imposes a burden on developing children. Once grown, the wounded inner children of adult children have a wish for revenge, a wish for their parents to be accountable for harm done and a wish to hear their parents say, "I am sorry." What is often forgotten is that these same adult children also have loyal inner children who wish for reunion, even if only with nonexistent fantasy parents rather than with their parents as they really are or were.

Although the stated intent of the ACoA movement has always been to describe rather than to blame, there has evolved a parent-bashing flavor as it has become quite fashionable to make us parents responsible for the shortfalls of our children's lives. This is not surprising. Social movements usually overstate their cases as part of the process whereby they correct an existing imbalance in the social order. Eventually what is valuable is absorbed into the culture, and the overstated or ill-conceived is discarded. ACoA is still in its infancy and, therefore, still in the process of developing healthy ways for the emotions expressed to lead to completion and resolution.

It is important for us to remember that part of the impetus for the ACoA movement was the myth in the recovering alcoholic community that the alcoholic, the spouse and the children would ride off into the sunset to live happily ever after once sobriety was achieved. In addition, according to the myth, the poor sick person had suffered enough and should not be made to suffer more with reminders of any damage done.

What we failed to take into account was that rather than happily riding off into the sunset, addicted families were in a world of hurt in early recovery. They had lost their central family member, the addiction, around which all responses had been organized. The recovering family member was often as emotionally inaccessible as before recovery began, if not more so, because he or she was emotionally fragile and at high risk of relapse. Small children in these newly recovering families certainly could not speak the truth about the harm that was done to them by their parent's active addiction.

Hence, there built up a need inside these children to tell their stories and release the pain. It is in the telling of these stories, in being witnessed by like-traumatized adult children and in having their feelings and truths validated, that adult children complete what I call the Child's Journey — the mourning for the wounded inner child.

A dilemma exists, however. A wounded inner child is not the exclusive province of our children. If we are parents recovering from a major addiction or dysfunction, it is highly likely that we, too, came from an addictive or dysfunctional family. We brought our own wounded inner children into adulthood and our own pent-up needs to tell our stories, to be witnessed and to grieve over the losses of childhood.

As a clinician and educator in both family therapy and addictions, I have met many people over the past few years who tell me that when they attend addictions conferences, inner child workshops or self-help meetings, such as Adult Children of Alcoholics, or when they read self-help books from the AcoA movement, they are unable to take in the information about their own inner children. Instead, they take in the information in their parental role. All they are able to feel is their own sorrow, shame, guilt, anguish and self-rebuke about the effect they have had on their children.

These parents experience the ACoA movement as an indictment of their sins of omission and commission as parents. Their shame and anguish, combined with the hurt and anger of their children, lead to an emotional cutoff instead of to healing. This shame is particularly harmful for parents in the first five years of recovery because it increases the potential for a return to addictive behavior.

I am reminded of a sign in the saloons in the 1800s: "Please don't shoot the piano player. He's doing the best he can." An unintended consequence of the AcoA movement is that we are in the process of shooting the piano player.

As a clinician, there is one thing I am quite sure of. Neither side intends harm. We parents and our children are doing the best we can in approaching what is a terrifying and very risky issue. Those of us who are filled with shame dread our children's rebuke, fantasizing it as a nuclear blast that will strip us bare, revealing all of our worthlessness, failure, defectiveness and inadequacy.

No wonder we are sometimes so defended against inviting and entertaining our children's point of view on harm done in the parent/child relationship. It's bad enough to be reproached by our children when we feel we have parented adequately, but if we feel there has been a seriously damaging shortfall because of our own dysfunction, it is nigh unto personal annihilation to be on the receiving end of such criticism.

This is possibly why we feel nervous when our children define themselves as wounded adult children and begin attending self-help meetings such as ACoA, reading self-help literature and seeing therapists. When they bring home the latest copy of some book like *Toxic Parents*, which our children may interpret as blaming parents unmercifully for all of their children's problems, we do not generally respond by saying, "Thank you for sharing. Could you get me a copy of this wonderful book that details how I ruined your life?"

Instead, we recoil in shock, hurt, dismay and anger, and in our defensiveness we cut off communication. We feel we would be fools to volunteer to be abused by our children. Often we end up saying things we don't really mean, but with our backs to the wall, we feel we are fighting for our lives and what's left of our parental dignity.

Instead of healing, more unintentional hurt has been inflicted. The barriers between us and our children have grown higher. We begin walking on eggshells with our children in an attempt to avert another explosion, carefully avoiding any real issues between us, especially those with a high potential for emotional reactivity.

We and our children face a very human problem: We all need our parents whether they have failed us or not. And if our parents have failed us, they usually came from parents who failed them. We parents are often untreated wounded adult children, and our parents were untreated wounded adult children. That is to say, neither we nor our parents had the opportunity to mourn or to heal wounds we received as children of addicted or dysfunctional parents.

I have said that this book is a journey. It is a journey that can take us from self-flagellation to self-love and compassion. It can take us from avoiding our children to reconnecting with them in caring ways. It is not an easy journey, so I suggest you take along all the support people you can muster. Take the old-time support system of family and friends. Talk with them at the kitchen table about what you are reading and feeling. Take the new support system of therapists and self-help groups.

It is a difficult journey, but you don't have to take it alone. You can surround yourself with supportive people who can remind you when the going gets tough, "Please don't shoot the piano player. He's doing the best he can." You did the best you could. You're doing the best you can.

# SECTION

# I

# OUR
# PARENTAL
# TOOLBOX

# CHAPTER

## 2

# What's In
# Our Toolbox?

All of us begin our journeys as parents with good intentions and high hopes. Many of us anticipate that parenting will be a source of happiness, fulfillment and gratification.

We may hope that we can re-create for our children all that was good in our own childhoods. We may hope we can be better parents to our children than our parents were to us.

On the level of magical thinking, we may see parenthood as a way either to honor our parents for a job well done or to rebuke them by tossing out the model by which they raised us and replacing it with one we hope will better meet our children's needs.

We may also, consciously or unconsciously, hope that our better parenting will help reparent our own wounded inner children.

How we treat our own children might give our inner children the message: "This is how you should have been treated."

Whether our parents did a parenting job we consider to be 90 percent good or 90 percent horrible, when we begin our own parenting journey, we do not reckon with the reality that *we can't know what we don't know, and we can't give what we didn't get.* Wherever our parents' model of parenting was bad, it gave us only a model for how not to be. It gave us no guidelines for how to be. We then embark on the journey of parenting with the exhausting task of making up the missing pieces as we go along.

If we are throwing out our parents' model completely, we must literally recreate each day our parenting model for ourselves. We have no support or validation from the past that we're doing it right. All we know is that we aren't doing it "wrong" in the same way we felt our parents did.

To the extent that we make it up as we go along, we carry with us a stew of often conflicting feelings. On the positive side, we feel happy we are giving our children a better start than we had, and we are happy to be reparenting our own inner children. On the negative side, we experience fairly high levels of anxiety because no one is reassuring us we are doing it right.

Also, although throwing out our parents' model allows us to release some of our hurt and our anger with them for having failed to meet our needs, doing so will evoke guilt feelings in us. Our loyal inner children will always remain inherently loyal to our parents, no matter what our parents' transgressions were. We may carry the thinly disguised wish to avenge our childhoods by besting our parents, but we will also unconsciously feel disloyal and fear retaliation from these giants of our past.

## The Parental Toolbox

No matter how well or ill prepared we feel we are for the task of parenting, we all draw on the same resource as we try to figure out how to do the most responsible job we can — our parental toolbox. This is the repository of all our experiences of having been parented, of having been soothed or unsoothed, protected or unprotected, nurtured or unnurtured, guided or unguided on our journey from birth to young adulthood.

It will be only years later, when we look back with 20/20 hindsight, that we will fully realize how well or ill prepared we were to be parents. But early on, when we take on this new role, we are protected by denial, blind faith and sheer optimism from knowing how little some of us received and how little there was to choose from in our parental toolbox. Had we realized it at the time, we might not have had the courage to become parents.

Develop compassion for the young adult you were when you embarked on the journey of becoming a parent. For some of us, it was like being asked to build a house, only to open our toolbox and discover we had been given few, if any, tools to do what we were expected to do.

Finding ourselves with few parenting tools, we may have discovered we also lacked the necessary tools to ask for support — to voice how frightened we were or how ill prepared we felt. If we grew up in a family where pain was abundant, we probably grew up with a "Don't Talk" rule and a history of little or no support for our feelings, especially negative ones such as fear, anger, sadness or confusion. "Fake It Till You Make It" may have been our motto. We may have told ourselves, "No one else seems to be having trouble with this. It must be me. I'm inadequate. I should know how to do this. I'd better not let on how dumb or frightened I feel. I certainly can't ask for help. There is no one who can help anyway."

We may have held our breath until we could leave home. Having left the past behind, we may have been relieved to get on with a life that finally belonged to us and that we would completely control. What a nasty surprise to find that the mere fact of getting close to another human being and having a child could open our unconscious computer file of our own childhood experiences.

## Model For Relatedness

As we enter adolescence, in our quest for intimacy, we begin the process of moving toward individuals unrelated to us. The quest for relatedness is natural to us as human beings and holds the potential for incredible joy and gratification, or indescribable grief if unfulfilled.

The blueprint we draw from as we attempt to form intimate relationships with others comes primarily from what we have seen modeled in our immediate family of parents and siblings. It comes secondarily from what we have seen modeled in our extended family of grandparents, aunts, uncles and cousins. We unconsciously absorb these models without being aware of the content of what we are learning. While we might think of relatedness as closeness, in some families what is modeled is how to be distant rather than how to be close.

As you come to the exercises in this book, I want to encourage you to take out a pencil and actually write your answers. Experience indicates that those who write their responses, as opposed to simply thinking about or talking about their answers, experience neurological healing. Also you will need to refer to the answers in these early chapters when you get to later ones.

## EXERCISE

Now think back for a moment to the immediate and extended family of your childhood, adolescence and early adult years. What adjectives would you use to describe the quality of relatedness you saw modeled? Look at this list of some of the ways in which people organize their need for relatedness and circle the adjectives that fit your family's style. Add any others that come to mind.

close/distant
open/closed
communicative/silent
warm/cold
public/private
pleasant/civil/rude
sensitive/insensitive
sexual/asexual
friendly/apathetic/hostile
physically demonstrative/stand-offish, rigid, withholding
calm/chaotic
affectionate/cold
lively/dead
respectful/abusive
including/excluding

connected/isolated
committed/indifferent
engulfed/separate
family is primary source of intimacy/secondary source
clinging/detached
uncontained/contained
direct/indirect
trusting/mistrustful

---

Our family's model for relatedness will define our unconscious comfort zone. Even if the way our family handled relatedness failed to meet our need for contact and left us relationally hungry, empty and unsatisfied, the style of intimacy between people in our childhood home will continue to be the style that feels most natural and comfortable to us.

Do we know about this unconscious patterning as we approach our first intimate relationship and our first child? Usually not. Usually we have traveled fairly far along the road of partnering and parenthood before we begin to recognize the pull of these patterns, before we can feel the yearning and sadness that stem from what our needs were as children and how often they were not adequately or appropriately met by our parents. It is as if we have needed to stay asleep and deny the wounding of our own inner children until we were grown up and more resourceful. Then, eventually, in our struggle to be close to our partner and our own children, we can let ourselves realize how painfully little we knew, or what unhelpful things we learned, about relatedness.

For some of us, this realization comes to full conscious awareness and leads us into the healing process of grieving over our own childhood losses and reclaiming our lost selves. For others of us, the pain and anguish of unmet needs from childhood remain out of conscious awareness and are acted out in a replay of our childhood experiences with closeness, using our partners or children as the screens onto which this drama is projected.

For example, we may relate to our partner in the same reserved way we saw our parents relate to one another, then turn toward one or several of our children as safe objects for closeness. They can become our cuddly teddy bears whose function is to give us an outlet for all the love we feel but have never been able to express. Our unconscious wish is that if we love them the way we always yearned to be loved, we will be loved in return — and that our own inner child will finally feel lovable, worthwhile and wanted.

What happens, though, if our new baby is colicky, inconsolable or unable to mirror the unconditional love and adoration for which we yearn? In response to feeling rejected, we may unconsciously retaliate by withholding warmth, affection or attention. Worse yet, we may actively punish our child for failing to meet our needs. It is as if we have a hungry wolf inside left by our own needs not having been sufficiently met in childhood, and that wolf turns mean when deprived again.

We are "monkey-see, monkey-do" people who repeat what we were taught about relatedness — in this case, that we can't get closeness from our partner. Yet at the same time, our yearning for relatedness and our anger at its absence in our lives remains to fall onto the only other likely source of relatedness nearby our children.

Let me give you another example: Our parents may have formed a couple relationship that was so close we were excluded. We grew up feeling abandoned and left out. We could see the warmth and affection of their love for one another, but we felt like the Little Match Girl freezing to death out on the sidewalk. While we watched our parents inside with their warm, toasty relationship shared only by one another, we were outside striking matches for warmth.

As we move into adulthood and begin the process of selecting a partner, we may gravitate toward someone who seems warm, toasty and cordial to others, much as Mom and Dad were toward each other. We may find, however, that our partner is incapable of letting us in. We will then re-experience feeling like the Little Match Girl as we watch our partner relate warmly to others, but not to us.

---
| EXERCISE |
---

Take a moment to look back over your adult relational history. How have you worked out the need for closeness with your partner or partners and children? Do you see any patterns that were set in motion in childhood — the hungry, voracious wolf; the freezing, uncomplaining Little Match Girl; the hungry chigger that wants to get under someone's skin to be close and loved; the tough guy who doesn't need anyone because he was alternately loved and rebuffed so many times he quit trying? These are just some of the relatedness patterns that might be in our toolbox as we begin forming the family that will eventually be the container within which we rear our children.

---

## The Dual Cassette Deal

Our parents' marriage/partnership was what I call a dual cassette deal. Our parents brought with them from their own families of origin videocassettes filled with their parents' beliefs, attitudes, values, myths, rituals, methods of communicating, lists of allowed and not-allowed feelings. These cassettes dictated which partner should lead, which should follow, when and within what dimensions. They determined each of our parents' comfort zones — how close or how distant they should be to each other, to their children, to their extended family and outside friends.

Our parents, in the process of working out their relationship, had to try to develop a synthesis of these cassettes of expectations. At any given time, the tune for how to be a family was piped by one or both cassettes from our parents' original families and the cassette they uniquely synthesized called "our family." To the degree that the cassettes from their families were similar, conflict was lessened. But if their social class, religion, race, ethnicity or financial backgrounds were dissimilar or if their families had different beliefs, rituals or ways of handling feelings and ideas about how to structure family life, they might have had a lot of trouble trying to make an amalgam that was comfortable for both of them.

If this wasn't confusing enough, they often had to deal with members of their immediate and extended families, with their judgments and unsolicited advice. Our parents had to reach compromises that would fit these people's expectations as well, or carry the discomfort of breaking family rules.

Also in the relationship, of course, were our parents' wonder children, loyal children and wounded children. Each of these inner children had ideas about how this new relationship and this new family should meet their needs.

Pleasing all these people and combining all these tapes was quite a job! We certainly might have received mixed messages about how to build relationships and how to be parents from parents who had to make so many compromises.

## Model For Parenting

Because marriage/partnership is a dual cassette deal, sometimes our parents couldn't agree on what was right for "our family," and for us as their children, because the models of parenting and family life they each brought were so different.

Dad may have felt a need out of his working class, male-dominated family to be strict and to make the children tough so they could cope in a dog-eat-dog world. Mom, out of her protected upper-middle-class background, and in rebellion against her distant, overbearing father, may have wanted to be more permissive, feeling that childhood should be free from the harshness inevitably encountered later.

You can see how these two models of parenting would clash. And you can speculate on how their inability to come to terms with their own backgrounds would get in the way of concurring on how their children were to be parented.

## EXERCISE

The list that follows contains some of the styles parents have to choose from when they develop their own parenting methods. As you look at the list, remember that each of your parents may have had a combination of styles. One parent's style may have been dramatically different from the other's.

First go through the list and put an *M* over or next to each word that fits your mom's parenting style, if you were raised by your mom. Then go through the list once for each significant parenting figure in your life and put letters at the words that fit their styles (*GM* for Grandmother, *D* for Dad, *SD* for Stepdad, etc.)

Remember to include the nontraditional people who parented you. Maybe your sister had a big role in raising you, or your mom had a long-term relationship with a woman who parented you. When all the letters are on the list, you will have a snapshot of the parenting styles that were modeled for you.

_____ permissive/strict _____

_____ democratic/authoritarian/anarchistic _____

_____ laissez-faire/highly structured _____

_____ unprotective/protective/abusive _____

_____ overprotective/appropriately involved/uninvolved _____
(smothering)                                        (detached)

_____ intrusive/respectful of boundaries _____

_____ over-giving/under-giving _____
(martyr)          (scrooge)

_____ over-receiving/under-receiving _____
(expects to be taken care of)/(you can never pay them back)

_____ consistent/inconsistent _____

_____ cooperative with you/competitive with you _____

_____ cooperative with other parent/
competitive with other parent_____

_____ unilateral/bilateral _____
(one does all the parenting,      (both give input and share
other gives no input)             responsibility)

_____ present/absent _____
(death, desertion, workaholism)

_____ oscillating presence _____
(drug addiction, mental illness, criminal arrests)

_____ one present/one absent _____

_____ both absent/surrogate parent figure(s) present _____
(e.g., grandparent, aunt, sibling, orphanage)

_____ passive/assertive/aggressive _____

_____ critical/accepting _____

_____ controlling/doormat _____

_____ responsible/irresponsible _____

---

I mentioned in the first chapter that we frequently judge ourselves as parents from a perspective of 20/20 hindsight, marshalling all the awareness and life experience it has taken us years to accumulate, and then treating ourselves as if we had all this information available to us when we began this journey with our children. It's important for us to remind ourselves repeatedly what models for relatedness and parenting we had available *then* — 20, 30, 40, or 50 years ago — when we set out on the course of raising children.

# CHAPTER

# 3

# What Winds Our Springs?

Our family is the most important learning environment to which we will ever be exposed. Within the confines of our family we are almost imprinted with the emotional, behavioral and spiritual designs of how to be as a person. Our family is so powerful that it is often not until adolescence that we notice that other families and individuals organize activity, emotions, values, beliefs and patterns of communication different from the way our family does.

I was 16 when I was literally hit by the fact that families are different. I was having dinner for the first time with my best friend's large, Swedish, Lutheran family. My friend's father sat in a big chair at the head of the table and her mother sat in a smaller chair at the foot of the table. Their four children and I sat along the sides.

In my family the unspoken rule was that we were to serve ourselves from whatever plate was directly in front of us and then pass it to the left. I reached for the bread plate in front of me at my friend's house, only to have my friend's father rap me across the knuckles with his table knife and sternly say to me, "In this family I serve everyone's plate, and no one eats until I say so." I sat in stunned, embarrassed silence as he said the prayers and then began filling a plate for each person at the table.

The atmosphere in this family at dinner was one of tense restraint. The power hierarchy and the status of women were clear. His wife, whom I absolutely adored, sat quietly and obediently at the end of the table, much like one of the children.

Dinner in my home was quite different. It was not sweetness and light, but no one in my family would ever have rapped me on the knuckles with a knife in front of other people. Nor would anyone in my family ever have been so presumptuous as to determine how much anyone ate, when, or how, as my friend's father did.

Incidentally, I don't know if my friend's father's chair was actually bigger than her mother's chair, but the discrepancy in power between them was so great that my memory tells me it was. This is an example of how all of us tell ourselves "stories" as a way of explaining our experiences to ourselves. Needless to say, if members of that family were to read this book, my version of reality might not match theirs at all. Their versions might not even match each others'. Such is the power of the filter we bring to the reality we experience, and the power of the need to understand, in some way, what is happening to us.

## "It's Not What We Say . . ."
## Our Family Emotional Process

In my friend's family, the obvious family rules could be stated, "Fathers serve all dinner plates. Fathers say the dinner prayers. Fathers say when everyone is to start eating." Because rules like these are obvious, they are easier to keep or to throw away when we start our own families. We may decide when we grow up that the father in our new family will not serve the plates.

The more powerful tools and rules we get from our family, however, do not come from the obvious content, but from the family emotional process. We pick up these tools unconsciously, not by listening to what our family says it is like, but by watching what is actually done.

For instance, it will be extremely difficult for my friend to recognize, let alone to change, the feeling that it is right for the father in the family to have the power, that it is right for him to enforce his power by physical force and public humiliation. This is an example of what we learn from family emotional process.

My friend's father and I had an interaction around a particular piece of content, and we acted as though that piece of content were in and of itself important. In fact, the content was merely a vehicle to reinforce the deeper family message: "Dad is on top; Dad has the power."

In the next few chapters, we are going to try to pull apart the different pieces we learned at the subtle level I call our family emotional process. Bear in mind, however, that these pieces are like the pieces of learning how to ride a bicycle. You can never explain completely how to ride a bicycle. You can explain discrete actions, but not how it is all put together to equal riding a bicycle. You can ride the bicycle, however, even if you can't explain how to do it.

We can pull out various parts of the family emotional process and describe them. We can look at what was done in our family, what was modeled and what was not commented on. But even in pulling out all of these pieces, we cannot comprehend the totality of it. We can do it perfectly well, but we can't perfectly explain it. Such is the nature of human behavior — it is always more than the sum total of its parts.

## Three Interpersonal Needs

William Schutz, in his book *The Interpersonal Underworld*, talks about three interpersonal needs that wind our springs as human beings:

- Who's in and who's out (inclusion, prominence)
- Who's on the top and who's on the bottom (power, dominance)
- Who's near and who's far, how near and how far (affection, closeness)

## Inclusion

We human beings are social animals. We need one another in order to feel vital, alive and filled up. My dilemma as an individual and my family's dilemma are the same: How do we include enough people so we can feel our vitality while at the same time keeping ourselves from being flooded with too much contact, especially too much contact with people we don't want around?

Creating a large enough family system is important for several reasons. We need people as sources of nurturance, support and succor during the good times and as shock absorbers for the stressors that come down the pike during the bad times. We also need to feel connected so we can access our own internal resources.

Studies have shown that no matter how bright particular school-aged children are, they cannot realize their full capacity until they feel socially well connected, liked and nurtured in an adequate support network.

The same is true for us as adults and for our families. No matter how delightful and wonderful we may be, no matter how resource rich we may be inside, no one will see evidence of that if we feel socially isolated and disconnected, because we will not be able to externalize that in our behavior.

Our family solves the inclusion dilemma by deciding who belongs to this family and who doesn't. Does our family include just the family of procreation — Mom, Dad and their children — or does it also include our parents' parents and siblings, our parents' grandparents and aunts and uncles and cousins? Does it include some people we are not biologically related to but who have been called Aunt Minny and Uncle Tim?

Once our family decides who is in, how does our family draw a boundary and maintain a boundary around itself? Once the boundary is there, how rigid is it?

| Unbounded | Semipermeable | Rigid |
| --- | --- | --- |

Rigid boundaries have labels that say, "No trespassing, strangers not allowed. Family business is family business. To go outside the family for anything is an act of disloyalty."

Some families have boundaries that are not so rigid, that have some degree of permeability. Let's say, for instance, we develop very close friendships, sibling-like relationships. If our family has a semipermeable boundary, our parents will say, "Because these people are your friends, they are our friends. Because you like them and they are important to you, you can bring them in and we will make them feel at home. We won't block them out and treat them like outsiders. We will respect them as important. We will see ourselves as enriched by having input from the larger world."

If you imagine the degree of permeability of the family boundary on a scale, this semipermeable position is moderate compared to the tightly drawn, no-trespassing-allowed, rigid position that would be on the far right. There is a parallel to that on the far left, which is the detached, unbounded family.

If the extreme right holds the enmeshed families where the bonds are fastened with Super Glue, where everyone seems stuck to everyone else and nobody is supposed to leave, then on the left is the detached family. When we grow up in a detached family we have a sense that if we drift away, no one will reach out and grab us and pull us back in. In the boundaryless family, there is no definition of who's in the family and who's not in the family, who belongs and who doesn't belong.

We saw classic examples of the unbounded family during the 1960s and '70s when the flower children and the hippies formed familylike groups. Families were crash pads; we had no idea who might be home any given night. People just came and went; it didn't matter if they were related or unrelated.

A family without a boundary is characterized by high degrees of anxiety and chaos and low degrees of safety, security, connectedness and sense of belonging.

## EXERCISE

Take a moment to think about your family. Did your family include lots of people (global) or few (narrow)? Was the boundary rigid, or was your family chaotic and nearly un-bounded? Who guarded the boundary and decided which people were allowed in and which were not? Was the boundary left unguarded? If there was a boundary guard or guards, did they guard ferociously, or were they flexible about how people were to come and go? Plot your family by making an X where they fall on each line.

Global                                                    Narrow

Chaotic, Unbounded                                          Rigid

Unguarded                                        Ferociously Guarded

Who was the guard? _____

List the people included in your family:

_____    _____

_____    _____

_____    _____

_____    _____

_____    _____

## Our Toolbox

Let me give an example of how our family's attitudes toward inclusion may have affected our parental toolbox. Let's say we were born to parents who put a narrow, rigid boundary around the family. They may have been under-social; that is, they may have lacked the skills to reach out to other people. Then, unless by inborn temperament we are more outgoing, we will not only put a narrow boundary around our own family, we will not know how to reach out to people because we never saw such behavior modeled. When we have children of our own, in all likelihood we will model the kind of narrowness, disconnectedness and social isolation our parents modeled.

Our adult inclusion tools will come not only from what our parents modeled but also from the emotional tone of the family in which we grew up, from our inborn temperament and from our experiences as latency-age children between the ages of seven and twelve. The ages from seven to twelve are the most critical ones for learning from other children how to connect. If we come into adulthood socially disabled and we pass that disability on to our children, in all likelihood they will have difficulty with their latency-age period because there is nothing in our toolbox we can teach them to use when they are attempting to acquire peer skills.

The implication for us when we are growing up is that, first, when we get to adulthood, we cannot establish enough social connectedness to access fully all of our inherent capacities. Second, without that connectedness, we cannot fully feel our aliveness. In a sense we are socially three quarts low and, by the way, may have a tendency to develop a substance abuse disorder so we can add to ourselves "a quart" at a time to make up for that deficit. Last, we will be impaired in our capacity to grieve when we experience losses because we will not know how to reach out to other people for comfort. Since grief is a socially facilitated process, we may end up passing on the unresolved sorrow of our own life to the next generation.

## Dual Cassettes Again

As we know, when two people come together to create a family, each of them brings a cassette from the family of origin that says how things are supposed to be. Well, each of those cassettes is encoded with instructions about inclusion — who is to be included and under what circumstances, who is to be excluded and under what circumstances.

Let's say, for instance, that Mom's cassette on the issue of inclusion says that in this family we are to include only the most immediate nuclear family in the inner circle. We will be simply cordial and friendly to our extended family. We will attend obligatory social functions, such as birthday parties and family celebrations, but we really will not consider those extended relations to be on the inside.

In order to make up for the paucity of family connectedness on Mom's cassette, Mom's family historically went outside the extended family for its connectedness. It formed extensive friendship networks with people to whom Mom's family was not related.

Mom's family might have done this in order to minimize conflict. There are often fewer unresolved emotional issues, losses, sad times or conflicts with outsiders than there are with insiders. Insiders are more likely to "have the goods" on one's family.

So Mom comes equipped with a cassette that says:

1. There is a limit to how much extended family is included actively in this family.
2. We make up for the absence of extended family members by an extensive social network of friends outside the family.
3. The boundary around this family is to be relatively tightly drawn, and Mom is to function as the gatekeeper. People are allowed in, but only when Mom wants them in. Mom really doesn't want people coming and going without her permission, either family members or members of Mom's friendship network.

Let's look at the cassette Dad brought from his family of origin. Dad's cassette says that happy family life includes all his extended family plus people to whom he is not related by blood or marriage — friends he has acquired over the years by virtue of being neighbors, and so on. These long-term friends become quasi-family members. Because the "family" is so large, however, Dad doesn't have an extrafamilial friendship network. Friendships are limited. Dad doesn't perceive himself as particularly social or as having much time to interact with people outside his own family system. But within what he defines as his family system, the boundaries are not only semipermeable, they are almost nonexistent.

Dad's point of view is, "If you're related to me, if you are family or quasi-family, come by any time under any circumstances and anything you ask of me will be given. What's mine is yours. On the other hand, if you are not part of my family, you are not welcome to drop by or to make any demands on me whatsoever."

When Mom and Dad put their cassettes together to create the unique synthesis called our family, you can see what problems they are likely to have. They're going to be pulling in somewhat opposite directions.

Mom is going to want to welcome only her closest kin and her pals, and to be totally in control of when and how often. Dad, on the other hand, will want all of his kin — as defined by him — to come and go as they want, but anyone else will be defined as a stranger and not welcome.

If we are the children of these two people, how do we discern who's in and who's out, who's okay with Mom and who's okay with Dad? There is a tremendous potential for conflict between Mom and Dad unless they can come to a compromise.

We kids will end up with a toolbox full of double messages from these two. We may conclude that males and females have different ideas about inclusion. We may come to our adult relationships equipped with ambivalence about including people at all since there was so much conflict in our home about it.

Think back for a minute to the wonderful Swedish family with whom I had dinner when I was 16. One of the things I remember with tremendous fondness was going to my friend's house when her mom was home and cooking fudge in her kitchen. Her mother was a warm, wonderful, welcoming, including woman who gave us lots of space to learn how to do things, and who was supportive and interested in each and every friend who came to the house. When she was there, the house had an air of informality, ease and comfort. We knew we could say and do things when Mama was home and Papa wasn't home that we couldn't say and do when Papa came home.

When Papa came home, things became more tense, more structured, more formal, and the hierarchy of who was powerful and who wasn't became very clear. I don't mean to characterize my friend's father as cold, because he was a beneficent dictator, but he was clearly a dictator. When he was home, it was clear that he would determine who was in and who was out and how long anyone could stay. Needless to say, when both Mama and Papa were around, it was Dad's cassette that predominated. The cassette marked "our family" had a heavy overlay of the rule system that he had brought from his family of origin.

The conflict between their cassettes was resolved by deciding that when Mama was home alone, she could live by her rules and that when Papa was home, everyone lived by his. Both value systems were respected.

---

## EXERCISE

Think for a moment about each person who parented you. Using different letters to represent different people, as we did in Chapter 2 (*GM* for Grandmother, *D* for Dad, etc.), plot on the following lines how they defined who was "in" your family. For example:

| **M** | **GM** | **D** |
|-------|--------|-------|

**Global**                                        **Narrow**

Now it's your turn:

---

**Global**                                        **Narrow**

---

**Unbounded**                                       **Rigid**

---

**Unguarded**                          **Ferociously Guarded**

Once you have completed these three scales, notice the discrepancies, if any, between the cassettes of the major parenting people in your life. How did your family resolve these discrepancies? What messages did you get about inclusion because of these discrepancies?

---

## What We Do And What We Want

The issue of inclusion is not just about what we do; it's also about what we want. Our parents may not have included very many people inside the family boundary because they didn't have good social skills. Or they may not have included very many people because they didn't want very many people inside. Each of the three family tasks — inclusion, control and closeness — has an expressed dimension (what we do) and a wanted dimension (what we want).

Let's look at the two dimensions on two lines. If Mom is on the far left of the expressed dimension, she is extremely undersocial; that is, she never does anything to get herself included or to include other people. If Dad is on the far right, he always engages in behavior to get included and to include other people all of the time. If they are in the middle, they will do things to get included and to include others sometimes, when it's appropriate.

**EXPRESSED** (what we do)

| M | | D |
|---|---|---|
| Never | Sometimes | Always |

The second dimension is what we want. If Mom is on the far left, the undersocial end, she doesn't want anybody to include her ever. If Dad is on the far right, the oversocial end, he wants people to always include him no matter what. If they are in the middle, they want to be included when it's appropriate, but it's not important that they be included if it's not appropriate.

**WANTED**

| M | | D |
|---|---|---|
| Never | Sometimes | Always |

Looking at where our parents fall on each of the lines may clear up some confusion we may have felt as children. For instance, let's say Dad was on the "Never" end of expressed inclusion and the "Always" end of wanted inclusion.

**EXPRESSED**

| D | | |
|---|---|---|
| Never | Sometimes | Always |

**WANTED**

| | | D |
|---|---|---|
| Never | Sometimes | Always |

He was socially reticent and socially unskilled. He longed to be included by other people, but he lacked the capacity to initiate contact with people or to signal to other people that he yearned for contact. His aloof behavior left people with the impression he wished to be alone when the opposite was true.

As children, we may end up not only lacking the tools to initiate contact and signal interest in contact with people ourselves, but we may also inherit a bitterness from Dad, who feels, "People are not as interested in me as I am in them. People are not interested in me and in my family." The truth is that even though we grow up with the sense that people are not interested in us, they have no way to know we want to be included because we have unconsciously learned to give the messages, *No trespassing allowed. Outsiders need not apply.*

Maybe Mom is high on expressed inclusion. She is socially skilled and good at getting herself noticed. But maybe she doesn't really want to be included very often, and she's selective about whom she wants to be with.

**EXPRESSED**

|  |  | M |
|---|---|---|
| Never | Sometimes | Always |

**WANTED**

|  | M |  |
|---|---|---|
| Never | Sometimes | Always |

In that case, we might feel encouraged to invite her in and then feel rebuffed and confused by her refusal. We may also have inherited in our toolbox her social behavior and/or her selectivity, confusing both our partners and our children.

## EXERCISE

Take a moment to plot the people who were significant parenting figures on the following lines. Again, use a letter to symbolize each one: *SM* might be Stepmom, *UT* might be Uncle Ted.

*PERSON 1*
**EXPRESSED**

---

Never                    Sometimes                    Always

**WANTED**

---

Never                    Sometimes                    Always

*PERSON 2*
**EXPRESSED**

---

Never                    Sometimes                    Always

**WANTED**

---

Never                    Sometimes                    Always

*PERSON 3*
**EXPRESSED**

---

Never                    Sometimes                    Always

**WANTED**

---

Never                    Sometimes                    Always

Now reflect on how each parent's Expressed inclusion needs and Wanted inclusion needs were played out in their relationships with each other. How did they resolve their differences? How were their needs played out in their relationships with you?

---

Let me give you some examples of how differences in our parents' inclusion needs might have affected both our parents' relationship with each other and what we learned about inclusion. Let's say we were raised by our dad, Sam, and his long-term partner, Jan.

## DAD
High expressed: "Hi, I'm Sam." (Dad's behavior says, "Notice me.")
High wanted: "Come on in." (To Jan, "You don't pay enough attention to me and you never want friends over.")

## JAN
Low expressed: "I'm invisible. I have no voice."
Low wanted: "I'm a recluse or very selective." (To Sam, "Why do we have to entertain so much?")

Why does Dad say to Jan, "You don't pay enough attention to me."? He has a high need for others to include him, but he is with a woman who lacks the capacity to initiate inclusive behavior. She also has a very low need to be included, so it would not occur to her to initiate this behavior toward him. It's natural for her to assume he wants the same thing she wants. She doesn't want him to initiate inclusive behavior with her, and so she doesn't initiate it with him.

Jan is very selective about the people she wants to be included by. She feels inundated by Dad's high expressed inclusion behavior, which keeps the house full of people. Thus, "Why do we have to entertain so much?"

Our toolbox may get filled with double messages because of the conflict between them, or we may pick one of them to model ourselves after.

If we had a closer relationship with Jan than with Dad, or had her temperament, we are likely to have picked up her style of being unassertive and selective. We may then end up marrying, because of our comfort zone, someone who has a high need for prominence and a high capacity to elicit including behavior from other people, just like Dad. We may end up with the same dilemma in our marriage we saw in the relationship between Dad and Jan.

Let's say we were raised by Mom, Jewel, and her long-term partner, Helen.

## MOM
High expressed: "Hi, I'm Jewel."
Low wanted: "Don't call me, I'll call you."

## HELEN
Intermediate expressed: "Hi, I'm Helen, but I can't possibly compete with Jewel."

High wanted: "Jewel doesn't want very many people in our lives, so I will let the kids and their friends in behind her back. I will live vicariously through the children."

From living with this couple, we children will get a fairly consistent message about the desirability of being noticed because we will have seen that in both Mom and Helen. But we will get mixed messages about when to include people and how much. Mom will be uncomfortable when we invite people over, and Helen will be delighted.

---

## E X E R C I S E

Plot yourself on the following lines as you were when you were a child.

**EXPRESSED**

| | | |
|---|---|---|
| Never | Sometimes | Always |

**WANTED**

| | | |
|---|---|---|
| Never | Sometimes | Always |

How well did your inclusion needs match each of your parent's inclusion needs? What areas of conflict do you notice? Can you see any ways your preferences reflect what you learned from your parents?

---

## Exclusion

When we talk about inclusion, we are also talking about exclusion. The family cassette on inclusion also determines exclusion — who, how and why.

I met a 17-year-old woman a few years ago who had been told by her father that when she turned 18, he would break her plate and burn her bed. This woman came from a family that extruded its family members at a particular age — in this instance at the age of 18. The message was, "You're only allowed here until the age of 18, and after that you're on your own. You're not included in this family after you're 18."

When this woman becomes a mother, I wouldn't expect her to be able to access her family as a resource to help her solve problems. She's already had the experience of feeling as if she was spat out, so why would she go back and ask these people for help?

This woman's family was also an isolated and suspicious family that thought human nature was basically bad, that people were not to be trusted. Therefore the family could not avail itself of resources in the larger community.

In all likelihood, this woman as an adult will not be able to reach back to her family for help when she faces a crisis, and she will not be able to reach out easily to resources in the larger community, such as friends, therapy, agencies, etc. She has been excluded and has learned too well how to exclude.

It's possible to be physically present in the family but psychologically excluded. A classic example occurs within addicted families when the nonaddicted spouse and the children psychologically exclude the addicted spouse. Often they close ranks and draw a new boundary with the addicted spouse on the outside.

When this spouse goes into recovery, he or she will have to earn the right to be re-included in the family. Usually he or she will have to establish a new track record of sobriety and sober behavior in order to do so.

## Healthy Families

Families have an almost infinite number of ways to handle the questions of who is included and who is excluded, how is the boundary drawn and by whom and how permeable is the boundary. How do we know if what we learned in our family was on the healthy end of the continuum and therefore potentially helpful to us when we grew up and began forming our own families?

Well, first and foremost, we know that what our family did was healthy if what our parents taught us worked. It was healthy if it helped us solve problems and deal with stress, if it helped us feel competent and resource-rich as we faced the challenges of partnering and having children.

The healthier our family was, the clearer and more flexible were its rules about inclusion. Our parents were willing to use both the internal resources of our extended family network and the external resources of a viable social network. Our parents made compromises between the cassettes they brought from their families of origin so that the inclusion rules were clear.

Healthier families fall in the middle range on the scales. They are neither too global, chaotic-unbounded and unguarded, nor are their boundaries too narrow, rigid and ferociously guarded. They are neither social recluses nor socially compulsive.

Inclusion is the first interpersonal need a new family must satisfy. Parents must decide who is in this family and who is not. Once the family group is formed, the next question is who makes the decisions in this family? Who has control?

## Control

We live in a culture that talks about control as though it were a dirty word. Yet in reality, all human beings are controlling in one way or another. Only in its extremes — either in its abdication or in its overuse — is control pathological. (An abdicator is someone who has power — like a parent or a king — but gives up that power and avoids the responsibility that goes with it.)

The nature of being human is to feel some degree of fear and anxiety. We deal with this fear and anxiety by attempting to organize our reality and our experiences in such a way that we feel competent and in control.

Control may manifest itself in subtle ways that look noncontrolling. For example, our chronically ill mother may use her illness to control us — just as Bugs Bunny fakes dying to get control when he is in trouble in the cartoons. Or control may manifest itself in obvious ways — like the heavy-fisted hand of our dad's violence. But control is always present.

Another way of talking about control, by the way, is to use the word structure. What is the amount of structure we need for ourselves, and what's the amount of structuring we need to impose on others in order to feel safe? We can also use the words *dominance, top, bottom.* Who's on top, who's on the bottom? Who's dominant, and who isn't?

A good example of control can be found in the Swedish, Lutheran family I introduced you to earlier. I wasn't sure whether the dad's chair was actually larger than the mom's chair, but the power differential — male to female, husband to wife and father to mother — was very clear. Giving one person all or most of the control is one way a family might work out the issue of control.

Our goal here is to identify the tools we brought from our family of origin into the family we then created which either helped or hindered us in the parenting of our own children. Often the tools we received for structure and control depended on our sex and where we were in the birth order.

In the Swedish, Lutheran family it would be relatively dangerous to be an eldest son because of the father's investment in control. An eldest son might have tremendous difficulty getting enough space to flex his muscles and develop his own sense of competence and autonomy because he would constantly be coming up against his father's high need for control.

The eldest son in such a family may resolve the dilemma by making a decision to avoid family life altogether. He may never want anyone in his life who can "tell him what to do" or to whom he has to be responsible. He may live out his life as a rebel, looking intimacy-phobic when he is actually control-phobic. Given his father's power and his own inborn temperament, he may have only the tools to be constantly at loggerheads with authority, particularly male authority.

If he does partner, his mother's complacence will put in his toolbox a likelihood of partnering with someone who is relatively uncomplaining. His partner will not be likely to give him any trouble, but also will not be likely to give him much support.

The eldest daughter in such a family may have some tools marked with the caveat: "Avoid males who are extremely powerful and controlling." She may be inclined to pick a man who will give her less trouble than she experienced with her father when, as a young woman, she attempted to develop her own autonomy. Her mother may give her a model for how not to be as a woman, if her mother was not someone she could admire.

The tools in the toolbox for children in this family could run in either direction. They may want partners who are strong and dominant just like Dad while they move into Mom's position of being controlled. Or they may want someone just the opposite of Dad and, in effect, move into Dad's position. This latter move is a phenomenon called identification with the aggressor — where we move into the position of the person who was the aggressor against us in childhood. That way, as adults, we get to be in the strong role this time, and someone else gets to be in the weak role.

We can get tools in our toolbox from watching our siblings as well as our parents. Let's say Dad is violent and controlling, and Mom is violent and controlling. Our oldest sibling, a boy, is born with a combination of firstborn maleness and inborn temperament to reach out to his environment and challenge it. We're secondborn, and we watch our brother get clobbered repeatedly by our parents. He has a high need for control, Dad has a high need for control and Mom has a high need for control.

We are not only secondborn; we have a more easygoing temperament. When we look up the birth order and watch what happens to our brother, three things happen. First, we are traumatized — we are a secondary trauma victim because we are powerless and shocked and hurt by his battering. Second, we learn how *not* to be from seeing what happens to him. Third, in adulthood we're going to carry survivor guilt about what happened to our brother that didn't happen to us. In a sense we are like the child born in the rain shadow of the mountain. All the water/anger/violence got dumped on our brother, and none of it got dumped on us.

## What We Do And What We Want

Whether we are using the word *control, structure* or *dominance,* there are two dimensions: expressed and wanted — just as there were with inclusion. Does Dad *behave* in ways that control others? Does he *want* control and structure from others?

Let me give you an example. Let's say that Dad is an abdicator. By that, I mean Dad does nothing to take over, to lead or to structure. He also doesn't want anyone else to take over, to lead or to structure. So Dad not only abdicates responsibility himself; Dad also wants no leadership or structure from others.

## DAD
Low expressed: "I'll never be bossy."
Low wanted: "Don't tell me what to do."

Maybe Dad got to be the way he is because he grew up in a home with a heavy-fisted, authoritarian father who was always structuring everyone and everything. Dad may have vowed that no one would ever tell him what to do, nor would he ever be bossy and controlling with others as his father had been. Dad has done a 180-degree pendulum swing on the issue of control.

The problem for us as children in this home is that we need boundaries, clear expectations and structure. The absence of this from Dad creates, first of all, chaos and, second of all, a vacuum. Since nature abhors a vacuum, it is a given that someone is going to step into the vacuum and begin manifesting control behavior. And who to our wondrous eyes, should appear but Mom?

## MOM
Moderate expressed: "I'll structure things if necessary."
Moderate wanted: "I don't want to live in complete chaos."

Mom abhors chaos. Mom can't tolerate the anxiety she feels when there is no leadership in the family. So Mom steps in and begins controlling to make up for the vacuum in leadership left by Dad. Mom structures for both of them. Mom structures everything all of the time in all dimensions. Mom is higher than Dad on both the expressed and the wanted dimensions of control, and that makes her the controlling parent.

At one level, we kids are going to be less anxious because Mom is reducing the chaos and providing some clear parameters within which we can function. On the other hand, Mom and Dad are in constant conflict with one another because Dad cannot tolerate anyone ever telling him what to do for any reason.

Who we blame for this fighting depends on our focus. Does Dad fight back because Mom is controlling, or is Mom controlling because Dad refuses to provide any leadership? In reality, it is like the dog chasing its own tail. The more the dog runs, the faster the tail goes; the faster the tail goes, the more the dog runs to catch it.

| EXERCISE |
| --- |

Take a moment to think about the parenting figures in your life again. Using different letters to represent different people, plot each of them on the two lines below. Remember that expressed control has to do with behavior. How often does this person take over being responsible, structuring? High expressed means this person takes over all the time. Low expressed means this person never takes over — if he or she were in a crowded theater on fire, he or she would do nothing to help organize people to get out of there.

Wanted control means how much does this person want someone else to provide structure and control? Maybe this person is a 52-year-old baby in diapers wanting the world always to take care of him or her. Or maybe this person never wants anyone to tell him or her what to do.

*PERSON 1*
**EXPRESSED**

| Never | Sometimes | Always |
| --- | --- | --- |

**WANTED**

| Never | Sometimes | Always |
| --- | --- | --- |

*PERSON 2*
**EXPRESSED**

| Never | Sometimes | Always |
| --- | --- | --- |

**WANTED**

| Never | Sometimes | Always |
| --- | --- | --- |

*PERSON 3*
**EXPRESSED**

| Never | Sometimes | Always |
| --- | --- | --- |

## WANTED

| Never | Sometimes | Always |
|-------|-----------|--------|

Take a moment to reflect on how each parent's control needs affected their relationships with each other. How did they resolve any conflicts that arose because of differing needs?

How did each parent's control needs affect their relationship with you?

---

Let me give you some examples. Let's say that in our family both Dad and his partner, Patrick, because of their own histories, are incapable of providing leadership. This is sometimes the case when both of our parents were youngest children who came from very chaotic dysfunctional families where they were basically unparented children. They come to adulthood with a need to be parented, a need for someone to provide them with leadership and structure. Their scales might look something like this:

**PATRICK**
Low expressed: "I won't take over anywhere ever."
High wanted: "Won't someone please do something?"

**DAD**
Low expressed: "I won't ever take over either."
High wanted: "Won't someone please do something?"

Now, bear in mind that Patrick and Dad can't give what they didn't get, and they can't know what they don't know. Neither Patrick nor Dad has been parented; so they don't have the capacity to assume the leadership and provide the structuring that their children need. They not only don't lead, their need to be led is high. Since nature abhors a vacuum, most likely one or more of us children will become parentified. Our childhood will be cut short, and we will function in the position of a surrogate parent. Our family will be pretty chaotic because both the children and the parents are being led by children.

When we begin parenting our own children, we will find some important tools missing. We will not have in our toolbox the experience of having been parented appropriately, and we will never have seen appropriate structure or limits set. We can expect that we will create a similar legacy in our own families once we are grown.

Let me give you an example in which our parents' Wanted and Expressed control were somewhat different. Let's say we were raised by our mom and our stepdad.

## MOM
High expressed: "I'm the captain; mind me."
High wanted: "I need structure to feel safe."

## STEPDAD
High expressed: "I'm the captain, too, but I'm indirect in getting my way. If I don't want to do something, I'll say I have a headache instead of fighting with you directly."
Low wanted: "Don't tell me what to do. I can defeat you with my indirect methods any day of the week."

Growing up in this family might put a tool in our toolbox that says, "Avoid conflict and control at all costs." Because both of our parents need to control, we will feel the tension of that in the air. We will also get in our toolbox the knowledge of how to defeat people in positions of power by using indirect methods. But we will not be clear about how two people might work things out in a healthy way on the issue of control.

---

## EXERCISE

Now take a moment to plot yourself on the two control lines below as you were when you were a child.

## EXPRESSED

| Never | Sometimes | Always |
| --- | --- | --- |

## WANTED

| Never | Sometimes | Always |
| --- | --- | --- |

How well did your control needs match each of your parent's control needs? What areas of conflict do you notice? Can you see any ways your preferences reflect what you learned from the ways your parents behaved toward you or toward each other?

## Healthy Families

How does a healthy family resolve the issue of control? Healthy families assume that it is the job of parents to be parents and the job of children to be children. Healthy families assume that there is some repository of wisdom in the parents by virtue of their chronological maturity and their life experience. Parents are expected to, and in fact do, provide structure in the form of rules for how we do things in this family.

Parents have worked out some complementarity between the two of them on their need to control and their need to be controlled. They will work this out initially in their intimate relationship and later in their parental relationship. In so doing, the parents will have an understanding about who takes control on which issues.

Parents will resolve the important parenting issues behind the scenes between the two of them. They will not undercut one another or create inappropriate alliances with any of the children as a way of covertly running their own agendas. They will not pull children into the conflict.

## Closeness

Closeness is the third primary need a family has to address. In *The Interpersonal Underworld*, William Schutz calls this the need for affection. I am using the term *closeness* here because the word *affection* calls up images of physical touching, whereas closeness gives images of either physical or emotional connection. We can feel close, for instance, by sharing our feelings in an intimate conversation.

How close do I want you to be to me? How close do I want to be to you? How much closeness is enough; how much is too much?

How long can I tolerate closeness? What do I do when I can't tolerate any more? What do I do when I'm not getting enough?

We learned about closeness from what we saw modeled in our families — how our parents acted toward one another. We also learned about it from how our parents behaved toward us.

## What We Do And What We Want

Once again, our family's *behavior* might have been different from what it *wanted* on the inside. Let's look at families on the two dimensions of expressed and wanted closeness. On the expressed dimension, our family may range from the far left of never being physically or emotionally close under any circumstances to the far right of being close all the time. It might fall in the middle — where family members are close sometimes and distant other times.

### EXPRESSED

| Never | Sometimes | Always |
|---|---|---|

Our family can also fall to the far left, the middle or the far right in how much affection is wanted. On the far left, our family never wants closeness; in the middle our family wants closeness some of the time when appropriate; on the far right our family wants closeness all the time from anyone who is in the environment.

### WANTED

| Never | Sometimes | Always |
|---|---|---|

Take a moment to plot your family on the lines above.

Let me give you some examples of families that represent the extremes on the issue of closeness. Let's say that Stepmom and Dad are the ice queen and the ice king. We grow up with them sitting at opposite ends of the living room reading their books.

One of the ways they discourage closeness is by choosing and arranging the furniture in such a way that our home is cold and sterile. A stranger might describe the house as stark and orderly, never warm, friendly or inviting.

When Stepmom and Dad are home, no music is to be played, and we children are to come and go quietly and respectfully. No displays of affection are allowed. To come in and touch, hug or kiss our parents or to be touched, hugged or kissed by them would be unthinkable.

In the process of growing up, we might secretly wonder if Stepmom and Dad yearn for closeness. When we become grown, we may test out this question by hugging them and telling them we love them whenever we see them. If they are, in reality, on the far left on both expressed and wanted closeness, we will get stiff, boardlike hugs in return and an uncomfortable silence whenever we touch them. Every time we say, "I love you," nothing will come back.

What if we grow up in a family on the far right on both closeness dimensions? Everyone in our family is always kissing everyone else with yucky-stucky kisses. We are always being hugged and pawed and told how important we are, how much we are loved. We have a sense that we can never have a moment of privacy under any circumstances. Nor can we ever have a negative thought or feeling because it is an act of treason not to be telling people we love them all the time. It also might be an act of treason to keep a diary. Everything has to be open and affectionate in our family.

At some level, all these displays of affection feel compulsive. It feels good to have all the closeness and togetherness, but there is also an underlying terror that if we aren't clumped together in an ongoing encounter group something bad will happen.

Our family is not only very expressive, it also wants expressive behavior back. If we come home on a given day and feel contemplative and private, that is not okay. Our family wants constant reassurance of closeness.

We don't have permission to be different from the rest of the family, and we don't have permission to be a private, separate person. We don't have the freedom to have a range of emotions at any given time. Although everything looks like sweetness, there is something very coercive in our family.

Violence is a distinct possibility in both the ice family and the sweet family. The ice family is cool, aloof, reserved, not inviting.

There is a sense that if someone attempts to be too close, there will be some kind of negative consequence. The negative consequence might be violence or criticism or silent stonewalling. But it is clear that if we don't behave the way we're supposed to, we're going to get it.

In the cotton candy family that clumps together and is overly affectionate, there is also the sense that if we fail to comply, something negative is going to happen. In either of these families violence might be stimulated by the anxiety created by too much closeness or too much distance. Violence is sometimes the way people establish parameters about how close is too close and how far is too far.

If we grew up in a family that was at either extreme of the closeness scale, we are likely to have only the tools in our toolbox that can replicate what our family did. We won't know how to let people move in and out of closeness.

In both the ice family and the cotton candy family, our parents are on the far end of the scale on both expressed and wanted affection. Let's look at some examples where expressed and wanted are different.

### DAD

Low expressed: "I'm cool and reserved."
High wanted: "I sure would like someone to be warm and close with me."

### MOM

Low expressed: "I'm cool and reserved too."
High wanted: "I hope someone will give me a hug."

Now, all children come into the world affectionate and wanting at least some closeness. When, as children, we express our affection to the kind of parents just described, we may find them incredibly responsive to our hugs, even though they don't give hugs much themselves.

We may get in our toolbox, then, the ability to be warm and to reach out to people even though we don't see that warmth modeled by our parents. On the other hand, we may not get the tools we need to know when someone is giving us honest back-off messages. After all, our parents were cool behaviorally but enjoyed our affection, so why shouldn't other cool people enjoy it too? We may be very surprised when our warmth is rebuffed.

Some of the tools we get from our parents will depend on our temperament, our birth order, our gender and with which parent we identify. For instance, let's say we are born to the parents outlined above, but we are relatively aloof by temperament — for even though all babies are naturally affectionate, some are more self-preoccupied than others.

If we are born to these parents who want closeness and we are aloof, we will be, temperamentally, a poor fit for our parents. They will be disappointed in our inability to generate closeness. They will not model affectionate behavior, so we will have no way of knowing that's what they want. We and our parents will consider one another unaffectionate.

Here's where birth order can make a big difference. Suppose we are the secondborn. We have an older sister who offers affection well. We sit and study her. We watch her get her way with our parents by being affectionate. We can learn to mimic her and glean from her the tools we need to be close.

Let's look at the issue of mixed messages. If Mom falls at the high end of the scale both in expressing and in wanting closeness, there is no mixed message. How Mom acts and how she feels are consistent.

On the other hand, if her expression is at the high end and her want at the low, we are going to be quite confused. Her affectionate behavior is going to generate affectionate behavior in us, and we will be quite puzzled when she is nonreceiving.

Here's another example in which differences on the expressed and wanted dimensions can be confusing for us as children. In this instance, our parents are Mom and her partner, Ray.

## RAY
Low expressed: "I'm frozen, but I'm not cold."
Moderate wanted: "I'm amenable to closeness. I can take it or leave it."

## MOM
High expressed: "I love to gush over you."
Low wanted: "But please stay away because closeness brings up horrible memories of having been sexually abused."

In this situation, the couple has one mismatch and one match. Mom's gushy expressed affection is going to make Ray very uncomfortable with his moderate wants. On the other hand, Ray's low expressed affection is perfect for Mom. Mom is not going to feel overwhelmed or scared by too much closeness as she was when she was sexually abused.

We kids are going to get a mixed bag of confusing tools from this couple. Ray's low expressed affection may cause us to think men are nonexpressive to the point of being near dead. Mom's gushiness may leave us with the conclusion that women are just too much. We may be confused about why Ray likes Mom's gushing some times and not others, because we don't know that Ray's position on wanting is moderate and Mom's expression is extreme.

We are going to be very puzzled about why Mom hangs in there with a man who seems so frozen. What we don't know is that Ray's coolness is just right to make Mom feel safe. Most of all, we will be left with a lot of confusion about how to be affectionate, how to receive affection and how much is too much.

---

## EXERCISE

Think about the major parenting figures in your life and plot them on the following lines.

*PERSON 1*
**EXPRESSED**

---

Never                    Sometimes                    Always

**WANTED**

---

Never                    Sometimes                    Always

*PERSON 2*
**EXPRESSED**

---

Never                    Sometimes                    Always

**WANTED**

| Never | Sometimes | Always |
|-------|-----------|--------|

*PERSON 3*
**EXPRESSED**

| Never | Sometimes | Always |
|-------|-----------|--------|

**WANTED**

| Never | Sometimes | Always |
|-------|-----------|--------|

How were each parent's closeness needs played out in their relationships with each other? With you?

Take a moment to look at some of the discrepancies. How did you, as a child, deal with the mixed messages, if there were any? How did your family deal with the differences, if there were any?

Plot yourself as you were when you were a child.

**EXPRESSED**

| Never | Sometimes | Always |
|-------|-----------|--------|

**WANTED**

| Never | Sometimes | Always |
|-------|-----------|--------|

How well did your closeness needs match each of your parent's needs? What areas of conflict do you notice? Can you see any ways your preferences reflect what you learned from your parents?

## Healthy Families

A healthy family has a warm, inviting, cordial atmosphere. The emotional tone in the house is pleasant. The range of feelings allowed is fairly broad.

Most important, a healthy family has a tremendous respect for individual differences. There is an implicit permission to move in and out of closeness based on what our individual needs are at any given time.

There is also an ongoing acknowledgment that we need connectedness. The family shows by its behavior its willingness to provide comfort, support, attention and affection.

There are clear ways to move in and out of closeness. In order to get some space, we don't have to get sick, we don't have to start a fight, we don't have to become violent or hysterical and we don't have to develop an addiction. We don't have to pull in one of the children. We don't have to be indirect.

In our culture most people don't have an awareness that we all have different needs for affection and closeness and that those needs shift quite normally from time to time within each individual. We don't have a recognized and accepted language to establish boundaries around closeness, so people find all sorts of indirect ways of saying, "You're too close." Classic examples of indirectness are the wife who has a headache, the daughter who gains too much weight and the husband who becomes a workaholic.

## Our Tools

The point of this exploration is not for us to chastise ourselves or beat up on ourselves. The point is for us to see more clearly what tools we got in our family of origin that we might have taken with us into the families we created as young adults, and to have some compassion for the young adults we were.

We did the best we could at the time with the information we had. We didn't have all this information back then. We may not have known how to determine who should be in and who should be out of our new family. Or we may have been unconsciously following unhealthy models from our family of origin.

We may have had no way of knowing how to structure our new family in a healthy way or determine the best division of power. We may not have known how to moderate closeness and distance except by using the tools we got in our own family of origin.

The more dysfunctional our family of origin was, and the more pain there was in our family of origin, the more likely it is that we will be on the extreme ends of the scales on inclusion, control and closeness. Either we trust no one ever, or we trust everyone all the time. We want either to let everyone in all the time or to let no one in ever. We want to control everybody all the time, or we never want any control or responsibility any of the time. We want to jump into somebody's pocket and be close all the time, or we want to avoid closeness at all costs because it's so painful.

The more painful our childhood family was, the more likely it is that we are going to want to control how our new family deals with inclusion, control and closeness. We will desperately want to create a family that does not replicate what was painful, frightening and overwhelming in our family of origin. And yet, because our comfort zones are unconscious and already set by our childhood family, we often end up creating families that are not so different on the dimensions of inclusion, control and closeness.

# 4

# Our Family
# Emotional Process

Think back for a moment to the Swedish, Lutheran family I ate dinner with as a teenager. In that family, the dad communicated the rules to me directly, enforcing them with physical punishment — a rap on my knuckles. If anyone at the table felt any anger about his rules or his methods, that conflict never came out into the open. Communication patterns, rule enforcement and conflict resolution are three more pieces of the family emotional process.

The family emotional process also includes what is allowed or not allowed in our family. What emotions are allowed expression? What differences are allowed between people? Are mistakes allowed? Are we allowed to process losses openly? Are we allowed to put more energy into our new family than we do into our family of origin?

Whatever family emotional process we grew up with, we repeat with our new family. It is possible to become consciously aware of the family emotional process we inherited and to change some of this process once we are adults. However, we must first become aware of our inheritance.

Remember, the point of looking at the family emotional process is twofold. First, we want to look at the tools we had available to us and at the gaps in our toolbox when we began our journey as parents many years ago. Second, we want to develop some compassion and understanding for ourselves as young parents, and possibly even for ourselves as parents at midlife. Only then can we mourn whatever we need to mourn in the past and change whatever we need to change in the present. Only then can we take the next steps toward healing our relationships with our children.

## Communication

Let's begin with the communication patterns in our family of origin. Did we grow up in a family where communication was direct: that is, did we grow up in a family where we were expected to speak directly to the family member we had an issue with? Or did we grow up in a family where communication was indirect? Communication in families falls on a continuum from direct on one end to indirect on the other.

---

Direct                                                              Indirect

If our family is indirect, most likely we experience "switchboarding" or "triangulation." Here's an example of switchboarding:

Let's say we have an issue with Mother. If our family uses triangulation we do not talk to her directly. Instead, we talk to our brother, who is the family switchboard operator. We tell him about the issue we have with Mom and he, in turn, expresses our concern to Mother. Mother then gives our brother her response and he passes it on to us.

You will notice that because we are growing up in a family that uses a switchboard, we are not learning to deal directly with people with whom we have issues. If we carry this pattern into our partner relationship and into our relationships with our children, we may be unable to deal directly with them when we have issues with them. Instead, we may draft our spouse or partner or one of our children into the switchboard role and send all the communications we feel uncomfortable with through this person.

Why would our family choose to switchboard instead of communicating directly? Whenever two individuals have an issue between them that has the potential for generating tension, they will look for ways to avoid the tension and unpleasantness. One way to reduce tension is to pull in a third party. Instead of there being two people in on the communication, there are three, and communication goes around the triangle. Switchboarding is a type of triangulation.

In the example above we probably often disagree with Mother, and our personalities probably clash. Maybe our brother is her favorite child. If we deal directly with Mother about something that we think might upset her, chances are we will get into a fight. By communicating through our brother, who can put things "more tactfully" and to whom mother is generally more responsive, we can lessen the real or expected tension with Mother. Switchboarding is a safety operation.

In a sense, we pass the tension on to our brother, but at least he has a less conflictual relationship with Mom. We are asking him to communicate with her on our behalf. However, we never ask him directly or make this request explicit. This is an implicit demand which he agrees to in order to lessen the overall tension in the family. The higher the level of anxiety in a family, the greater the likelihood that a family will use triangulation.

A switchboard is a persistent triangle that does not change. That is to say, our brother is almost always the person through whom all family members send communications to Mother. He has had that role from a relatively early age and, should that pattern not be deliberately changed, he will continue to play that role even when he and Mother are both elderly.

Another common switchboard pattern happens sometimes in stepfamilies. If Mom doesn't allow Stepdad full latitude to make decisions about us or to discipline us, he will always have to communicate his wishes about us to her instead of directly to us. Mom will be the switchboard. Such a triangle can create tremendous potential for conflict between our parents, tremendous potential for our parents to act out their personal conflicts in their relationships with us, and it can make it impossible for Stepdad ever to become a legitimate parent co-parenting with Mother.

Unlike switchboard triangles, ordinary triangles shift, depending upon what is going on in the family system. For instance, if the touchy issue involves my brother the switchboard, we cannot communicate through him to our mother. In that case, we will try to create a temporary triangle. Maybe we tell our other brother our concern, hoping he will carry the information to Mom, but if he doesn't, we will look for another family member to do it and create a triangle with that person.

Communication in families also falls on a continuum from sparse to overly abundant.

| Sparse | Overly Abundant |
|---|---|

There are families that fail to communicate as much by the profusion of communication as by the paucity of communication. If we grow up in a family that never shuts up, this overly prolific talking is most likely a defense against feeling uncomfortable feelings and a way of avoiding sensitive topics.

Living in our family may be like being educated in a one-room school where everyone recites the lesson out loud at the same time. No one listens to anyone. No one really feels seen or valued or respected or attuned to. Each of us feels caught up in the babble of our family.

We may be the child who is perched on the edge of our chair at dinner, always waiting for an opening to get into the conversation. We may end up in adulthood feeling as though we do not have a voice. We may, in fact, become an adult who is always perching and waiting and never finding an opening, never being seen or heard, never feeling we have a voice, feeling invisible and disempowered.

If we try to make a 180-degree pendulum swing in our new family, we may create a silent family and become silent parents. We may maintain the silence that was forced on us as children. We may also be emotionally overreactive to a surplus of talk from our spouse and our children because it feels to us like the babble of our childhood. We may select a spouse or a partner who tends to be terse and noncommunicative. Little do we realize that our partner's lack of communication avoids and denies emotionally sensitive topics in the same way that our family of origin's babble avoided emotionally sensitive topics. We will have replicated a similar avoidance pattern of communication even though it is now avoidance by silence rather than avoidance by babble.

What if we grow up in a family on the other end of the quantity scale? What if our family does not communicate at all?

I am the first to acknowledge that it is impossible not to communicate. Even when we think we're not communicating, we're communicating. But in some families, most of what *is* communicated is a lack of aliveness, a lack of externalization, a lack of information.

An uncommunicative family feels dead and ahistorical. We get no sense of where we fit into the history of our family because our parents do not talk about themselves, their past or what they feel or think. It is as if we sit at the dinner table with Neanderthals who merely grunt and squeak, giving us few external clues to what is going on within them. We then have to guess at the content. We have to become extraordinarily sharp at watching the process by which information — the little that there is — is communicated, because the process of communication seems almost nonexistent.

This process of guessing about what is being communicated also happens in families where there is mental illness or addiction. Messages are unclear, contradictory or full of gaps created by denial. Remember that one of the rules in an addicted family is: "There's nothing wrong here. Don't talk about it."

In most of our families there are disallowed topics adding to the paucity of communication. What if we grow up in a family where it is not okay to talk about any topic that is considered touchy or conflictual?

Maybe we cannot talk about an illegitimate birth or alcoholism or poverty or criminality. Maybe we cannot talk about someone our parents did not like or did not approve of. Maybe we cannot talk about someone with whom our parents are in conflict — one of our grandparents or uncles or our parents' business partner. As children, we know which topics and patterns of communication are allowed and which ones are not allowed, even if no one tells us specifically. Our parents model how to communicate and we fall in line. We also, fortunately or unfortunately, may carry that model of communication into our adult life.

If we never see people talk directly to each other about sensitive issues, if we never see anyone talk about the topics that are disallowed in our family, we will be ill prepared to model those communication skills for our children. Again, we can't give what we didn't get.

In a sense, expecting ourselves to be able to model these skills for our children is like asking ourselves to replicate the sound of a tuba if we have never heard a tuba, never heard of a tuba and thus have no idea what a tuba sounds like.

Remember that many of us are the 180-degree-pendulum-swing parents who decided we wanted things in our new family to be different from the way they were in our own family of origin. And yet, ironically, we tend to replicate the communication patterns of our family of origin and also to select partners who have communication styles that are familiar to us. If we heard grunts and squeaks at the dinner table, we are likely to select a partner who grunts and squeaks. We are likely to grunt and squeak and guess what our children mean, and feel that that is communication.

Family communication patterns also fall on a continuum from reactive on one end to responsive on the other.

---

Reactive                                                      Responsive

Reactive communication is often explosive — "Step on a crack and you'll break your mother's back." If we do something small — step on a crack — by inadvertently mentioning a topic that is sensitive for Mom, it's like stepping on a mine in a minefield — or like breaking our mother's back. It's a big deal. When we grow up in a family that is reactive, there is a lot of denial. Therefore, a whole series of minefield topics cannot be discussed.

Responsive communication, on the other hand, is respectful. Even if the topic is loaded, our parents have dealt with some of their feelings about the issue and can respond appropriately. They can allow us to talk about whatever the issue is.

In a reactive family we are spoken for. We are interrupted, preempted and talked over. We experience our parents as insensitive to us and unreceptive to what we have to say. Some of the unresolved conflicts in our family may have less to do with the topic of conflict itself than with the reactive process of communication. When communication is chronically cut off and left incomplete, misunderstandings are inevitable, and only partial resolution of conflict is ever possible.

In a responsive communication pattern we are allowed to speak for ourselves. We are allowed to complete a communication sequence. We are given enough space to resolve any tension, anxiety or conflict over the subject about which we are communicating. We are encouraged to be direct, clear and concise. Our parents, in turn, are direct, clear and concise, as well as receptive and sensitive to what we have to say. When we grow up with this kind of communication we have a sense of being heard, seen, acknowledged and validated.

When we become adults and start our own families, we are likely to repeat the same patterns of reactive or responsive communication with which we grew up. Either listening well and being listened to feels familiar, or cutting off and being cut off feels familiar. Either sudden explosions or calm responses feel like home.

As you read this, you may end up thinking, "Oh my God, I don't communicate any better now than I did 20 or 30 years ago when I began my family. How am I going to communicate with my adult children — which is the reason I am reading this book?" Relax, if you will. We are going to talk about how to listen to your children and how to be a more effective communicator with your children. Please trust that there will be help when the time is right.

## EXERCISE

Take a moment to think about your family of origin. Plot their communication style on the following line.

Direct                                                              Indirect

Did your family have a switchboard operator? Who was it?

Did your family have other triangles or other ways to communicate indirectly?

Plot your family on the quantity-of-communication line that follows.

Sparse                                                    Overly Abundant

How did you react to the amount of communication in your family? Did you become silent, join in, try to fill the silences?

What topics were not allowed in your family?

In your family were you allowed to finish your thoughts, or were you interrupted or talked over? Did you feel as though there were hidden mines that might blow up if you said the wrong thing, or did you feel comfortable bringing up even sensitive topics? Plot your family on the reactive/ responsive continuum that follows.

Reactive                                                        Responsive

## Enforcement

All families have rules. All families must decide what is to be punished and what is to be rewarded. Just as important as the content of the rules themselves is the process by which rules are made known and enforced.

In some families, most of the rules are overt, directly spoken and clear. In other families, most of the rules are covert, unspoken, and we only find out about them after we have violated them.

Think again about the children's rhyme, "Step on a crack and you'll break your mother's back." In some families we only discover we have stepped on a crack because our mother acts as if we have broken her back.

For example, when I was five, I traded a box of chocolate pudding with a little boy up the street for a peek at his penis. His mother caught us as we were trading peeks at one another's genitalia. His mother was aghast at my behavior. Although her son was exactly the same age I was and was as interested in seeing what I had as I was in seeing what he had, I was treated like the perpetrator.

I was literally dragged home by the scruff of my neck and delivered to my mother and my aunts and my uncles, who were all sitting on the back porch. My shameful act was reported to them, and I found out this was not something I should have done. Although I had never been told about this crack, I had broken my mother's back.

How were rules enforced in our family? Probably the most powerful enforcement tool, and the most potent shaper of behavior, was shame. I cannot recall exactly the words that were said to me as I stood in that circle of my mother and my aunts and my uncles, but I can tell you that the shame I felt was severe. As that ring of giants stood around me pointing fingers at me, saying I should be ashamed of myself, I felt even smaller than my five-year-old size.

Incidentally, the shaming did not stop me from being curious about little boys' penises. It simply drove the behavior underground. But it did teach me that sexuality and curiosity about sexuality is shameful. Even more important, however, the shaming made me feel I was a bad person.

When we are shamed we feel exposed and humiliated to the core of our being. We feel reduced to the ashes of nothingness. We feel that who we are is inherently bad, evil, malevolent, unlovable, unvaluable.

Sometimes our family rules are enforced not by overt punishment that is shaming, but by a silence that is equally shaming. I come down the stairway dressed up and looking pretty. My father, whose attention I want, turns away without a word. I have been told, without a word being spoken, that I am not worth commenting upon.

Family rules may also be enforced by comparisons that are shaming: "Little Susie down the street doesn't do such and such."

There can be an emotionally or physically abusive aspect to rule enforcement in the family. If, for instance, whenever Dad is displeased with us, he flicks us in the temple with his finger and says, "You dummy, you dummy, you dummy," we will not come away with high self-esteem.

The extreme of rule enforcement and punishment, of course, is serious physical abuse. Many of us have come from such abusive families that simply making it into adulthood is a statement of our incredible resilience and ability to survive and adapt.

Rule enforcement and punishment can leave us with either damaged self-esteem or intact self-esteem. If we come from a family where there is empathy and sensitivity and respect for our individuality, in all likelihood we will be talked with when we break a rule, and we will not be shamed. We will be both supported and corrected at the same time.

There is an important difference between enforcement that attacks the child's self and enforcement that attacks the child's behavior.

Enforcement attacks the child's self when it says, "You are a bad person, a bad little boy, a bad little girl. You should be ashamed of yourself. You're a dummy."

Enforcement does *not* attack the child's self when it says, "You got into the cookie jar when you know that is not allowable behavior. You have to ask Grandpa when you want a cookie. I am disappointed in your behavior, but I love you as a person."

If we grow up in a family where the enforcement methods are harsh or shaming, it will affect the toolbox we bring to our new family in two ways. First, we may have deep emotional wounds and a sense of diminished personhood in our toolbox. Second, we will probably have a blank space where there should be healthy models of enforcement.

We may not want to replicate our family's enforcement methods, but we may have no other models that can guide us when our children are difficult. We all know that children are not just magical children. They can try the patience of a saint.

We are likely to do one of two things in our new family. We may do the 180-degree pendulum swing and vow never to be the shaming parent. Instead we may become the laissez-faire, permissive parent who never shames, but who also never intervenes or gives direction.

Or we may, in fact, act out the defense mechanism of identification with the aggressor. Though we do not consciously intend to do so, we become the shaming parent to our children that our parents once were to us.

---

## EXERCISE

Each of the parenting figures in your childhood may have used different methods to enforce the family rules. Think for a moment of times when each of them corrected or punished you. What methods did each one use?

Which methods were shaming, and which were not shaming?

---

## Conflict

What process does our family use to handle conflict? Probably no emotion is handled more poorly in our culture than the emotion of anger, and anger goes hand in hand with conflict. When we talk about conflict resolution, we are also talking about anger.

How is anger handled in our family? Who is allowed to be angry and who is not? Maybe in our family children are not allowed to be angry, but parents are. Or maybe one of our parents is allowed to be angry and the other parent isn't.

For instance, if Dad is physically and verbally abusive and seems angry all the time about everything, it is highly likely that

Mom is relatively passive, silent and nonconflictual. Clearly Dad is allowed the emotion of anger. Mom is not allowed the open expression of anger, but we might ask ourselves, "Where does Mother's anger go?"

For reasons buried in her own childhood, Mother may not feel she has permission to express her anger openly. She may have married Dad so that he could express open anger for both of them. This does not mean Mother is never angry. Mom expresses anger for both of them in the sneaky, silent way which is her style. And in conflicts between Mom and Dad, Mom will use an indirect style and Dad will use a direct one.

For instance, when we are adolescents, Dad wants our rooms to be clean. Dad's standard for cleanliness includes making our bed, putting away our clothes, vacuuming the carpet once a week and keeping large objects, such as rotten food, off our dresser and desk. Dad comes into our room to see if we have done our chores as ordered by him. Our room does not pass muster. Dad furiously goes to Mom and complains to her about our room being dirty.

Mom, however, does not agree with Dad's standard for cleanliness for us as adolescents. Nor does she agree he should be the one to make the rules for us. She may even have said to us behind the scenes, "You know how your father is: He expects the house to look like a museum. You really don't have to keep your room as clean as your father insists. I'll take care of your dad."

When Mom and Dad have this conflict over our messy rooms, Mom's anger will not come out directly. She will say to Dad, "Their rooms aren't that bad. I'm sure they vacuumed some time in the last week. I'm sure they have cleaned the tops of their dressers and the tops of their desks some time in the last month. They're boys. Boys will be boys. I'll get them to clean it up tomorrow."

The issue, by the way, is not just our dirty rooms. The issue is the inability of Mom and Dad to resolve the question of who's in control. Their conflict about control gets played out over our rooms, giving us one message from Dad and one message from Mom.

Mom's and Dad's inability to resolve their conflict about control will affect our relationship with them. In this example, we will feel somewhat estranged from Dad, and we may feel angry about this estrangement. Since Mom has covertly allied herself with us against Dad and used us in her battle with Dad, she will foster our anger at Dad and will get in the way of our having a direct, nonconflictual relationship with him.

In the section on communication, I talked about functional communication as direct, person-to-person communication. In an instance such as this, where we are in alliance with Mom against Dad, we do not have an opportunity to have a direct, person-to-person relationship with Dad. Nor do we have an opportunity to work out our conflict with Dad directly without Mom as an intervening variable.

We also don't see our parents working out conflict in a direct way. Since we generally see Mom win with her indirect methods, we may learn her method of "conflict resolution": Be indirect, and pull in your children as allies.

Most families have some conflicts that seem unresolvable. What does our family do with its "unresolvable" conflicts?

One method of dealing with these conflicts is to deny the conflicts; they simply are not there. The classic example of denial is called "the elephant in the living room." In an alcoholic family, even though the alcoholism is as obvious as an elephant standing in the middle of the living room, everyone acts as though the elephant is not there.

Our family can also handle a conflict they cannot resolve by acting the conflict out. Mom and Dad fighting over our dirty rooms to avoid their conflict over control is an example of how a conflict can be acted out. Acting out the conflict provides a way to discharge the anger and the energy while at the same time avoiding the real issue.

Sometimes we children become the scapegoats, the targets, the whipping boys or girls for the issues our parents cannot resolve. Acting out their anger toward us scapegoats distracts them and reduces the tension between them.

Let's say, for example, Stepdad feels relatively small and powerless out in the world of grown-ups. He can't tolerate being seen as small and powerless in Mom's eyes; he adores her. He can't speak about his feelings. Instead, there is an unnamed tension between Mom and Stepdad about his lack of success, his shame over his lack of success and her feared or real criticism of his lack of success. He takes out on us his feelings about what he cannot resolve in the outside world and what he cannot speak about with Mom. He becomes a petty tyrant, demanding that we be perfect. In so doing, he feels big and powerful with these little people who cannot resist his demands. He acts out his frustration on us, his scapegoats.

Let's look at another example. I am a 16-year-old boy, and I have asked Dad if I can borrow the car tonight to take my girl-friend on a date. Dad has said yes. Dad then notices I have not done my chores correctly. Dad forbids me to use the car.

I cannot possibly tell my girlfriend that I cannot go out tonight because "my mommy and my daddy" won't let me. Since my family has no conflict resolution process I can turn to, I act out what seems to me an unresolvable conflict.

I sneak out the window and steal the family car. I go out on my date. At 2:00 A.M. I come home and brazenly beat on the front door, demanding to be let in, even though I know this will result in a direct confrontation with my father.

My father is enraged. He beats me, shames me, grounds me, prohibits me from talking on the telephone or doing anything but going to school for a two-week period. There is no chance my father will give me room to state my point of view. I will never be able to tell him what it feels like to be a 16-year-old male facing the prospect of being shamed in the eyes of my girlfriend. There is no way this episode will do anything but leave a scar on me and a scar on my dad.

What Dad and I have not learned is how to resolve conflict. Nor have we learned how to hear one another's points of view. My dad has a valid point of view; I have a valid point of view. Both of those points of view got lost in how the conflict was handled.

Addictions are a way of dealing with conflict that cannot be resolved. It has often been said that substance abuse addictions in men have to do with conflicts they cannot resolve in the larger world and that substance abuse addictions in women have to do with conflicts they cannot resolve in their intimate relationships. This is, of course, a gross generalization, and there are many, many exceptions to it. But let's take an example that fits the pattern.

Let's say, for instance, that our stepmother does not feel she has a voice. She grew up in her own family of origin as the last born, an unwanted, disempowered child. We would expect her to put herself in a marital situation where she can replicate feeling unwanted, disempowered and voiceless, which, in fact, she has done with our dad.

Because she has no sense of personal power or personal efficacy, because she has never seen conflict resolution modeled and because anger for her is a disallowed emotion, she will feel powerless in the face of an "unresolvable" conflict between her and Dad. Her anger may come out by her being unconscious on the kitchen floor, drunk with alcohol.

Those of us who are proponents of the disease and the genetic concept of alcoholism may take umbrage at what I am saying. But bear in mind that alcoholism is more than just a genetically mediated disorder. Alcoholism often serves a function and often provides a secondary gain for the alcoholic.

In this instance, our stepmom's alcoholism, though possibly genetic in origin, serves the relational function of saying to Dad, "I'm angry with you. I feel disempowered. Let's see how powerful you feel trying to get me off the kitchen floor." Our stepmother uses her addiction as a way of dealing with what seems to her an unresolvable conflict.

Our stepmother, for instance, might want to leave her marriage. Because of the beliefs of her Catholic family, she cannot tolerate being the first person in her family to ask for a divorce. If she can become sufficiently obnoxious, maybe Dad will leave her and resolve this conflict.

## Cutoffs

One of the most common ways families handle an unresolvable conflict is by using a cutoff. When we use a cutoff, we terminate our relationship with the person with whom we have a conflict. When Mom hasn't seen or spoken to her older sister for 30 years, she has used an extreme form of cutoff.

Cutoffs don't have to be physical, however. Earlier I used the term *fixed-distance, perfunctory relationships*. Those are relationships in which family members maintain physical contact but have cut off relational contact. That is to say, nothing important is allowed to happen in those relationships. There is no intimacy, and there is no potential for conflict.

For example, Joseph's mother has a very limited tolerance for any kind of intense emotion. If Joseph tries to talk to her about anything that is emotional or controversial or in any way disturbing to her, she will become very upset and say, "I don't need this. I don't need to be upset like this. I don't need to talk about this."

If Joseph continues to push the issue, she'll become either confused or mute. Obviously, he can't force her to talk about anything she doesn't want to talk about because, by going mute or presenting herself as confused, she'll cut him off.

Here's another example. Roberta and her stepfather despise each other. But the rule in the family is that Roberta and her stepdad can't fight openly because it will upset Mother. So although she and her stepfather are often the only two people awake and in the kitchen in the early morning, they do not acknowledge each other's physical presence.

At night at the dinner table, they make polite conversation. She and her older brother polish off dinner in three minutes flat and then say, "Mother, that was an absolutely wonderful dinner. May we be excused?" Mother says, "Thank you. Yes, you may be excused," and they bolt from the table. That's a relational cutoff.

What do we learn when we grow up in a family where emotional cutoffs are the name of the game? If Mom stopped speaking to her sister 30 years ago or if our older sibling was cast out of the family for some unspoken crime, we will learn to avoid conflict. We will naturally be afraid that if we cross Mom or if we say something she does not like, she will cut us off for 30 years as well.

Our greatest fear as children is that we will be abandoned or annihilated — and *annihilated* means not only being killed; it means going into relational nothingness with the people to whom we have to be attached in order to survive. We will avoid conflict to avoid this ultimate cutoff.

We might pick up the cutoff pattern ourselves. If Joseph is in an intimate relationship and his partner starts pushing him to talk about something he doesn't want to talk about, he may hear himself say, "I don't need this. I don't need to talk about this right now."

Suddenly, halfway through the sentence, Joseph may think, "Oh my God, this is exactly what my mother did that drove me crazy. I've learned to do cutoffs too." Then he has to stop himself and remember that relationships are labor-intensive endeavors that require a commitment to be there with another human being around the hard issues. But that was never modeled in his family; so it's a stretch for him to do that.

In *Family Therapy In Clinical Practice*, Murray Bowen defines certain individuals as relational nomads. These are people who yearn for intimacy but also fear it. When they get to the point in a relationship where they are about to have real intimacy, they cut off the relationship. Then they move not only into a new relationship, but also into a totally different life. In the course of a lifetime, a relational nomad may create totally new relational networks three or four times. They sever the past as if it no longer exists. They live histories of emotional incompletion and unfinished grief work. They do not resolve conflict. They just move on and on and on and on.

In healthy families conflict is dealt with directly in respectful, person-to-person exchanges. The conflict is not buried or avoided. It is not allowed to fester or to continue unattended.

A healthy family recognizes that the resolution of conflict has the potential to lead to deeper, more intimate and more respectful relationships between the people involved. Conflict resolution implies sensitivity and respect. People are expected to develop empathy and a willingness to put themselves in the other person's shoes. Family members are willing to really see, hear and validate each other. The point of conflict resolution is to look for ways to resolve the problem, not to find ways to blame the other person or to make the other person wrong and ourselves right.

Healthy families recognize that all individuals within the group contribute to the strength of the group as a whole. If any person feels disallowed, invalidated or extruded by virtue of an issue that goes unresolved, not only is the position of that person weakened; the position of the family as a whole is weakened.

If a conflict appears to be unresolvable, the family may reach for outside help, such as a counselor, a minister or an attorney. They may pull in their extended family system or friends. A Native American family may call a meeting of their entire social network, extended family and elders for a discussion of the problem.

In a healthy family, a conflict that seems unresolvable stays out in the open and continues to be a subject for discussion. The family is willing to experiment with various solutions and to go through a process of trial and error as it attempts to resolve the conflict.

## EXERCISE

List the members of your family of origin in the first column. In the Anger column write "yes" or "no" to indicate whether or not this family member was allowed to express anger openly. Since we know that anger that is not expressed openly will still come out somehow, in the Indirect Methods column write the ways in which each person's anger came out indirectly. Include yourself as a child or a teen on the list as well.

| Name | Anger | Indirect Methods |
| --- | --- | --- |
| | | |
| | | |
| | | |
| | | |
| | | |
| | | |

How would you describe your family's method of conflict resolution?

What did your family consider unresolvable conflicts?

What did your family do about these conflicts?

If you have trouble identifying specific "unresolvable" issues, think back to any addictions, cutoffs, abuse or scapegoating you remember in your family. Then ask yourself, "What might have been the underlying issue when my parents used cutoffs or scapegoating?"

Were the children in your family asked, or forced, to play a role in these conflicts between your parents?

Did your family call in outside support to help with the most difficult issues?

Did your family encourage empathy, good listening, validating the other's point of view, experimenting with various solutions?

---

## What Is Allowed?

All families have rules that tell us what is allowed and what is not allowed in "our family." In my friend's Swedish, Lutheran family, for example, no one but Dad was allowed to serve the plates. That was an obvious rule.

There are rules that are much more subtle, however, that settle into our bones and make us feel that certain behaviors are "good and safe" or "bad and dangerous." These rules are not usually communicated directly, but they are enforced.

We are going to look at some of these subtle, but extremely vital, rules to see what was modeled for us. We need to find out which ones ended up in our toolbox, unconsciously telling us what should be allowed and what should not be allowed in our new family.

### Are Mistakes And Human Fallibility Allowed?

Are mistakes and human fallibility allowed in our family of origin? Or to phrase the question differently: Are our parents realistic? Do they have realistic expectations, or are their standards too high or too low?

If our parents expect too much of us, we may become perfectionistic children — depression-prone, always feeling defeated, always feeling like failures. Or we may become children who never try because the standard is set too high. We look at the goal and say, "What an order! I can't go through with it."

If our parents' standards are set too low, our parents may fail to encourage us. Perhaps they came from families where their weaknesses were never acknowledged. If they then became 180-degree-pendulum-swing parents who swore they would support their children when their children felt afraid or weak, they may inadvertently fail to reinforce our strengths. Instead, they undermine our autonomy and our developing sense of identity.

How are mistakes seen in our family of origin? Does a mistake mean that one of our parents goes ballistic? Or is a mistake merely something to learn from and correct?

Remember that we are all "monkey-see, monkey-do" people. Our parents will often either repeat with us what happened with them or attempt to be 180 degrees different from their own parents.

If Mom came from a brutalizing, sadistic, Nazi-like, punishing family where mistakes were capital offenses, then Mom is likely to respond to our mistakes in a similar way. For instance, Mom may send us to our room when we are six years old to straighten up our toys. Because we are six, we most likely will not stack our toys perfectly. When Mom comes back to check on our work, she may knock all of the books and toys off our bookcase and make us start all over again because we didn't do it "right." We may repeat this process four or five times with her until we finally get it right, until we finally get it perfect.

What we learn is that mistakes are capital offenses. We also learn either to be paralyzed, frightened children who will not try anything or to be perfection-seeking adults who not only expect perfection from ourselves, but also knock the toys off the shelves of every other person around us who fails to perform to our unrealistic standards.

This attitude about mistakes ties in with another piece of the family emotional process: What is the basic attitude our parents have about human beings? Are human beings basically good or are they basically evil? Are humans trustworthy or untrustworthy?

If our parents consider humans untrustworthy, they may assume that when we make a mistake, we are making that mistake on purpose — deliberately being bad or acting out the evil inside us. They may teach us to be suspicious — to watch out for guns and bogeymen and people who are going to get us. They may impair our naive, loving, open-hearted, trusting wonder child.

If our parents see humans as basically good, most likely they see mistakes as inevitable and necessary for growth. Mistakes are part of trial-and-error learning; they are aids to self-correction and examples our parents can use to help us learn to be healthy, self-directing human beings.

Making mistakes is human. Needing help is also human. In our family, are we allowed or expected to ask for help? Is help given?

Those of us who come from highly dysfunctional families may learn to become what I call defensively self-reliant. In families where there is little clear communication but severe punishment for rules broken, in families where we are expected to be perfect, we learn we cannot rely on our parents for help. We become afraid to admit we don't know something, to ask for help. In fact, we learn to not even know we need help, let alone ask for it. To ask for help means being vulnerable and running the risk of being rejected or shamed or punished or met with silence.

We may also learn not to ask for help because we see our parents as fragile. When we ask for help, we face our parents' incompetence or our fear that they will fall apart in the face of their own inability to help us. We will avoid anything that might shame or embarrass them.

In our family of origin, are we allowed to acknowledge illness or addiction or human frailty? Is it all right to be subject to the human condition? Or are we members of a family attempting to heal intergenerational shame through silence and perfection? In such an instance, we cannot acknowledge imperfection, even if imperfection includes disability, addiction or illness.

In healthy families, there is an acknowledgment that we are fallible human beings, that we are imperfect people in an imperfect world. Our parents have realistic expectations of what is or is not possible. Our family does not think in terms of black and white, but understands that much of life is middling gray.

In healthy families, human beings are seen as basically good, as basically trustworthy. Our parents acknowledge that there is evil in the world, and that we must learn to discern good from evil and people who are trustworthy from people who are not trustworthy. But there is an underlying belief in the basic goodness of human beings.

In healthy families, mistakes are seen as necessary for growth. In order for us to avoid becoming Johnny One-Notes who only do what we do well, and do that compulsively, we need to try many different things so we can discover what we are good at and master what we are not good at. It is all just seen as learning. Making mistakes has nothing to do with our goodness or our badness, our stupidness or our smartness.

In healthy families, we are not only allowed to ask for help, but also expected to ask for help. We are given help based on our level of development. When we are little, we are not expected to do more than we realistically can do. When we are older, we are given less help in areas where we are developing autonomy and more help in ways that are appropriate to us as fledgling adults.

We are allowed to acknowledge and expected to acknowledge our fallibility. It is all right to say, "I can't. I don't know how." It is all right to say, "I'm sick. I feel scared." It is all right to say, "I have a problem. I have an addiction, and I don't know how to deal with it. I need your help."

------------------------------| **E X E R C I S E** |------------------------------

Plot each of the people who parented you on the following scale. How realistic or unrealistic were your parents in what they expected as you were growing up? Did they expect perfection (expectations too high), or did they expect failure or nothing (expectations too low)?

Too high                                                                    Too low

What did each parent do when you made a mistake?
What did each parent do when you asked for help?
How did your parents react when you had an illness, an addiction, a disability?

How would you describe each of your parents' attitudes toward human beings? Would they say humans are basically good and trustworthy or basically bad and untrustworthy? Plot each one on the line that follows.

---

Basically good                                                      Basically bad

---

## Are We Allowed To Process Losses?

One of the most important things we learn or fail to learn in our family of origin is how to deal with loss. As children, are we allowed to acknowledge and process loss?

If we find a dead sparrow, how do our parents explain death? Do they help us put the sparrow in a cigarbox and dig a little grave and say a eulogy for the sparrow? Or do they ridicule our feelings of sadness? Do our parents throw it in the garbage or put it in the incinerator and feed our negative fantasies about what happens to dead things?

When the little girl next door and her family move away — the little girl who is our best friend and her parents who are our beloved surrogate parents — how do our parents help us deal with our feelings of loss and sadness? Is our sadness acknowledged? Are we held and allowed to cry? Are we helped to talk about how sad we feel? Or do our parents act as if the little girl never lived next door, as if her parents had never been important to us? How our family deals with loss, separation and mourning teaches us how to grieve and how to complete relationships as they come to a natural or unnatural end.

Grief has been called the pain that heals itself if we do not get in the way. That is to say, if we can allow ourselves the full range of emotions that go with grief, and if others do not shame us or otherwise impede our grief process, we will heal.

If losses cannot be acknowledged openly, particularly the loss of a central family member or losses that have catastrophic effects on our family system, we send our feelings underground and end up with an enormous fund of uncompleted grief.

In the film *Harold and Maude*, Maude is an old woman who may still be carrying unresolved grief from her childhood, which was not worked through at the time the losses occurred. We see her going from funeral to funeral, graveyard to graveyard, vicariously grieving over the loss of people to whom she is not related.

It is as if there is a pent-up demand for grief energy to be expressed. It will be expressed either appropriately in grieving that is supported at the time of the loss, or inappropriately in vicarious grieving, depression, aggression, psychosomatic illness or through some other avenue of incomplete mourning.

What do we do with grief that is not allowed? What do we do with loss that cannot be acknowledged?

When we are children, unless we can get reassurance and a realistic perspective from someone older, we often assume inappropriate responsibility for the loss. Remember that, as children, we can be quite grandiose, tremendously overestimating our capacity to affect things.

Let's say we lose a sibling with whom we had a fight or a sibling with whom we were competitive and whom we occasionally wished dead. If we cannot air our feelings about this sibling's death, we may be plagued by the fantasy that our wish caused the death.

We can attribute all kinds of malice and evil to ourselves, particularly between the ages of three and six, which are the critical times for conscience formation. We desperately need our parents to teach us how to deal with loss in order for us not to attribute such powerful malevolence to ourselves.

We desperately need our parents to help us understand what is written in Ecclesiastes — that there is a season for all things. There is a season for sorrow and grieving; there is a season to begin again. They must teach us that when any attachment is severed, if we do the work of grieving, we will be free to attach again, to trust again and to begin the next stage of a growth process.

We may have come from a family that has experienced what I call "unspeakable" losses or socially negated losses. Maybe one of our parents was murdered, and we cannot talk about that loss because of the tremendous shame inherent in murder itself. Maybe our father was jailed for child molestation. We cannot speak of the loss we feel or of how much we miss our father because he has committed what is seen as a socially heinous crime. There will be no sympathy for our grief.

We may not be able to speak about our grandfather who was homosexual and who died in the arms of his lover. We may not be able to talk about our beloved father who was repeatedly unfaithful to our mother and whose infidelity is such a source of shame to our family. We may learn not to mention our aunt who died as the end result of syphilitic infection. We may have a parent who died of an addiction, a form of suicide that cannot be discussed because of the shame attendant upon that kind of death.

There is a phenomenon called the multigenerational shock wave. When a family does not process a major loss completely, a shock wave travels down the generations and affects family members who weren't even alive at the time of the loss.

Let's say our mother never grieved over the loss she experienced when she moved away from her family of origin. She has managed to avoid this grief by psychologically never leaving home. Her family of origin is still more important to her than the family she has created with her spouse. Her allegiance is to her own family of origin, particularly to her mother.

When we are 13 years old, our mother's mother dies. Again, instead of grieving over this loss, she avoids it. This time, she goes "crazy" for a number of years. She behaves toward us in very inappropriate ways, as if we were both her lover and some hated object. Her behavior is extremely confusing. In effect, she is acting out her pain and confusion on us, instead of working through her internal anguish over losing her mother.

We, at 13 years old, have no way of making sense out of our mother's behavior. Her actions give us a very confused and anguished adolescence at a time when we need her help in making the transition from childhood to young adulthood. We may get physically or psychologically stuck at home in much the same way that our mother was stuck at home with her mother, still trying to resolve our relationship with our mother before we are free enough to move on and create a life and relationship of our own.

The loss in our mother's generation affects the tools we take to our adult life. One tool may be a confusion about our gender identity, that is to say, who we are sexually. If we are female, are we our mother's surrogate husband? Are we male or female?

Our intimacy tools may be affected also. Maybe we can't let anyone get close to us because one of our closest relationships felt frightening and terribly confusing. We might set off on a course of being a loner.

We may make the transition into young adulthood and intimacy but act out this confusion about gender and intimacy with our own children in much the same way our mother acted out her confusion with us. Thus our mother's unmourned loss has traveled down the generations in a shock wave that affects our children.

We need tremendous help as children in learning to deal with loss. In healthy families, losses are acknowledged and worked through. We are given support to have a full range of emotions about the loss. We are not shamed for our feelings. We are helped to talk about the loss and to put the loss in perspective. We are taught that it takes time to work through loss. Most important, we learn the wound will heal if we have support; we will be stronger for the experience; we will go on with our lives.

---

## EXERCISE

Think back to your first experiences with loss. Did your parents help you understand the loss? Did they comfort you and allow you to express your feelings and thoughts?

How did your parents explain death to you?

How did your parents deal with losses that happened to them?

Were there "unspeakable" losses in your family? What were they?

---

## Are Differences And Autonomy Allowed?

In our family of origin, is it all right to be unique, to be different from the other family members, to be separate? Are differences respected, or are differences ridiculed, shamed and punished? How much autonomy are we allowed to have?

Some of our families had a rule about difference: "In order to be a member of this family, we all have to be the same. Children have to be carbon copies of their parents. If they are not carbon copies, they will be considered Benedict Arnolds, disloyal to the family."

In these families, any difference may be seen as competitive. A difference may, in fact, bring to the fore our parents' sense of incompetency or inadequacy. If our "different" dream or ability went undeveloped in our parents' lives, it may be punished in its nascent form in our life.

In these families, we may be expected to have a relationship with only one parent. Particularly if our family has experienced desertion or divorce, we may be expected to be loyal to our remaining parent. We may be considered disloyal if we have feelings of yearning, love or longing for our absent parent, because our feelings are different from the feelings of our custodial parent.

In other families, differences are fostered. We are encouraged to find our own spot in the sun. We are encouraged to develop our own unique abilities. We are allowed to have our own feelings and our own voice. Since differences are respected and we are not tied to a hidebound family loyalty code, we are allowed and expected to have a different relationship with each parent without feeling as if we are alienating the other parent.

If our family allows us to be different, it is more likely to allow us to develop our autonomy as well. If family members are separate, autonomous people, each of us is expected to take responsibility for our own actions. Responsibility goes hand in hand with autonomy.

Do our parents take responsibility for their actions, their errors? Do they promptly admit when they are wrong? Or do they assume they are always right and put all the blame on us children?

Blaming is often an intergenerational issue. If our parents came from families where there was too much blame put on the children, our parents probably did not learn how to take responsibility because they didn't see it modeled by their parents. Our parents, in turn, become blamers and expect themselves to be perfect. Any criticism is taken as more blame and more shame, as if it were again handed out by their powerful parents to them as powerless children.

We, then, being overblamed by them, may not know the difference between blame and responsibility when we rear our own children. We may overblame our children because we have internalized so much childhood shame from being blamed that this shame is triggered when we are asked to take responsibility.

If we come from an overblaming family, to learn to say, "I'm sorry, I'm wrong," is excruciating work. When we come into adulthood, we may not have in our toolbox an ability to say we are wrong, just as our parents had no ability to say they were wrong.

It's possible, by the way, for our parents to say they are wrong in words, but still not apologize. We may grow up with parents who were so blamed and shamed that they learned to defend themselves by saying something like, "All right, all right, I'm a no-good S.O.B. You know I'm a no-good S.O.B; all the world knows I'm a no-good S.O.B. You're always right; I'm always wrong."

This kind of defusing, disarming, self-defensive statement does not lead to conflict resolution. It gives everyone involved, including the parent who talks that way, a feeling of impotence.

In either the overblaming or the totally self-blaming family, we do not learn about real apologies or amends. We do not learn how to take responsibility for our actions.

Healthy families support their members' autonomy by teaching them how to take responsibility for harm done. They know the difference between blame and responsibility and can apologize and make amends when it is appropriate.

The ultimate family rules about autonomy have to do with our leaving home. Our family needs to give us roots to grow and wings to leave. Deep in the family emotional process are embedded the unspoken expectations about how deep our roots should go, how long our roots should stay attached, how big our wings should grow, when or if we should leave home and how we should leave home.

Are we expected to leave home, or are we expected to stay home and take care of our elderly parents? Is it considered an act of disloyalty to grow up and leave home? If there is a "Don't separate" message in our family of origin, it will have implications for us in our later spousal or partnered relationships, because that rule requires that we be more loyal to our family of origin than we are to our new family.

---

### EXERCISE

Were you expected to be different from your parents and siblings or the same? Plot each of your parent's attitudes on the following line.

---

Different                                                    Same

Were there particular differences your parents had strong reactions to? What were they? Do you know why your parents reacted so strongly to these differences?

Were you allowed to have a different relationship with each parent?

Do you remember your parents apologizing or admitting mistakes? Do you remember your parents making amends?

Do you remember your parents blaming?

---

## Are All Emotions Allowed?

One of the critically important parts of the family emotional process has to do with which emotions are allowed and which are disallowed. Ideally, each of us should be gifted with a family that can allow the full range of human emotions. Ideally, each of us should be gifted with a background that tells us that, just as it is written in Ecclesiastes, there is a season for all things, there is also a season for all feelings.

No emotion is inherently bad. Feelings are just feelings. Feelings are not stupid; they do not have IQs. We can use feelings in bad, stupid or irresponsible ways by doing things that are damaging to ourselves or to others, but feelings in themselves are not bad or stupid.

If healthily supported, feelings should not be a source of shame, but a source of personal growth and self-awareness. They should give us guidelines for appropriate action.

Many of us did not grow up in the fantasy-land family I have just described. Most of us grew up in families where certain feelings were forbidden.

In many of our families, anger is a forbidden emotion. I think that, particularly, we Americans are anger-phobic. Our country is one of the most violent, dangerous and destructive nations in the world — it is probably more dangerous to be in downtown Los Angeles than to be in a Third World terrorist country, for instance. On one hand we disavow anger and talk about how peace-loving we are, and on the other we act out our anger enormously. So anger in many families is a forbidden emotion.

In other families, fear, weakness and vulnerability are forbidden. Male children, in particular, may have the experience of being brutally punished for what is seen as unmanly or cowardly behavior. The message may be, "Hide your fear at all costs. Men don't do that."

Little boys, of course, have all the same feelings that little girls have. Unfortunately, if fear gets driven underground, it can come out in adulthood in macho bravado or risk-taking behavior that is both dangerous and aversive to others.

In some of our families, sadness is a forbidden emotion. It is not all right for us to be sad, to be hurt, to whine or to complain. These emotions are punished and driven underground.

In other families, it is not okay to be lonely or to feel empty or bereft. We must always feel, or appear to feel, fine.

In some of our families, the joyous emotions are forbidden: laughter, fun, play, expansiveness, joyousness. This is not difficult to understand, by the way, in a country in which many of the founders were Puritans — or criminals. When you look at it from that point of view, it makes sense that sinfulness and joyousness are often considered to be next-door neighbors.

We learn that the forbidden emotions are sources of shame. We will be shamed if we allow these emotions to emerge. Eventually, with enough practice, we learn not to notice when we feel these feelings.

Since all emotions are part of the normal range of human feelings, when any emotion is not allowed, it will be pushed underground, leading to an emotional poverty in our family. It will leave us with a somewhat constricted personality, a personality that is lopsided in the direction of grimness or anger or playfulness and irreverence, or fear or sadness.

When I was a small child, I was called the terrible-tempered Mr. Bang by my family. My anger was recognized, but it was shamed. Other emotions were so forbidden they were not even named. I was not allowed to be the anxious, frightened child that I was, nor was I allowed to be the terribly sad and fretful child that I was. All of these emotions simply got rolled into one lump, and I was called temperamental and difficult.

As an adult, I have learned to stop when I feel angry — the one emotion I had been allowed to name and acknowledge — and see if any of the emotions I hadn't been allowed to name or acknowledge are present. I ask myself, "Is this anger a primary or a secondary emotion? That is, am I really angry, or is this my habitual response when I am frightened, sad, empty or hurt?"

You can see from this example what might happen to emotions we are forbidden to acknowledge in childhood. We may bury them under other feelings as I sometimes do. We also may act them out; we may project them; we may be indirect with them, or we may turn them into illnesses.

For instance, one of our parents may act out anger. The cords in our parent's neck may be straining almost to the point of popping while our parent screams at us, "If you don't behave, I'm going to get angry at you." Our parent is completely unaware that he or she is already angry and acting out that anger.

If our parents were treated sadistically by their parents, they may act out the hurt and anger they were never allowed to express by behaving in torturous ways toward us. They may have no conscious awareness that they have put together hurt and power and combined them in a toxic, sadistic cocktail for us.

Feelings that have been forbidden can be projected onto other people. If our parents are carrying buried grief, our sadness may be intolerable to them. They will see mirrored in our sad face their own sad inner child of the past. Our sad face has the potential for triggering their own grief over their own unmourned losses, and they may find themselves saying, "Wipe that look off your face or I'll give you something to be sad about." They may punish us as a way of vicariously punishing the sad child within themselves who is beginning to feel the forbidden emotion. They may fear that our sadness will be as huge and overwhelming as their own.

Forbidden emotions may come up in indirect ways. Passive-aggressive behavior is a good example of indirect anger, for instance. Let me give you an example.

Let's say my partner asks me to pick up the dry cleaning and I resent the request. Maybe I see it as an unreasonable demand being made on my time.

I may not feel free to say to my partner, "I don't want to pick up the dry cleaning; pick it up yourself. I feel like you are making an unreasonable demand on my time." Instead I say, "Yes, I'd be delighted to pick up the dry cleaning." Then I forget to pick it up.

When I get home, my partner says to me, "I thought you said you'd pick up the dry cleaning."

I can say, "I forgot. What do you want to do, kill me? I forgot. It's not a capital offense."

What I have failed to do, first with myself and then with my partner, is to own the extent to which I felt angry at the request. Rather than dealing in a direct, person-to-person way with my partner, I have instead acted out the anger in an indirect, passive way. This is called passive-aggressive behavior.

Forbidden emotions can show up in several other ways. Sometimes an unexpressed emotion comes out through an addiction or a psychosomatic illness.

Let's go back to the example in which our grandmother dies when we are 13 and our mother goes crazy. As part of mother's craziness, she develops hypochondriasis. She develops a whole series of nonorganically based, mythical illnesses.

Even though her family rules say she is not allowed to mourn this loss, her internal signal system is trying to tell her there is something wrong here that she needs some help with. If she doesn't attend to the signal, she may, in fact, end up with a real illness caused, or aided, by the stress of the suppressed emotions.

Let's look for a moment at how these allowed and disallowed emotions from our family of origin affect the tools we take to intimacy and parenting. If we come from a family with a fairly large range of forbidden emotions, those are likely to be the emotions with which we are least comfortable and most unfamiliar. We may pick as a partner someone who is within our emotional comfort range, someone who has the same restricted range of emotion that we have. We therefore role model and allow a very narrow emotional range for our children.

Or we may pick as a partner someone who looks exciting because he or she carries the emotional range that has been disallowed for us. The irony is that the more time we spend with a partner who has all these "exciting" emotions, the more fault we are likely to find with his or her emotions. Our childhood discomfort is still with us.

In this case, we not only will bring emotional limitations to our children, but also create conflict for them. They will have to choose between our constricted emotional range and our partner's wide emotional range — a range which has become scary for them because of our discomfort and conflict with it. We have provided our children with two models for how to deal with emotions, but we have left them with the feeling that emotions are dangerous. They have not seen how to stand in emotions, deal with emotions, acknowledge emotions and work through emotions.

---

## EXERCISE

Take a moment to look at the following list of emotions. Circle any that were not allowed in your childhood family. Add any others to the list that your family did not allow.

| | |
|---|---|
| Anger | Grief |
| Fear | Anxiety |
| Weakness | Vulnerability |
| Sadness | Hurt |
| Loneliness | Emptiness |
| Playfulness | Joy |

Others _____

What did each of your parents do with the feelings that were not allowed in your childhood family? What did you do with the feelings that were not allowed? Here are some possibilities:

Buried them under other emotions
Acted them out
Projected them onto other people
Expressed them indirectly
Got addictions or psychosomatic illnesses

Others _____

---

## Are We Allowed To Prioritize Ourselves Before Our Family Of Origin?

We all need parents who have a healthy self-focus. Having a healthy self-focus means our parents can put themselves first. They can put their relationship with their spouse or partner second. And finally, they can put the needs of their partner and their children above the needs of their family of origin. In so doing, they model a healthy self-focus.

They give us this message: "Until and unless I have a healthy sense of my own separateness and completeness, I have nothing to give someone else. When I have a healthy self-focus and little unfinished business from my childhood, I can come together with another relatively complete person and be ready to be intimate. I can then provide a holding environment for children. I can appropriately parent them and put their needs before the needs of my family of origin. It is not that I am not caring or concerned about my family of origin, but my priorities have shifted. My allegiance is now to this family I have created."

Now, let me explain the difference between healthy self-focus and narcissism. A number of us came from families where we had narcissistic parents. Narcissism is not healthy self-focus.

Narcissism is a kind of self-focus wherein the rest of the world does not exist. If I am narcissistic, I am never able to see my partner's or my children's point of view or to have empathy with them. My needs always come first. That is very different from healthy self-focus.

Having a healthy self-focus means I know that if I attend to my own needs, and if I take responsibility for my own completeness, I will fill myself up in such a way that I am then available to be empathic, to see others' points of view and to attend to others' needs.

Many of us have parents whose allegiance is still to their families of origin or to one or both of their parents. Maybe Mom's heart still belongs to her daddy. Her allegiance is to her father and therefore cannot be transferred to her partner. Maybe Dad is still his mommy's little boy. With his primary allegiance pledged to his mother, that allegiance is not available for his spouse or partner.

There is a finite amount of energy available to invest in family life. Prior to emancipating, most of our family-life energy is invested in our family of origin. In adolescence, we begin withdrawing small sums of our energy from the family energy bank, and we begin investing that energy in peer relationships and in banks outside the family.

If our family expects us to emancipate, they expect us to make more and more withdrawals of energy from the family energy bank to invest in banks outside the family as we approach young adulthood. When we become intimate and form a union, the family acknowledges that most of what is invested in the family energy bank will now be transferred to an outside bank called "new couple."

With the birth of each child we are expected to remove more and more deposits to invest in the bank that is now called "new family." We still have a small amount invested in the original family energy bank, but the lion's share is now invested in our new family. That is as it should be.

Some of our families, however, expect us to keep all of our family-life energy in the family of origin bank forever. We are not supposed to remove any in adolescence. We are not supposed to remove any in young adulthood. In fact, some of our families have the perverse belief that we, as a new couple, and our new young family should take energy from our own bank and invest it in the family of origin.

This poses a tremendous dilemma for us as a new couple and a new family. The dilemma may be compounded when one of us in this couple believes we should take energy back into our original family bank and the other believes we should withdraw energy from the original family bank. One of us is still stuck in our family of origin, and one of us is trying to tug our partner into the present and the future.

---
## EXERCISE
---

List the priorities your parents had for their family-life energy as you were growing up. If Parent 1 put his or her family of origin first and the new couple second, for instance, write *family of origin* on line 1 and *couple* on line 2.

| Ideal | Parent 1 | Parent 2 | Parent 3 |
|---|---|---|---|
| 1. Self | 1. _____ | 1. _____ | 1. _____ |
| 2. Couple | 2. _____ | 2. _____ | 2. _____ |
| 3. New Family | 3. _____ | 3. _____ | 3. _____ |
| 4. Other | 4. _____ | 4. _____ | 4. _____ |
| (including | _____ | _____ | _____ |
| family of | _____ | _____ | _____ |
| origin) | _____ | _____ | _____ |

How did these priorities affect your family?

Are there differences in your parents' priorities? How did these differences affect your family?

---

## Family Emotional Process As Energy

We need our parents to have energy and skills enough to be present for us. If our parents have good communication skills and good conflict resolution skills, they can have clear relationships between themselves, with us and with their parents. This means they have more energy for us and can teach us the skills we need to build our own families some day.

If our parents allow mistakes and human fallibility, we all have less energy tied up in fear and in hopeless attempts to be perfect. If they allow losses to be grieved over and all feelings to be acknowledged, we use up less energy trying to suppress feelings or trying to find indirect ways to express them. If they allow us to be different and autonomous, we can use for our own development the energy it would take to pretend to be the same or to fight for our right to be separate. If they prioritize themselves, their partnership and our family before their family of origin, they have more energy for us.

We, in turn, will have enough energy to be present for the new family we create when we reach adulthood. And we will have the skills they modeled in our toolbox.

# CHAPTER

# 5

# Who's
# On First?

## Our Role, Our Gender, Our Birth Order

Our gender, our birth order and the role we played in our family of origin will also affect what's in our parental toolbox. Perhaps we are the classic example of the *oldest* child who is a *female* and who is put into the *role of caretaker* for our younger siblings and/or our alcoholic parent. Clearly we will get from this experience certain parenting attitudes and skills to take into our new family when we have children.

The tools we take with us from this experience will vary according to our inborn temperament and our family. We may take an emptiness to the family we create because the burdensome parental role denied us the experience of siblinghood. We may approach the prospect of parenting our own children from an out-of-gas, I've-already-done-that position.

Roles, gender and birth order can affect what is in our parental toolbox in a host of more subtle ways as well. Let's look at the roles we might play in our childhood family. Then we can speculate about their effect on our adult family. The role we played for so many years in our family of origin can easily stick with us as we choose our partner, relate to our partner and parent our children.

One way a family can solve problems or reduce anxiety is to allocate roles to the children based on their birth order, inborn temperament and gender. These roles have been delineated and described by many different authors, but there is some agreement that individuals emerge in families to fulfill the following functional roles:

1. clown/distracter/pleaser
2. hero/caretaker/responsible one
3. mediator/lost child
4. scapegoat/acting-out child

Each role seems to carry a predominant feeling. Clowns and scapegoats carry the anger for the family; lost children carry sadness; the hero/caretakers carry depression.

All of the roles carry fear because the roles we play serve to defend us as children against our fears that the family will disintegrate and that we will be abandoned. We fear that family disintegration will bring our personal annihilation.

If our family has trouble dealing with conflict directly and productively, or if it has declared that anger is not allowed, we may be the child who has got the job of putting oil on the waters of conflict. We may jump in by being a clown to distract the angry person, or we may jump in and try to mediate. If anger is disallowed in our family, anger then pushes an anxiety button in us and we go into action. In effect, we give the "Don't-be-angry, let's-stop-this, let's-all-be-happy" message for the whole family.

Scapegoats also have a specialized function. If we are the family scapegoat, we will draw the fire onto ourselves to protect everybody else in the family. We become the container for family anger either by acting out the anger or by attracting the anger.

If we are the caretaker or hero, we are overly responsible and therefore prone to depression. We are too good for our own good, out of touch with our own wounded child, our own vulnerability.

We caretakers are depression-prone because we end up feeling like the sow with four teats and 13 piglets — we face constant and impossible demands with not enough resources at our disposal. We try to rescue the family honor and dispel the family shame with our over-responsibility.

We are often the parentified child when there is a vacuum in the intimacy system of the adults or a vacuum in the parental system. At the expense of our own inner child and our own childhood development, we move into a pseudomature, hyper-responsible role as a surrogate spouse to one of our parents or as a surrogate parent to ourselves, our siblings or one or both of our parents.

Our gender can affect the role we play in our family. Males are more likely to be in the scapegoat role; females are more likely to be in the hero/caretaker or parentified role. Lost children can be either sex.

Birth order also affects our role. For instance, if we are the oldest child, we will frequently be the hero/caretaker. If, however, we are also a male in a family where it's dangerous to be male, we may become the lost child, while the secondborn, a female, may end up being the caretaker and the responsible child.

If we are a middle or a younger child, we are more likely than the oldest to be a lost child. As an interesting sidelight, younger and middle children are more often referred for psychiatric help between the ages of seven and twelve than anybody else in the birth order.

Oldest children are less likely to show up in therapy as children because of a need to stay in the strong role and deny vulnerability. We oldest children are much more likely to have a tremendous amount invested in being strong and autonomous and unneedy. Inside we are lonely and in pain, with a convincing external veneer of strength and competence.

We middle children are like the back wheels of a car. No matter how fast we go, we can never catch up with the firstborn. We never have the same privileges the older children have; we are never as coordinated; we never know as much. We also never experience the relaxation of parental rules that youngest children do. We are squeezed from the bottom and squeezed from the top.

If we are the middle child in a dysfunctional family of five kids, we might try to hold onto the two above and the two below, desperately attempting to hold the family together in order to have a family. Our fear is, "If I let go, I'll get abandoned or lost. I will literally be nowhere." Sometimes we can't hold onto the children on either side of us, and we have to go outside the family to find our connectedness.

Falling in the middle of the birth order, we may feel connected to no one. We may isolate. Our siblings above us, who are close in age, are connected to one another for better or worse by friendship or rivalry. The siblings below us may be so far away in age and/or gender we may not feel close to them, important to them. As one man positioned in the middle of many siblings told me, "Water, water everywhere, and not a drop to drink."

If we are the youngest, we are more likely to be infantalized. We are likely to feel irrelevant and discounted: "Nothing I do gets noticed or makes a difference." We may be turned into the family pet, the mascot, the placater, the clown. We might become lost children. If we are not only the youngest but also physically the smallest, we may feel like a barking Chihuahua, underfoot but not to be taken seriously.

If we are an only child, we literally play all the roles. We don't have a sister who can major in caretaking and minor in clowning, or a brother who can major in scapegoating. As an only child, we have to change our role according to the needs in the family. We may be the hero when we are the straight-A student and the scapegoat when we are so audacious as to leave home. We may move into the lost child role or the clown role when our parents are fighting.

Being the only child is like being the Levis in the advertisement showing two sets of mules pulling on the pants from opposite directions. The needs and expectations of both parents pull on us. The ad demonstrates that Levis are so strong they won't tear, but only children will tear. What if one parent says, "Love me, be disloyal to your father," and the other parent says, "Love me, be disloyal to your mother"? How can we resolve that kind of dilemma?

There is also a great likelihood that we, as an only child, may break down in adulthood if we come from a severely dysfunctional family of origin. If we absorb and internalize too much family junk, if we don't have some very important alternate attachment figures available to us, we may not develop enough resiliency.

Spacing makes an enormous difference in the effect our birth order has on us. If there are more than five years between one child and another, the younger child basically starts a new family.

Let's say we have a family where there is an oldest brother; then eighteen months later, a sister; five years later, a brother and five years after that, another sister:

Carl, age 13
Alexandra, age 11½
Willie, age 6½
Tammy, age 1½

The first two children will face the birth order issues and the gender issues. If maleness is preferred in that family, the second-born, a daughter, may be close to her brother because they are close in birth order but also competitive with him because she can never quite catch up.

The youngest two children are what I call "de facto onlies." They are basically isolates in the birth order because there is nobody close to either one of them. They are more likely to be parented by a sibling than by their own parents because their parents may have run out of interest in and energy for parenting.

One or both of the two older siblings may end up being enraged over having to parent their younger siblings. They may feel as though they are being robbed of their own childhoods, robbed of the chance to be siblings with these siblings and robbed of the credit legitimate parents would get.

Our birth order, our gender and our childhood roles have implications for a lifetime. Let's say my sister is the oldest female child and absolutely adorable. Let's say I am the secondborn female who is not particularly attractive and not so bright as my sister. If my sister is my father's favorite and he relates to her appropriately, while I am not his favorite and I am sexually abused by him, what are the implications for my adulthood? How will this constellation of birth order, gender and role affect me when I form my own intimate relationships and parent my own children?

When we begin selecting a partner for our adulthood, the degree of "fit" we feel with the person we choose will be based in part on gender and birth order complementarity.

For instance, if I am the oldest brother of sisters, and I marry/partner with a woman younger than myself who was the oldest sister of sisters, I am gender compatible with my partner. That is to say, I, as an older male, know something about females younger than I. But I know nothing about females in the same birth-order position (oldest) as mine. I am compatible male to female, but not oldest to oldest.

On the other hand, my partner is neither gender-compatible with me, since she has no history with brothers, nor birth-order compatible with me. She will tend to compete with me as an oldest with an oldest. If I had a younger sister, close in age to me and highly competitive with me, something about this union would ring bells or resonate for me from my childhood history.

Let's take another example. Suppose I am the youngest brother of a dominant older sister and the son of a beautiful, sexy mother. If I marry a strong, smart, beautiful, sexy older woman, who is the oldest sister of brothers, we have a potential marriage made in heaven. We match on both age and birth-order dimensions, and I get resonance with my sexy, beautiful mother as well.

---

## EXERCISE

Think for a moment about the families your parents grew up in, and fill out the following chart. You may be surprised to find blanks in your knowledge of your parents' families. At some point you may decide to do some research to fill in those blanks.

Look at the lines under Birth Order. Write the name of one child in your parents' families on each line, starting with the oldest. Next to each name put the child's gender. Between the children write the number of years between them.

For example:

Carl   male
18 months
Alexandra   female
5 years
Willie   male
5 years
Tammy   female

If you had more than two major parenting figures, or if your parents had more siblings than will fit on these lines, please use another piece of paper.

**PARENT 1:**                    **PARENT 2:**

**Gender:** _____    _____

**Role(s):** _____    _____

**Birth Order:**

_____    _____

_____    _____

_____    _____

_____    _____

_____    _____

_____    _____

_____    _____

_____    _____

_____    _____

_____    _____

_____    _____

Do you know how the gender of your parents affected the way they were treated in their families?

Do you know what roles they played in the families in which they grew up? Can you see any way those roles affected the way they acted as partners to each other? As parents to you?

Can you see any personality traits or patterns of relating they have that might arise from their birth order?

Now look at your own childhood. Fill out a chart for yourself and see if you notice ways that your gender, your birth order and the role(s) you played affected the way you were treated and the things that were expected of you. How might they have affected your adult life, intimate relationships and parenting?

Fill out a chart for each person who parented your children as well. If your children had more than one parent, use another sheet of paper.

**MYSELF**                         **PARENT 1**

**Gender:** _____

**Role(s):** _____

**Birth Order:**

Can you see ways these parents' gender, role and birth order may have affected their relationships with you? With your children?

_____

These charts will come in handy when we talk more about your gender, role and birth order.

## Little Families, Big Families, Gender-Skewed Families

The size of our family of origin can have a great impact on the tools we take to parenting. Medium-sized families have the possibility of creating a home where there are sufficient time and attention available for us to feel special and people available to learn from and get nurturing from. If we grew up in a very small family or a very large family, however, we are likely to be missing some essential tools.

Maybe the nuclear family of our childhood has a small, nonexistent or nonfunctioning extended family. Maybe we are geographically isolated from our extended family and we don't have any other close adults who can act as support for our family. The smaller our extended family system is, the fewer people our nuclear family has to draw on for support and the greater the likelihood that there will not be resources and buffers enough to absorb the shock of anything traumatic that happens.

When any kind of trauma happens, the anxiety in a family increases. The function of our extended family system — our lateral supports — is to drain off some of the emotionality, to act like shock absorbers.

Lateral supports are like the flying buttresses on a medieval cathedral. Medieval cathedrals are magnificent buildings cut out of huge blocks of stone that are incredibly heavy. The weight of these stones is carried in two ways. All the arches on a Gothic cathedral thrust their weight into the keystone — the arch of the roof — and then back out on the ridge of the ceiling and down through the sides of the walls into the flying buttresses. The flying buttresses are beautiful, delicate lateral supports that come out from the sides of the building.

If you pull the keystone out of a Gothic cathedral, the whole ceiling will collapse. If you knock down the flying buttresses, as happened during World War II, the weight of the church cannot hold itself and the walls will collapse.

Families are very much like Gothic cathedrals with their own internal stresses and external flying buttresses. If a family has strong flying buttresses — extended family and other lateral supports — then some of the pressure of the weight of hard times in a family can be thrust outward and shared with the extended family system.

Lateral supports are particularly important when a family is withstanding tremendous pressure, like the birth of a disabled child, the unexpected illness or death of a parent, the birth of too many children in the face of too few resources or even a giant cultural catastrophe like the Great Depression. Families that have lateral supports to help absorb and drain off some of the weight of what's going on are more likely to be resilient and to remain standing under the pressure.

In the face of any major stress or major change, all families become dysfunctional for a while. Healthy families have the internal and external resources to move out of this temporary period of dysfunction and on to a successful resolution of the problem.

Unhealthy families, on the other hand, lack the internal and external resources to resolve first the stress and then the dysfunction. They stay in the dysfunctional behavior so long that it becomes normalized, absorbed into the structure of the family and "how it is in our family."

It's important for us to remember that families that are not able to resolve problems are not bad families. They are simply families that reach into their toolboxes in the face of major stress and find that the tools and supports are either absent or inadequate. They then have to create makeshift solutions which, unfortunately, become problems and problem generators in and of themselves.

Lateral support systems provide people who will calm us and soothe us when our parents can't. They provide people who will calm and soothe our parents. Developmentally, when our parents can't soothe us and no one else is around to do it, we don't learn how to soothe or calm ourselves.

Addiction, by the way, is viewed by some as a misfired attempt at self-soothing. If we didn't get soothing in our family and didn't learn how to soothe ourselves, we do the best we can to find some way to do so. Addictions and compulsions feel like things that will soothe us.

The literature concerned with resiliency puts forth the idea that the presence of someone in our environment who can give us direct interpersonal contact and attention will make us feel calmed and soothed by being seen, being heard, being reflected and being valued. The person who gives us this support doesn't even have to be a primary caregiver. We will internalize those feelings and make them part of our personal toolbox. If our family system is too small, no one will be there to offer that soothing.

Another hazard of growing up in a small family system, or of being a de facto only child in a large family, is that we miss out on what children learn from growing up with siblings. If we have siblings who are close enough in age, we learn things like how to fight, how to divide labor, how to tease. Even if we are made the parentified child and have to take care of lots of siblings, we have the advantage — not shared by only children — of developing competencies in organizing, being responsible for and teaching our siblings.

For instance, at Christmastime I went away with two friends of mine, both of whom have sisters. I have no sisters. My two friends kept doing what looked like bickering to me. Alarmed, I would jump in and say, "Come on you guys, we're on vacation. Stop fighting."

They told me two things that opened my eyes. First, they said, "We're just acting like sisters." One of my friends was an older sister in her family, and the other was a younger sister in hers. "We're just doing our younger sister/older sister dance," they said.

Then they said, "You don't know how to kid. You don't know how not to take this seriously." So I'm missing a developmental piece that you get with siblings about kidding — that it can be good-natured, that it can be a way of using humor to lighten things up.

Families that are too large have their drawbacks too. In a large family we are more likely to be the victim of one of our siblings than just to be teased kindly. We can be unmercifully bullied, shamed and tormented by a sibling. Our parents may simply not have enough energy to notice or take care of what's happening. Or if our parents are out of gas or overwhelmed, we siblings may act out the problems of our parents and won't be protected from one another.

Sibling incest can occur under such circumstances. Incest between siblings is five times more common than father/daughter incest and reflects an absence of appropriate protection from parents. Sometimes the siblings turn toward one another to act out sexual stuff that's going on in the parent generation. Sometimes the incest is seen as nurturance-oriented, a way of trying to soothe or co-parent each other. Sometimes the incest is extremely violent and sociopathic. I have worked with a number of women clients who, as adults, are still afraid to let their older brothers know where they live because they had been so brutalized by them as children.

Physical violence can occur in any dysfunctional family, but it is generally worse when we grow up in a large dysfunctional family. If there are unresolved conflicts between our parents, they are likely to be acted out in physical violence between us and our siblings. I'm not talking about normal childhood teasing, hitting and bickering. I'm talking about home as being a dangerous and frightening place.

This childhood experience may set us up to require that our own children never fight. Or we may replay our family drama, ignoring manifestations of violence between our children and using the same words to deny reality that our parents used — "Kids will be kids." Thus we perpetuate in another generation the abuse of children by their siblings.

A big family system may have lots of lateral supports, but unfortunately, not all lateral support systems are helpful. If our extended family is burdensome or toxic, then it adds stress to our family instead of relieving stress.

For example, imagine our parents as a young couple having their first child. If members of both extended families of origin suffer from active serious addictions, those extended families cannot act as flying buttresses for this new family, and they also add stress. Our parents can't invest their energy in their new family if they focus on the crises in their families of origin, and they can't rely on their families for help and support.

Large families put a particular stress on middle children. If we are a middle child in a very large family, how do we find our place in the sun? How do we carve out a unique identity? If we are the fourth of six children, the identities of oldest, prettiest, smartest, most athletic, funniest and one-who-makes-the-most-trouble may already be taken. So what roles are available to us?

In large families there are more comparisons. We are more likely to end up with a self-image that includes words like biggest or littlest, prettiest or ugliest, fattest or thinnest, most masculine or least masculine, most feminine or least feminine.

It is easy to get lost in a large family. We may feel as if we are part of a "huddle group" or "the kids" if our parents are unable to focus attention on each of us individually. If we are the "quiet one," we may be unnoticed by both siblings and parents. Big families potentially make for big comparisons, big competitions and greatly important sibling relationships — whether nurturing, torturing or isolating.

If all or most of the children in our family of origin are of the same sex, we have a gender-skewed family. Growing up in a gender-skewed family can affect how we feel about our own gender. If we grow up as the only boy in an all-girl family, what supports Dad's male energy and our male energy? If we grow up as the only girl in a family that has a gender bias against girls, our family is a dangerous place for us, and we may learn that being female is dangerous.

Let's say we grow up in a family where there are four sons, and Mom has a gender bias against boys. She has always longed for a girl. Mom's longing and bias are going to dramatically affect what we internalize about being male. Since our siblings are all boys, we may also have trouble carving out a sense of individuality. We may always be clumped into the category of "the boys."

## EXERCISE

What size were the families in which your parents grew up? Did they grow up in gender-skewed families? How did the size and gender configurations of their families affect how they parented you and your siblings? Did their families have helpful, detrimental or nonexistent lateral supports?

Look for a moment at your own childhood family. How did its size affect you? Was there enough support in the family system to soothe and absorb shocks? Did you have a chance to both learn from siblings and carve out your own unique niche? What did you learn about family size and lateral supports that you may have taken with you to your new family?

Did you grow up in a gender-skewed family? How did that affect your feelings about your own gender? About the opposite gender? What attitudes about gender might you have taken with you into your new family?

---

## A Life Of Their Own

As you know, one of my motivations in writing this book is my concern about the parent-bashing flavor of the ACoA movement. My hope is that this chapter has given you some idea about the host of variables that shaped your behavior as a child and your children's behavior, variables over which your parents, and similarly you as a parent, had no control. Birth order, only-ness, sibling relationships, gender, parental birth order and family size are all potent shapers of behavior. Regardless of the adequacy or inadequacy of the parenting we receive and the parenting we provide, these variables have lives of their own. Their effect can be augmented in positive or negative directions by the input we make as parents, but they cannot be erased.

# CHAPTER

# 6

# The Hopes And Fears Of All The Years . . .

Imagine our parents gazing down at us as newborns and wondering, "Who will you be, little one?" They are aware, from that first moment, that they hold in their arms a unique individual they will be getting to know over the next ten, twenty, forty years.

And yet even as they look forward to learning about us, they confront a task much more complicated than they can imagine. It will be difficult for them to see exactly who we are because they come to parenting with a music box in their toolbox that is playing over and over the refrain, "The hopes and fears of all the years are met in thee tonight." Being human, our parents can't help but hope we will fulfill the dreams they spun when they were growing up and the dreams they were handed by their parents and grandparents.

This music box comes with a companion tool that also makes it difficult for them to see who we really are. The tool is called resonance.

## Resonance

The concept of resonance comes from the field of music. If you are holding a tuning fork that is tuned to the note G, when you play a G on the piano, the tuning fork will resonate. You will hear the tone of G ringing from the tuning fork and feel vibrations running through it, even though it has not been directly struck.

We all have emotional tuning forks inside that resonate when some experience (like the G on the piano) is similar to an experience we have had before (the G of the tuning fork). For example, when our parents see us take our first ride on a swing, their memories of swinging resonate inside them. They may have vivid, full-color memories as they push us, or they may merely have emotional memories — delight or fear, perhaps.

The problem with resonance is that it keeps people from seeing each other clearly. If our parents are feeling the fear they experienced when they swung as children, they may not notice that we are having a great time and feeling fearless. They may urge us to hold on tight and ask, "Is it too scary?"

Our parents have good intentions. They intend to see us clearly, but they, like all humans, carry the music box of hopes and the tuning forks of past experiences that make it impossible to see 100 percent clearly.

## Physical Appearance

The most obvious feature our parents will react to in us is our physical appearance. If we look like one of their beloved parents, they are likely to develop a positive relationship with us. They will respond favorably and be reinforcing to us.

If, on the other hand, we look like someone with whom they've had considerable conflict, such as a sibling, parent, grandparent, aunt or even a spouse or partner, we will evoke negative associations. Their relationship with us is likely to be difficult.

This can be heartbreaking for parents. No parents want to have a negative reaction to one of their children. Our parents may have promised themselves, when they began this journey of parenting, that they would love all of their children equally, that they'd always be fair and patient. They'd be responsive and able to listen and communicate clearly. They'd never be rejecting or punitive.

Then, suddenly, they find themselves wanting to move away from us. They feel punishing and hostile toward us; they want to withhold affection. They are puzzled by their own responses because the reasons for their negative reactions may be out of their conscious awareness. They may not know our physical appearance is evoking painful memories of someone else. So without their being aware of why they are doing it, they begin to see us as a problem, and they begin to respond to us as if we were a problem.

## Temperament

Throughout this century, we have heard a lot about what is called the nature/nurture question. To what extent are personality and behavior affected by inborn, genetically determined factors (nature) and to what extent are they a result of learning, modeling and unconscious family processes (nurture)?

There have been studies of identical twins who were reared apart with no knowledge of one another — and it has been concluded that approximately 50 percent of our personality comes from our genetics and 50 percent from learning.

For our parents it can be pretty difficult to figure out whether a certain annoying behavior we are displaying is an inborn trait or a reaction to the environment, but let's put that part of it aside for the moment. Let's focus on the simple fact that there is at least 50 percent of our personality our parents can't do anything about. This 50 percent will evoke different reactions from them depending upon how well it fits in with their own temperament.

For instance, if our parents are depressed for any reason when their first child is born, and if that child is a passive, nontemperamental, easily soothed, self-entertaining youngster, the fit between their depression and that child's style is relatively good. I'm not saying it is good for their child's development that they are depressed, but they are not likely to feel incompetent, inadequate, stressed or overwhelmed by that child's demands.

Then, let's say they are still depressed when we are born, the second child. Unlike their firstborn, we are full of curiosity, vitality, energy and responsiveness to the environment. In this case, the fit between our parents' temperaments and our temperament is not so good. We may evoke in them feelings of emptiness, incompetence, failure, hostility and resentment by wanting attention and energy they don't have to give.

When there is a mismatch, our parents may define us as a problem child. Instead of them seeing their own depression as the problem, or the mismatch in our temperaments as the problem, we are called "too demanding, too needy." Even though they may be careful never to say this directly to us, the message may still get across.

For example, in my own family, one of my mother's most characteristic statements is, "David was such an easy baby." For many years, I did not ask her what she meant by that because I feared she would say I had been a difficult child. When I was middleaged, I finally mustered up the courage to ask her, "What do you mean when you say, 'David was such an easy baby'?"

My mother said, "Your brother was a very easy child to care for as an infant because he would spend much of his time playing with his own feet, toes, hands and fingers, examining them minutely." For her personality and needs at the time, he was easy. An interesting aside is that my brother's babyhood activities parallel in some ways what he now does as an adult. He's a research scientist, still spending lots of time alone, entertaining himself by minutely examining phenomena in the universe.

When I asked what I had been like as a child, my mother said, "You were a child who arrived with your mouth open, registering a protest. You were a very high energy child: curious, demanding, precocious and into everything."

Now, I will never know if I was actually "very high energy and demanding," or if I simply had ordinary demands and energy that she felt overwhelmed by because my personality didn't match her own. Her feeling that I was a very demanding child does not necessarily reflect the truth; it is simply her truth. Another mother may have found my personality exciting and my brother's boring.

What I do know is that I carried with me the impression that I was a difficult child. I interpreted my mother's favorite statement to mean that I was difficult and my brother was easy. It's important to remember that my sense of being a difficult child is also not necessarily the truth, but my truth. It's my own projection of my mother's experience of me as a difficult child.

## Names

Earlier I talked about marriage/partnership as a dual cassette deal — the challenge for our parents as a new couple being to integrate the similarities and differences they bring from their families of origin and create a synthesis for their new family.

Let's say they haven't been able to work through some of the differences between them. Maybe Mom still has negative feelings about someone in Dad's family of origin, and Dad still has negative feelings about someone in Mom's family of origin.

On top of that, let's say the conflict-resolution style both of our parents developed in their families of origin was the same: "Avoid anything that isn't pleasant. Don't talk about it and, magically, it will somehow go away."

When we are born, they unconsciously feel an opportunity to resolve these conflicting feelings about their in-laws. Without knowing why, they give us as first and middle names the names of the most hated family member on each side of their families of origin.

Each time they say our name, on one level there is an unconscious resonance of their experiences with the person we were named after. They may be surprised to find themselves repelled by us.

In addition, as soon as we have this name, we also have a ready-made mythology. The mythology might go something like this: "I'm named after my Aunt Margaret, so I must be like Aunt Margaret. Since everyone in the family says Aunt Margaret is crazier than a bedbug, how do people feel about me, and what do people expect of me?"

We might unconsciously decide, at some point, that we might as well play the game. We may end up resolving what, for us, is a lose-lose situation by ending our attempts to be good, ending our attempts to prove we're not like Aunt Margaret. We may instead protect ourselves from our feelings of powerlessness by trying to prove we can be even crazier than Aunt Margaret.

Our parents may give us the name of a beloved person, perhaps Dad's maternal grandmother, who was like a parent to him. She was the person from whom he got "good stuff."

Every time he looks at us and uses our name, the projection onto us is positive. The feelings that well up in him are feelings of fullness and love and gratitude.

Rather than being rejecting and negative toward us, Dad may go to the other extreme and see us in globally positive terms. He may be overpermissive. He may fail to see the negative behaviors we have that need some intervention and correction from him as a parent. Even when our parents give us the name of a beloved person, rather than a hated one, that name may still prevent them from seeing who we really are.

Molly is a composite character created from many people's histories. You'll be getting to know her throughout the rest of this book. Molly had both an appearance and a temperament that affected her mother. After Molly's father died, her mother used to tell Molly how fortunate she was that her father had died. "If he had lived, your life would have been full of grief because your father's temper was so terrible."

She would then go on to tell Molly how much like her father Molly was and how much Molly's temper was like her father's temper. "Your father had such a bad temper that if he had lived, he would have killed someone someday. Your anger is so much like his that if you're not careful, you'll kill someone with yours."

On top of the temperament similarity, Molly was also the spitting image of her father. While her mother was a petite 5 feet, 3 inches tall and weighed only 110 pounds, Molly was tall and stocky like her father, who had towered over her mother at a height of 6 feet, 4 inches and weighed 220 pounds. Since Molly's mother had divorced Molly's father shortly before he was killed overseas in WWII, every time she looked at Molly she saw a miniature replica of a man about whom she had mixed feelings. She could never look at Molly except through the lenses of guilt, hurt, anger, sadness, anxiety and disappointment about her failed relationship.

---

| **E X E R C I S E** |
| :---: |

Take some time to think about each of your parents in turn. Who do they most look like in their parents' families? Whose temperament is theirs most like? Who were they named after? How did their appearance, temperament and name affect how they were treated in their family of origin?

Now look at yourself. Who do you most look like in your parents' families? Whose temperament is most similar to yours? Who were you named after? How did these characteristics play a role in the way you were treated?

---

## Disability

If there is a genetically transmitted disorder in our family tree — alcoholism, juvenile diabetes, heart defect, etc. — our parents may overreact to a characteristic in us that looks like a symptom of that disorder. They may have seen that characteristic in their own parents or siblings, and when they did, it meant big trouble.

For instance, if they came from a family where there was mental illness, they may overreact to normal emotional displays in us because they have a higher sensitivity to emotional outbursts than people who have had no mental illness in their family of origin. They may lack the ability to differentiate normal from abnormal emotionality.

If they had a parent who had a psychotic break in their childhood and we are daydreamers — forgetful, inattentive and spaced out — they may overrespond to us as if our behavior is a precursor of psychosis. The irony is that our behavior may be in the range of normal, but because of their overreactivity, we may end up developing an expectation that we will have emotional problems later in life.

I think of a friend who couldn't wait to turn 35. His mother had been manic-depressive. My friend had read that after the age of 35, there was no longer a danger of becoming manic-depressive. So until he reached 35, he was hypersensitive every time he became anxious or couldn't sleep well, afraid those were the pre-cursors of the illness. You can be sure he will also watch his children closely until they turn 35.

## Obesity

When obesity is present in our family system, we internalize two things. First, we internalize our culture's fatness phobia; second, our family's fatness phobia.

Our parents may have spent much of their childhood, adoles-cence and young adulthood starving themselves in order not to be fat. They were afraid fatness would bring all the bad things to them that happen to overweight people in their family and in this culture.

When they see us move from being thin, wiry small children to being lumpy at 11, 12 or 13, they may become frantically alarmed. Suddenly we are lethargic, not so physically active as they think we should be, and we eat voraciously. They think, "Oh my God, this kid's going to be fat. Over my dead body is this kid going to be fat."

They may then embark upon a crusade to rehabilitate us. They may fail to recognize that many 12-year-olds become shapeless and pudgy. It is a normal part of development. We are at an age when our physiological demands for growth fuel are at a rate comparable only to those in infancy and early childhood. They may also forget that pudginess itself is not necessarily a precursor of obesity in late adolescence or adulthood.

So here they are, trying to curtail our eating, feeling constantly critical of us and repelled by us, failing to recognize that what drives their feelings is the culture, fear of their own fat and all their unfinished business with their own family of origin about fatness. They are sure they are concerned only for our own good because they know what a world of grief we are going to have being fat in a thin world.

Woe be unto us under these circumstances. We are caught between the imperatives of our physiology and the anger of our parents.

| EXERCISE |
| --- |

Is there a history of genetically transmitted illness in any of your parents' families? Is there a history of obesity? If so, how did this history affect the way your parents were treated in their families? How did this history affect the way your parents reacted to your weight? To any traits they may have seen as a precursor of a family illness?

## Birth Order

What might our birth order evoke for our parents? If they were firstborn children and experienced being the firstborn as difficult and burdensome, they may respond to us — if we are also firstborn children — as if we also experience being firstborn as burdensome. They may respond to us with an unconscious decision that we will not have to go through what they went through as the oldest, that we will not have to be overresponsible as they were.

In this example, they may project being burdened onto us. We may not necessarily feel burdened, but we may learn to react as though we are burdened out of our loyalty to them. Then they may be so permissive they do not allow us to develop an appropriate sense of responsibility. They may also unconsciously respond to us in a more positive and reinforcing way than they respond to any of their other children simply because they identify with us.

Maybe we don't have a physical appearance that would evoke a negative response, a name or a temperament or a feared quality or characteristic that might evoke a negative response, but still our parents have negative feelings toward us. It may be that we are in a birth-order position that is parallel to the birth-order position of the sibling with whom they had the most difficulty. Without its being in their conscious awareness, they are projecting onto us the characteristics of their own sibling.

You may think I'm stretching the point here, but I'm not. Studies have shown that teachers will respond more positively to, and give better grades to, a child who is in the same birth-order position as that of the teacher. A teacher will respond more negatively to, and grade more poorly, children who are in the same birth-order position as the sibling the teacher had the most difficulty with in childhood.

Let's say Dad was the secondborn in a family of three. He had a sister above him and a brother below him. No matter what he did, he could never earn the same adoration, respect and attention his younger brother got, even though it seemed to him his brother did very little to merit such royal treatment. Dad's wounded inner child harbored feelings of resentment because he felt as if he was the most worthy, most loyal and most loving child, even though he was never recognized as such.

Dad may be surprised when he has difficulty with us, his third child. The way we walk irritates him; the way we talk irritates him; the way we want attention irritates him. He is not aware that the mere fact of our birth order is evoking these feelings in him.

## Gender

Over the past two decades we have heard a lot about how we treat boys and girls differently, simply because of their gender. Our cultural conditioning has trained us to hold and carry girl babies and boy babies differently from the moment of their birth. But aside from this cultural conditioning, there are other reasons why our gender may evoke reactions in our parents.

For instance, one of my clients treated her son as though he were the crown prince. This bias was based not so much on favoring males over females as on the fact that the people who were kindest to her in her family of origin were her brothers and her father. The least kind people to her were her mother and her sister. She expects kindness from males and extends a kind of solicitousness toward them that she does not extend toward females.

Another client, Harriet, grew up without a father in a female-centered family where there was a generational absence of men. She then married and now has a family of sons. In spite of a reasonably good relationship with her husband, she feels uncomfortable with her sons. It's not so much that Harriet dislikes or feels hostile toward men; they simply seem foreign and unfamiliar to her.

Rather than being able to celebrate the maleness of her sons and the maleness of her husband, she is always communicating her discomfort on a less-than-conscious level. Her sons may have some difficulty knowing what the message is from Mom. They may not know how the absence of her own father and the generational history of absent males has affected Mom. They may simply pick up Mom's discomfort and decide Mom doesn't like men. They may also personalize it and decide Mom doesn't like them.

How we manifest our gender can evoke reactions from our parents as well. Sarah's mother was a handsome woman, but was not "pretty." Sarah's sister was a combination of both handsome and pretty and was her mother's favorite daughter. Sarah, on the other hand, was petite and beautiful — and her mother's least favorite daughter.

It wasn't until years later that Sarah suspected her mother's preference for her older sister arose from her sister's having a kind of femaleness her mother could embrace. Her sister was close enough in appearance to her mother so that her mother could identify with her and also enjoy the prettiness she herself had not been gifted with. Sarah's petite beauty, on the other hand, was a reminder of how her mother didn't measure up to the cultural ideals of femininity.

Sarah, in turn, married a tall, stocky man with whom she now has a daughter who is handsome. Right on cue, history repeats itself, and the child has a kind of femaleness Sarah can't embrace because it is so different from her own. Though petite, frilly dresses do not match her daughter's style or body, Sarah continues to push her to lose weight and dress in the "pretty" way Sarah feels more comfortable with.

Paul grew up in a family of powerful women. Even though he had brothers, he had a very powerful mother and very powerful older sisters — and he ended up with a family of girls.

Even though his stepdaughters aren't powerful in the way his mother and sisters were powerful, even though they are more like the cultural stereotype of women, unassertive and dependent, he may feel just as puzzled and powerless in the face of his stepdaughters' emotions as he felt in the face of his mother's and his sisters' emotions. In his powerlessness, he will parallel what men in our culture feel in general: "Women are a conundrum, and men will never understand them."

He is puzzled by women as the relational sex. He is impatient with them. He thinks they talk around things, cry too much, feel too much, complain too much. So when he becomes a stepfather to this family of girls, their gender is going to evoke for him not only the feelings that were evoked with his mother and sisters but also the feelings he has as a man about women in general.

By the way, during the emerging era of feminism, many dads felt it was pretty dangerous to be a man to begin with, but even worse to be a man marooned in a family of women. When daughters became adolescents and began holding their fathers, as males, responsible for every rape and every report of sexual harassment, many dads wanted to take to drink or take to the road. Dads experienced their daughters' femaleness as noxious and confusing, and they didn't want to deal with it.

Therefore, their daughters may have experienced their dads as becoming the enemy the girls had said they were in the first place. Their dads may have become terse, less communicative, more withdrawn and more defensive. As they became more beleaguered, they became caricatures of exactly what their daughters said men were.

Many dads are now suffering a tremendous sense of estrangement from their female children and haven't the foggiest idea what they did wrong or what their daughters want. Many are also carrying the scars and bruises of the feminist revolution and are not willing to wade into their families of daughters and let them have at it again. Yet they long for relatedness with their children.

---

## EXERCISE

How did your parents' birth order and gender affect the way they were treated in their family of origin?

List your parents and their siblings in their proper birth order in the columns below. Put the firstborn child next to number 1, the secondborn child next to number 2 and so forth. Then in the Myself column, list yourself and your siblings in birth order.

| Parent 1 | Parent 2 | Parent 3 | Myself |
|----------|----------|----------|--------|
| 1. _____ | _____ | _____ | _____ |
| 2. _____ | _____ | _____ | _____ |
| 3. _____ | _____ | _____ | _____ |
| 4. _____ | _____ | _____ | _____ |
| 5. _____ | _____ | _____ | _____ |
| 6. _____ | _____ | _____ | _____ |

Are you in the same birth-order position as either of your parents? Which of their siblings are in the same birth-order position you are in? How did your parents feel about those siblings? Can you see any similarities between how your parents felt about siblings in various positions and how your parents felt about you or your siblings in similar positions?

What were the ways in which boys and girls were treated differently in your family? How did your parents react to your gender, in particular?

---

## The Ongoing Drama

We were not born into a vacuum. We were born into an ongoing drama where the characters already had particular temperaments, preferences about gender and physical appearance and also histories with people who had certain names. All of these affected how we were treated and how we would, in turn, treat our children.

# CHAPTER

---

# 7

# ... Are Met
# In Thee Tonight

Our physical characteristics and our birth order are obvious. We can see how they might activate our parents' internal tuning forks and make it difficult for our parents to see us as we really are through the resonance inside themselves.

Our parents' unmet childhood needs, and the needs they can't fill in their adult lives, also make it hard for our parents to see us. These unmet needs are harder to identify. They push our parents to treat us in ways that are not based on who we really are or what we really need.

We'll look first at how unmet needs in childhood leave all of us with unfinished business. Then we'll examine some of the ways our parents may have asked us to meet both their unmet childhood needs and their unmet adult needs. Whenever their needs clashed with ours, whenever they asked us to forgo a normal task of childhood to fill a need of theirs, we lost a tool for our toolbox.

## Unfinished Business From Childhood

When I talk about unfinished emotional business, I'm referring to the ways in which our needs were inadequately met in childhood. If our needs were adequately met, we have a sense of being emotionally completed and filled up. If they weren't, we have a sense of hunger, yearning and deprivation.

Unfinished emotional business can be the end result either of not having our needs met, or of having our needs met so excessively that our developing sense of separateness, autonomy and competence were undermined. Both too much of a good thing and not enough of a good thing create damage — unfinished business. To the extent that our emotional needs were unmet or inappropriately met in childhood, we then carry into our adult relationships a feeling of neediness. We're like a hungry chigger that is always looking for something, but often we're not quite sure what.

Most of us had some of our needs met, some of them unmet and some of them "overmet." We will, therefore, have particular spots in our emotional makeup that are yearning to be healed, and other spots that are just fine.

It is unavoidable for human beings to experience some wounding as children. Since parents are human and therefore fallible, they can never meet children's needs perfectly. And, to quote M. Scott Peck, "Life is difficult." Life itself wounds us. Hence we and our parents all have wounded children inside who are to some extent angry, hurt, fearful, sad and empty.

The concept of unfinished business is important in this section of the book because one of the "safe" ways in which our parents probably tried to complete their emotional business from their own childhoods — heal their wounded inner children — was to reach to us, their children, for that completion. In so doing, they may have violated what was developmentally appropriate for us as children; they may have been completely out of sync with what our childhood needs were at any given time. This, then, created unfinished business for us that we carried in our toolboxes to our adult relationships and parenting.

## Resonance Again

Let's go back to the example of our parents' pushing us on a swing for the first time. If swinging in childhood was frightening for our parents, they may ignore the fact that we are having a great time and are feeling fearless. Their old fear may be resonating inside and urging them to ask, "Is it too scary?" On the other extreme, if swinging was joyous for them, they may ignore any fears we are expressing and say, "Isn't this great fun?"

The danger, obviously, is that our parents can easily fail to differentiate between us, their real three-year-olds, and their re-stimulated inner three-year-olds. They may protect us from experiences they feared or attempt to provide experiences for which they yearned, but in which we are not at all interested.

When our parents are pushing us on the swing, trying to comfort the fears they imagine we have, they may have a whole range of feelings. They may feel pleased to be able to comfort us, and they may feel rage or jealousy or competitiveness because their own parents never comforted them so well.

Our culture considers it abnormal for parents to have negative feelings like rage and jealousy toward their children. "Abnormal" feelings are kept secret and therefore go unacknowledged.

The irony is that it is totally normal to have some negative feelings toward our children. To be consciously aware of these feelings, and to be able to acknowledge them, takes the sting out of them. They become dangerous only when they have to be denied. When "unacceptable" feelings are pushed underground, into our unconscious, they fester and acquire great power to harm because they become so feared.

Can you see how the task of parenting is made impossibly complex by the completely human reactions of resonance and unfinished business? The simple act of pushing a child on a swing can set off a whole chain reaction of feelings.

Let me give you another example of resonance. What if Mother grew up during the Depression, hungry and poorly taken care of? During her difficult childhood, she may have had fantasies of someday feeding her own children all the things she never had available to eat as a child. She may have had fantasies of her children as snug, toasty warm, well clothed, rosy cheeked, chubby and well fed.

Once we are actually born, woe be unto us if we are finicky eaters, have food allergies or are not able to take in the food that Mother is able to provide. Woe be unto us if we take in the food Mother offers and then spit it back at her because the food doesn't taste good or makes us sick.

What no one ever told our mother is that, in the process of feeding her children, she is going to feel jealous of her biological children because they are getting the food she never got, getting the warmth and care she never got, getting the safety and security she never got. If she also has to face our rejection of her food for whatever reason, she will not only take it as a rejection of her and her nurturing; she will also feel furious with us for interfering with her being able to feed the wounded child within herself.

I don't want to characterize our Depression-raised mother as having only negative feelings when she feeds us. In all likelihood, she also feels a tremendous positive feeling of power because she has the capacity to feed us and keep us from being hungry. As a child, she had been helpless and dependent. She couldn't have said to her parents, "Feed me or else." She couldn't have said, "Take better care of me."

As a child, Mom might not have allowed herself to acknowledge the extent to which the parenting she received was inadequate. In fact, her loyal inner child may not have allowed her to see, until adulthood, that she wasn't well cared for. Even in adulthood, she may still be in some degree of denial about the inadequacy of the parenting she received. Ironically, she may not even be curious about why she feels so compelled to provide an ideal environment for her children.

So Mom may have negative feelings about what we're getting that she didn't get, and she may have positive feelings about finally being powerful; she may feel quite confused. If we, in adulthood, have eating disorders, we might look back to our own childhood and make note of the fact that our mother was a child who was hungry when she was growing up. When we were growing up, did Mom feed us not only well but also abundantly, elaborately and frequently? As we moved into adolescence and began developing adolescent fat, did Mother respond by saying, "You have such a pretty face, you would be so pretty if you weren't chubby"? Then, when we went on a diet, did Mother say, "I didn't spend all those hours cooking you good meals to have you ruin your health with this crazy diet"?

This, incidentally, is called a double bind and a no-win situation for a child. We are damned if we do and damned if we don't. If we comply with one side, of her request, "Eat, eat, eat," we will be chubby, unattractive and unacceptable in Mom's eyes. If we comply with the other side, her need and possibly our own need for us to be slender and attractive, we run the risk of being disloyal to Mother and possibly being attacked by her.

## Pent-Up Demands

I would like to introduce another idea that I think helps explain some of what happens in childhood with our parents. This is the concept of pent-up demands.

All of us, when we were little, thought of a million things we wanted to do that our parents wouldn't let us do. We all longed for the day when we could be the bosses of our own lives and satisfy these yearnings, these pent-up demands, in our way, on our own nickel and in our own time frame.

For instance, many of us, when we first began earning money, bought things that might not have looked very practical to our parents, such as elaborate stereo systems. Finally we could spend our money in any way we wanted without being judged by our parents as being frivolous. We were satisfying a pent-up demand to exercise our own power and to do as we pleased.

Pent-up demands come in many forms, not just in terms of how we spend money. When we were born, we provided an outlet for some of the pent-up demands left over from our parents' childhoods. Doing something as simple as giving us what they didn't get could relieve a pent-up demand for them.

For instance, as a child growing up, I never doubted I would get an education. In fact, it was not an option for me not to get an education. My mother had completed high school, but for a host of reasons had been unable to go on to the university. Although she was an extraordinarily bright, creative, talented woman, all of her life she felt a sense of shame about not having a college education. She never felt she was as good as other people.

Obviously, my older brother and I had to go to college. At the end of my freshman year in college, I wanted to quit school and work for a year or two. I felt I was not emotionally mature enough to go to college yet, and I wasn't clear about why I wanted a college education. From my mother's point of view, because of her own pent-up demands, it was absolutely out of the question that I might leave college.

Because the education was for my mother, and not for me, I ended up flunking out of college three times and taking ten years to get my degree. It was not until I could take ownership of my education and get it for myself that I could complete it.

I am ever grateful to have a college education. I feel sad for people who have received educational roadblocks instead of encouragement from their parents. On the other hand, it would have spared me a good deal of trauma if my mother had given me some space and some help in working through my ambivalence about being in college so young, rather than just pushing to get her own needs met.

Somebody once said, by the way, that we spend the first half of our life acquiring baggage from our parents, our family of origin and our culture, and the second half unloading that baggage and becoming who we truly are. For me, it took ten years to unload the baggage labeled, "My education belongs to my mother."

## To Be Someone They Didn't Have

If our parents' pent-up demand from childhood was for a playmate or for a sibling, we may be someone other than their child to them. Our parents may literally cross the boundary between the generations and attempt, at some unconscious level, to make us their siblings or their playmates.

Maybe our dad, in talking to his friends, says that his son is his best friend. As his 19-year-old son, we're in a position of being Dad's confidant, Dad's fishing buddy. We're not Dad's child, but somehow the playmate or sibling that Dad didn't have in his own childhood. It puts us in a position that denies us the opportunity of just being who we are. We feel as if we have to act in Dad's play in some peculiar way that we don't quite understand.

We can also be a surrogate parent to Mom or Dad. If either of our parents experienced themselves as unparented, when we are born, they may at some unconscious level say to us, "I'm glad you're here. Take care of me." It creates a tremendous dilemma for us if we feel as if we have to be Mom's mom or Dad's mom or Dad's dad.

I think of a man I once knew whose mother unconsciously said to him when he was born, "I'm glad you're here. You're the cuddly teddy bear I never had." When his mother held him, she wasn't holding him to comfort him, she was holding him to comfort herself. There was an implicit message from this mother to her child that her pent-up demand was for a cuddling, soothing presence — a "cookie person," a teddy-bear person. It was clear that her son was to serve this function.

## Powerlessness

If our parents were on the receiving end of behavior from their parents that left them feeling powerless and terrified, they may use the unconscious defense mechanism of identification with the aggressor on us when we're children. Our parents may protect themselves from ever being the terrified, powerless, frightened child again by being the powerful one this time. Their pent-up demand is to feel powerful, to be able to treat someone else the way someone once treated them. They may also have the wish for revenge as a pent-up demand, but they can't focus that revenge on their parents; it is focused on the children.

## To Fill The Lacks

What do we evoke in our parents from the unfinished emotional business of their childhoods? What pent-up demands do we meet? What role do we play, both in terms of their past histories and in terms of their current dramas, that has little to do with us and our needs?

One of the roles we can play is helper. We can help our parents fill up parts of themselves that feel empty, or we can help our parents avoid confronting lacks in themselves.

Bear in mind that the loyal child in us always wants to help our parents. Our loyal child is exquisitely sensitive to what our parents are able to do or not able to do, and to what our parents need us to do for them. Our loyal child hopes, by the way, that by helping our parents, we will make them more complete, and competent.

If our parents, as children, were taught never to be angry, never to fight back, they may have inside themselves an angry part they refuse to acknowledge. We might say they have disowned this angry part. When someone hurts them and anger is appropriate, they are powerless.

One of the ways our loyal inner child can step up to the plate and help our parents in a case like this is to carry our parents' anger. We can become the avenger on behalf of our parents.

You may remember a case that hit the press a number of years ago, in which a brother and sister murdered their father. When the family's story emerged during the trial, it was shown that the father had repeatedly brutalized the mother and the children, but particularly the mother.

The mother, out of her own passivity and sense of powerlessness, let her children act out her disowned anger and rage. You might say she unconsciously put out a contract on her husband through her children. As an act of loyalty to their mother, and in order to protect their mother, they may have murdered their father on her behalf without her ever murmuring a word asking them to do so.

By the way, the people on trial for murder were the children. The people who will potentially go to jail in an instance like this are the children. The mother was never on trial. The mother not only went free; she was never accused of wrongdoing.

## Fault Absorbers

We all know people who, when they tell their family history, will say something like, "Everything was okay in my family until shortly after I was born. Then everything fell apart." These people are the children I call the "fault absorbers," the children who are scapegoated or blamed whenever their parents want to disown responsibility for hard times.

If we are fault absorbers, we are children on the receiving end of a parenting message that goes something like this: "You make me sick/kill me/drive me crazy. Everything was okay until you were born/became an adolescent/grew up and left home." Rather than taking responsibility for their own lacks or assessing the events in their lives and in the culture that may be contributing to their difficulties, our parents make us the repository for blame, the scapegoat, the fault absorber.

Bear in mind, by the way, that each of us abhors feeling powerless. Assigning blame is a powerful defense against feeling powerlessness.

If things fall apart in our childhood family, it's highly unlikely we, as children, caused it. The falling apart is probably in response to a major loss the family can't process and from which the family is not able to rebound. Maybe Grandpa died. Or maybe our family lost a business or financial stability. Loss from any source — serious illness, the Great Depression, the flu epidemic of 1918 — has a tremendous impact on a family. If the family cannot make the connection between the problem it is having and the loss, if it can't see the problem as the acting out of the unresolved sadness over the loss, someone is going to be the fault absorber. Someone is going to be the donkey on which the tail is pinned.

I want us to remind ourselves at this point, lest we get into our own remorse and regret as parents, that we're reading this section to get back in touch with what we had in our parental toolbox at the time we began parenting. A theme of this book is: We can't know what we don't know, and we can't give what we didn't get. Pause for a moment and remember that we're looking at ourselves as children and what we did or didn't get in the process of growing up. We're looking at what some of the unmet needs of our parents were that might have been acted out on us.

If we find ourselves focusing on our feeling that we did the same things to our children, well, we probably did. Why wouldn't we have done the same things? Remember that we are "monkey-see, monkey-do" people. We learn from experience. When we began our journey as parents, the tools we had available to us in our toolboxes were tools that came from just the experiences I'm talking about right now. Let's ease up our criticism of ourselves for a moment and remember that we're really looking at what was in our toolboxes when we began the journey as parents, rather than looking specifically yet at ourselves as parents.

Let's go back to work. We're looking at how our parents may have inadvertently used us to avoid something lacking in themselves or to help fill up their empty parts.

Some of us have parents who are lacking in social skills. We all know people who, no matter how much they try, are too shy, too hesitant, too wounded to reach out to people outside their family to make friends. Perhaps they themselves had shy parents and simply never learned how to reach out.

Such people, when they have children, will often look at their children and say, "Thank God, I have a ready-made social network. Thank God, I have people to interact with on an ongoing basis." Then, rather than reaching out to other adults, they use their children as their friends and confidants. Their children become the people with whom they share their secrets, the people who assuage their loneliness.

If we are an only child and Dad's "best friend," it's highly likely that it will be very difficult for us to leave home when we reach adulthood. How can we possibly leave home and leave Dad behind? We see Dad as a poor, bereft person who will die if we aren't there for him.

We may never leave home, or we may take Dad along with us into our adult relationships. Our lucky partner not only acquires us in an intimate relationship but also acquires our dad, from whom we have never separated.

If our parents avoided areas in which they were incompetent by exploiting our competencies, we may have become a pseudo-adult, or what we often call the parentified child. This prematurely adult child does for the parent what the parent cannot or will not do for himself.

For example, Sam's mother had a terrible time saying no to people. If someone came to the door, Mom would run into the bathroom, jump into the empty bathtub fully clothed, and tell

Sam to go to the door and say, "Mother is in the tub." Sam then did not have to lie while he protected her from possibly having to say yes to someone's request if she wanted to say no. One of Sam's major issues in adulthood, not surprisingly, was that he had trouble saying no to people.

The example I just gave, though certainly having lifetime implications for Sam, is relatively benign compared to some of the ways in which this mechanism works.

Sharon was very bright and had graduated from high school quite early, but she had two whimsical, self-indulgent parents who literally refused to function as breadwinners. Her parents were more than capable of working and earning an income but, recognizing at a conscious or less-than-conscious level how capable she was, they basically sat down in helplessness and let her support the family. Sharon began working long before she was ready to be emancipated, long before she was ready to take on the financial burden of support. Her parents relied upon her until she married.

Another manifestation of this mechanism, particularly in highly dysfunctional families, is the child who is put in the position of meeting the bill collectors, making late payments and explaining why a payment has not been forthcoming. Children in that position feel tremendous shame while "helping" their parents.

Kent had parents who were financially irresponsible. When his parents ran off owing money, he was left behind as the only person in that small town who bore their name. Of course, all the bill collectors came to Kent, and Kent was left with the job of trying to cover for his missing, irresponsible parents.

To protect themselves our parents may have needed us to behave in certain ways so that we would not stimulate any of their unresolved feelings of sadness or anxiety or any memories they needed to keep out of conscious awareness.

Let's say we were raised by Grandma and Grandpa. If Grandpa grew up with siblings that were near-murderous to one another, and Grandpa's parents failed to protect him and his siblings from one another, the last thing in the world Grandpa is going to allow is fighting among his own children. If we argue, Grandpa will begin to feel that nauseating, clenching fist in the pit of his gut that reminds him of the chaos, turmoil, rage, anxiety, confusion and terror he felt as a kid when he and his siblings savaged one another. So Grandpa will say to us, "You're going to be friends if it kills you." We will be commanded to like one another, never to quarrel with one another, not to be rivalrous with one another. We will have to maintain a kind of pseudoharmony in order not to upset Grandpa.

Think about the hundreds of times we heard our parents say, "Don't say that; you will upset your mother. Don't do that; you will upset your grandfather." Oftentimes what "will upset Mother" is something that triggers unfinished business from her childhood.

Our parents may have been prohibited from grieving over losses when they were children. Maybe they needed to be brave little soldiers who didn't cry, didn't complain and didn't look sad, even in the face of major losses. Maybe there simply wasn't any support for their grief.

If, as their children, we grieve over our own losses, if we display the entire range of normal emotions and behaviors that go with grieving, we may function as a mirror and a trigger for their unresolved grief. We may be asked, consciously or unconsciously, to protect our parents from their unresolved grief by not being sad, not crying, not displaying any emotionality around losses. We may be asked to behave in much the same way they had been taught to behave in the face of losses in their own childhoods. If we have difficulty suppressing our emotionality and our grief, we may be called the crybaby or the Sarah Bernhardt of the family.

Just as some of us are asked to be avengers, confidants or pseudoadults, others of us are asked to carry the emotionality that the family cannot carry for itself. Then we are scapegoated for doing so — we are called crybabies. If this is our lot, we come to adulthood equipped with a sense of shame about our emotionality — a sense that somehow our feelings or any outward signs of our feelings are always inappropriate.

| EXERCISE |

How did your parents' unfinished business affect what they expected of you? Put an X by each item that applies to you and a + by any item that applies to one of your siblings. Your parents' expectations of your siblings may have affected their parenting of you as well.

Did your parents seem to hope you would be someone who could take the place of a "missing person" in their childhood?

a sibling      a parent
a playmate      a cuddly teddy bear
a friend      an outlet for their anger/revenge
a victim that let them be the powerful one

Did either of your parents seem to hope you would fill in their lacks? Did they seem to expect you would —:

carry the anger they weren't allowed to have
carry any other feeling they weren't allowed to have
be assertive/say no for them
be their social network
be a pseudoadult/parent, be competent where they were not
be the scapegoat, take the blame for family pain and problems?

Did your parents ask you to protect them from any of the following:

seeing feelings that might trigger their own feelings (sadness, anger)
seeing behaviors (teasing) that might trigger old feelings for them
"upsetting" them
"upsetting" a partner or grandparent
feeling powerless (you should not bring unsolvable problems to them)?

Take a moment to think and feel about the items you just marked and the items you didn't mark. How might your parents' expectations and your reactions to their expectations have affected the tools you eventually took to your own parenting?

## To Triangulate

Triangulation has been described as a method of communication two people can use to decrease the tension between them by pulling in a third person. The third person creates a temporary "solution" to the problem; that is, a decrease in tension, a distraction from the problem and a timeout from having to deal directly with the problem.

When two people are having difficulty in their marriage, they can use triangulation to mitigate that difficulty in a number of ways. They can triangulate a therapist. They can go to a therapist to complain about their marriage, but never take the energy back into the marriage to deal directly with the problem. Therapy can be a wonderful way to avoid working on a relationship. It can drain off just enough tension so the problems never reach a crisis stage that might demand change. Some people will stay in bad marriages for the rest of their lives as long as they are in therapy.

Another way couples can triangulate to try to avoid marital problems is to complain to their siblings, their parents and their best friends about each other. This is far cheaper than seeing a therapist. However, it has its down side too. At least the therapist agrees not to leak the information back into their network or community. Family members and friends tend to be far less trustworthy in this regard.

One classic way partners try to solve relationship problems is to have an affair. They sexually and emotionally triangulate in someone else. Unfortunately, they often then leave their original relationship and re-create with the new person the problems they had in the former relationship until they have to triangulate in someone new again.

The other classic way of trying to solve marital problems is to triangulate in the children. Let's look at how we as children may have been triangulated into our parents' relationship to help them avoid or "solve" problems they felt they couldn't deal with some other way.

Many of us grew up in families where there was considerable tension and conflict, either direct or indirect. Some of us were drafted into the role of family clown. We became the person who, when the tension rose in the family, would kid, joke or serve as a distraction.

Not only can there be a clown pulled in to help our parents with their marriage; there also can be a scapegoat. If we, as the scapegoat, provide our family with sufficient diversion — let's say we become a heroin addict — much time and energy can be spent chasing us and our addiction, so that our parents can avoid looking at the difficulties between them.

A number of times I have talked about how sensitive we are, as children, to the feelings with which our parents are burdened, whether our parents talk about those feelings or not. If we are particularly sensitive to feelings of pain, it is likely we will be triangulated into the role of the family hero, caretaker or emissary. As the hero or caretaker, we attempt to lighten our parents' load by being the overly responsible, overly adult child. In so doing, we forfeit being a child. If we are our family emissary, we dispel the family shame and restore the family name by distinguishing ourselves in the larger world.

If we are an only child or the oldest child, we are likely to move into the emissary role. If we grow up in a family where there is criminality, battery, sexual abuse, alcoholism or poverty, our family is especially likely to need a family emissary.

Whenever we are triangulated by our parents, we are being given the role of keeping our parents' marriage together. If we are the clown, we attempt to keep our parents' marriage together in one way. If we are the scapegoat, we attempt to keep our parents' marriage together in another way. If we are our parents' emissary to the world, we are also attempting to keep their marriage together. But the triangulated child who carries the most onerous burden is the child who is born in order to be the glue.

If we are born as the glue child, we were conceived specifically to glue together a fragile alliance or to create an obligation of such proportion that it will not be possible for one person in that union to abandon the other. If we are born into a second or subsequent marriage, we may have a feeling that we were born for some reason other than that Mom and Dad wanted some issue from their union. Our preassigned job may have been to so indebt Dad to Mom that he will not abandon her and her other children. We may feel like a child who is unwanted, and yet has a very specific function. Unfortunately that function has nothing to do with who we are as a person and what our own wants and needs are. We feel like a function, not a person, in our family.

Another way in which we may be triangulated into our parents' relationship is as a part of the ongoing drama of their marriage. We may be used as a pawn in a power battle between our parents, or we may be used as a mouthpiece in their struggles with one another.

Let's say we have a same-sex sibling particularly close in age to us. We may try to avoid or dilute the natural competition between us by saying, "I'm not like him. I'm not like her." We literally "de-identify" with one another as a way of having our own spot in the sun and our own unique sense of identity. This process can be exacerbated if our parents have conflict in their marital relationship that they are unable to resolve directly and decide to triangulate us in. In such an instance, one of us may be captured by Mom to be used as a pawn in her battle with Dad, and the other may be captured by Dad.

Suddenly, the parental battle is overlaid on the disidentification we have already established with one another — and Mom and Dad get to derail their conflict. Thirty years after Mom and Dad are dead, we siblings may still be carrying on Mom's and Dad's fight in our relationship with one another, with no conscious awareness that the fight has nothing to do with any substantive issue that ever existed between us.

We can also be triangulated in by acting out and verbalizing the agenda of one of our parents with the other parent. When we are children, we tend to see the world in terms of good and bad, villains and victims.

If Dad abdicates all responsibility, Mom may step into the power vacuum. If Dad is gentle and soft-spoken, and Mom is assertive, bordering on aggressive, we will tend to see Dad's soft-spoken-ness as caused by Mom's aggressiveness — Mom is bad. In truth, it's more likely that the interaction between our parents is circular, like the dog chasing its own tail. Mom may have become over-bearing to fill the vacuum of Dad's lack of assertiveness, and Dad may have responded by becoming less assertive, more "gentle."

When we, as children, experience one parent as unfairly ex-ploiting the other, we can be unconsciously induced by the "ex-ploited" parent to step in to fight the battle. So each time Mom begins a potential conflict with Dad, our anxiety goes sky high and we step into the fray to "protect" Dad from Mom.

Ironically Dad never needs to learn to fight his own battles. He has Mom talking for him some of the time and filling his asser-tiveness vacuum, and he now has us talking for him the rest of the time.

The tragic ending to this scenario is that when we grow up, we may avoid the "bad" assertive types and partner with someone "gentle" just like Dad — someone for whom we then will have to do the talking. The more we talk for our partner, the more frus-trated and exasperated we will get and the more "overbearing" we will become — just like Mom. Our partner, of course, will become more "gentle." And so it goes ad nauseum.

If we are the firstborn child, our birth automatically creates a triangle between Dad and Mom. For instance, Mom and Dad may have been cooking along pretty well in their intimate relationship. They may have come from similar families of origin and may have had similar beliefs, attitudes and values. Their visions for themselves and their lives may have been quite similar. They may have had the sense that they had established a solid base from which to "live happily ever after." Then we come along.

No one tells new parents how incredibly disruptive the addition of a new child into their lives will be to their romance, to the new life they are forming together and to their relationships with their in-laws or out-laws. In fact, even before we are born, Mom and Dad's relationship begins to change.

One of the "Don't talk" messages in our culture is that men are never allowed to talk about the terror/anxiety they feel in assuming financial responsibility for their spouses and children. They are never allowed to talk about the terror/burden they feel when adulthood is defined by a willingness to get in the harness every day for the rest of their lives and pull the load — never complaining, never noticing how heavy the load is and never commenting on how long they have to pull the load.

Here's Mom, pregnant with us, and Dad's anxiety level goes sky high, but he can't talk about it. Dad relieves his anxiety by beginning to drink more, by spending more time with "the boys," by being more and more preoccupied with his business. At some level he's responding to what feels like a lifetime sentence of being in the harness and pulling the load, but he isn't supposed to notice or complain about it.

Mom, on the other hand, has been sold a bill of goods by a culture that tells her she has a maternal instinct. She should not have a single ambivalent feeling about being pregnant and being a mother. She should long for a pregnancy and a baby with every fiber of her being. She should in no way, shape or form resent the way in which our arrival will dramatically alter her life.

Many mothers will secretly acknowledge in therapy that they immediately thought of having an abortion when they discovered they were pregnant, even mothers who struggled with infertility and went to elaborate lengths to get pregnant. Many moms feel a moment of panic at the actual confirmation of a pregnancy, but they, too, are not supposed to talk about it.

The classic triangle that Mom and Dad in all likelihood experience with the revelation that we are to arrive is that Mother begins falling in love with having a baby. When we do arrive, Mother's love affair with us deepens.

Father is supposed to be as ecstatic as mother when we arrive. He, however, gets a rude awakening. Mother is having a love affair with us, and Dad feels abandoned. Mom's and Dad's romantic and sexual relationship often goes out the window. After all, Mom is absolutely exhausted. She's getting very little sleep and has taken on a 24-hour-a-day, 7-day-a-week job. Meanwhile, Dad may be relatively absent because he's out in the world in harness, pulling the load and feeling anxious about his capacity to provide for this new family.

Note that Mom and Dad are no longer a couple. Mom and Dad are now a family, and with that comes a major shift in their relationship. They will not be just a couple again, if their marriage in fact survives, until the last one of us leaves home. So Mom and Dad begin a mourning that is usually out of conscious awareness and usually not talked about. They are mourning the loss of their early romantic couplehood.

Mom and Dad may not have conceived us in order to triangulate us into any relationship problem of theirs. Nevertheless, we three are now a triangle, which means that feelings from old triangles Mom and Dad were in as children may be reawakened.

Mom is experiencing a lot of deprivation. She is deprived of quality time with Dad and quality time with herself. She is giving us a lot more than she is getting from us in the early months of our infancy. This feeling of deprivation can restimulate unconscious memories of a childhood triangle in which Mom felt deprived. Those feelings of childhood deprivation will rise to the surface and may cause Mom to feel as if she will always be deprived in relationships, always give more than she gets.

Dad also may have been in a triangle with a parent and one of his siblings, feeling abandoned the same way he feels abandoned now.

Let's say that Dad got three years of "babyhood" before another sibling arrived to displace him. With the arrival of another child, the unspoken message in the family was, "You're a big boy now; babyhood is over. There's another baby here who needs our time and attention." Those feelings of abandonment are going to be restimulated for Dad when we are born and he hears Mom saying, "There's a baby now who needs my time and attention."

Dad doesn't know some of his feelings are stimulated by memories. All Dad knows is that having a baby is not so much fun. He is hurt, angry and lonely. He may even blame Mom and say, "This was all your idea. I didn't want to have children in the first place."

The arrival of a child may cause other triangles in a family as well, both visible and invisible. An invisible triangle may occur when our parents have us, not because they want us, but because someone else wants us. Then a triangle is formed between us, our parents and the religion or culture or person that is "making" our parents have children.

Sometimes Mom and Dad have children for the church. Think about the number of religious belief systems where contraception is forbidden and where our parents' obligation is to produce another generation of true believers. Often both male and female authorities in the church have sworn vows of celibacy — they themselves are not having much truck with this baby-making business at a personal level — but they tell our parents they don't have the right to prevent the conception of any child.

I grew up in the Southwest where, in certain Roman Catholic families, there is an unspoken rule that one child is to become a nun or priest, one is to marry and have children and one is to be given to the grandparents. The given-away child is supposed to be company for, and to take care of, the grandparents and then the parents.

This child is usually female. The unspoken rule is that she is not to marry or be sexual with men. If this girl child happens to become a lesbian, she may be able to comply with both of those injunctions pretty easily. After all, there is no injunction against "marrying" a woman. Being a lesbian is not a threat to the parents because the daughter does not have a husband who might compete with her filial obligations to parents and grandparents, particularly if her partner is willing to be absorbed into the family as "one of the girls."

We may be born to take care of our grandparents another way. Our parents may feel pressure to produce a grandchild to make their parents feel okay about the parenting job they did. Imagine our grandparents, sitting around a bridge table with a no-trump hand but no grandchildren. Imagine their feelings as their confederates tell about the exploits of their own grandchildren. At some level our grandparents feel indicted as having been inadequate parents if our parents do not fulfill the cultural expectation of having children on schedule.

As children, we may have been aware that we were triangulated into the battle between a parent and an in-law — say, between our mother and our father's mother. We may have been our grandmother's pride and our mother's enemy, or the reverse, depending upon which generation we felt a loyalty and an obligation to.

One of my clients, Grace, was the firstborn in her family. Her father had never separated from his mother, and Grace knew his mother was the one who had decided she should be born. Her grandmother did not actually create Grace, but was pulling the strings in the background.

Grace's mother felt furious that her mother-in-law was piping the tune about when she was to have a child. The day Grace's mother came home from the hospital with her new baby, the grandmother was waiting at the door of the apartment. She took Grace out of her mother's arms, and Grace's mother walked into her bedroom and shut the door. In effect, that was the last Grace's mother had to do with her.

Grace was born for her grandmother. Her mother, in a powerless position in relation to her husband and mother-in-law, abrogated any say over what was to become of Grace. Grace literally became her grandmother's baby.

In Grace's parental reservoir then, when she began the journey of parenting, she had a considerable feeling of abandonment. She was confused about her mother's distance and her grandmother's position in the place of her parents in her life. What model would she draw from in the parenting of her own children — the fragility of the connection to her own mother or the overinvolvement of her grandmother?

We can also be triangulated with our parents and their siblings. If our parents are in competition with their siblings, having a child may be our parents' way of winning the competition.

Let's say the middle sibling in Mom's family was the most admired child because of her beauty and her accomplishments. If this sibling is infertile, Mom may feel that the only way in which she can best her sister is to have children. On the other hand, if her sister does have children of her own, then the competition may not just be about who has children, but about who has the most accomplished, the prettiest and the most obedient children.

## EXERCISE

There are lots of ways your parents might have triangulated you, asking you to play roles that had nothing to do with who you were or what you needed. The following questions will help you inventory possible triangles in your family of origin.

Did your parents act as though you were the glue child who should hold their marriage or relationship together? Or any of your siblings?

Did either of your parents directly or indirectly ask you to be his or her spokesperson or ally in marital conflicts?

Did it seem as though a third party was so deeply involved in your parents' lives and your life that your parents may have had you for that third party — the church, their parents, in competition with a sibling?

---

Again, take some time to think and feel about your answers to these questions. What attitudes about triangulation and what patterns of triangulation might you have taken in your toolbox to your new family from these experiences?

## To Make Them A Success/Worthwhile

Our parents may need us to demonstrate their success as human beings, as sons and daughters and as parents. I gave the example of our grandparents sitting at a bridge table wanting to brag about their grandchildren. Well, our parents also sit at bridge tables wanting to brag about their children.

There is mighty competition among parents, whether it's parents of small children, latency-age children, adolescents or grown-up children. "My son, the doctor" is not a joke by accident.

If our mother was the scapegoated child in her own family, the family idiot, our mother may need us to be inordinately successful at what we do. And *successful* means different things to different parents.

Some of our parents will feel they are a success if we marry early; some will feel successful if we marry late. Others of our parents measure success by occupational achievement or attractiveness or the capacity to control others and wield power.

Success will be determined by the coin of the realm in our parents' families of origin. Woe be unto us if we lack the capacity to repay our parents in the denomination in which they need to be repaid.

If Mom needs to be esteemed in her family of origin and her siblings are occupationally distinguished, she will need us to be occupationally distinguished. She will need us to be an attorney, a stock broker, a ballet dancer, whatever counts as success in her family.

Our parents' standings in their own families of origin may be determined by what we do or don't do with our lives as their children. If we end up with an addictive disorder, or with any stigmatized identity that our parents' families find unacceptable, we lose value in our parents' eyes because our parents lose value in the eyes of their families. We may inadvertently give our parents' families additional ammunition in their ongoing war against our parents.

Imagine for a moment that we're three years old and run out into the street. Dad immediately dashes after us, grabs us and pulls us to safety. Dad is enormously relieved that we have not been hurt, but Dad is relieved not just because we might have been killed. Our dad has an audience in his head throughout that entire transaction.

What would his parents think about the kind of care he took of his children if we got hit by a car? What would his ferocious father-in-law and cold mother-in-law think about his parenting? What would the guy across the street, who is the perfect parent, whose kids never do anything wrong, think about him? Would his boss, who thinks he is the perfect family man, still give him that promotion? Would the culture label him a negligent and irresponsible parent? That moment determines our dad's success as a parent with a multitude of people. Often our parents' reactions to us have much less to do with us than with the scores of the judges in their heads.

Children who are adopted often report looking in crowds for their genetic reflections. They long to hear a voice that sounds like theirs, to see a stance or a gesture they recognize as their own.

Adoptees are not the only ones who wish to see themselves reflected. Our parents may have children in order to have people who mirror them, who are like them and who therefore validate their worth. The favorite child of a career woman will be the daughter who grows up to be a career woman. The favorite child of a housewife will be the daughter who becomes a housewife. By their choices, these children are saying that their mothers are good enough to be imitated.

Our parents may also have us in order finally to have someone in their lives who agrees with them. We are to be cherished for standing on the edge of the stage of our parents' lives murmuring confirmatory responses.

Our parents also may have us to have someone who belongs to them. Finally they have someone who is completely within their control, who can't be "messed with" by someone else.

## To Compensate

If we are the end result of an unplanned, unwanted pregnancy or a lousy marriage, we may be expected to compensate for our parents' unhappiness. Our parents may unconsciously project the message that we'd better be good because they have paid a high price for our existence.

We may also be asked to compensate our parents for their unhappy childhoods. If our parents were unparented children, they may come to adulthood feeling empty. They then look to us to make up for what they didn't get in their own childhoods.

One such parent might actually say, "You're my only reason for living. If it weren't for you, I would have killed myself or died. But you make life worthwhile." What our parent may be saying is, "I got so little in childhood, I felt so empty, that I was thinking of hanging it up. But you fill me up, and thanks to you, life is worth living." What we may tell ourselves is, "I have to keep my parents from killing themselves. I've got to restore meaning and hopefulness to their lives because they are empty and full of despair. I have to be very good and very talented because I don't just carry the weight of my own life; I carry the weight of my parents' lives too."

Maybe Mom divorced Dad, even though she still loved him, because he was violent or sexually abusive to us kids. Maybe Dad divorced Mom and took us to live with him because she was an alcoholic and a dangerously neglectful parent. We may feel we have to compensate them for what they gave up and what they went through "because of us."

Let's say Mom got pregnant when Dad was 15 and Mom was 14. Dad was honorable and shouldered his responsibility and married Mom. Mom was virtuous and bore us full term and didn't relinquish us. Mom and Dad will never forget that the price they paid for intercourse was us. They will never forget that they lost their adolescence and possibly the aspirations they had for themselves as adults because of us.

Let's complicate this scenario a bit. Let's say that Dad lost his father at the age of eight and that Dad's dream up until that time had been to become a doctor. Now Dad knew, even at the age of eight, that there would be no money for him to go to medical school. Dad and all of his siblings had their childhoods cut short because they all had to go to work to help support the family.

When Dad turned toward our mother to form a romantic and physical relationship, it was, in part, to find some warmth, some compensation for the hardness and early responsibility of his life. With Mom's early pregnancy, Dad received even more responsibility and more hardness. Even though he may love Mother dearly and us dearly, we may still feel we have to compensate him.

Maybe first and foremost we have to compensate for the death of his father and of his dream of being a doctor. Then, second, we may feel we have to compensate for Mom's early pregnancy, for her loss of a less burdened young adulthood and for Dad's becoming a father sooner than he had wished.

The degree to which our father was able to grieve over his losses, to feel hopefulness rather than despair and to restore meaning in his life will have a great deal to do with whether he views us as a premature gift or a premature burden.

Molly's story is a good example of what children may feel they need to compensate for.

Molly's mother, Eva, had an empty childhood. She was not only unparented but also unwanted and actively abused by her mother.

When Eva married, she was moving away from her dangerous mother; not necessarily moving toward her husband. She knew so little about her new husband that she had no way of knowing whether he would be dangerous or safe. Unconsciously Eva chose someone who was both a noncommunicator like her own father and an abuser like her mother, but to a milder degree.

When her husband had an affair, Eva fled to her brother's house, taking three-year-old Molly with her. It took great courage for timid Eva to buck tradition and strike out on her own. Eva's husband was killed shortly thereafter. Both Eva's family and her husband's family blamed Eva for his death from that day forward.

Molly grew up knowing she was to compensate for whatever had gone wrong in her parents' marriage and to be grateful to her mother for having left such an awful man. Molly was to compensate for Eva's terrible childhood, widowhood and rejection by both families.

Molly was also not to mourn her father's death or make demands on her mother, because her mother became so depressed that she was nonfunctional. Despite the fact that Molly had essentially lost both her parents — her father to death and her mother to depression — she was not to be anxious, fearful, mournful or complaining. She was to be the perfect child so that she could compensate her mother and protect her from being blamed by her family for any symptoms Molly might show.

## EXERCISE

Before you were even born, your parents had an idea of what you would be like if they were successful parents. They may have also been aware of their own parents' ideas about what successfully parented grandchildren would be like. In order that your parents might feel successful, did they ask you to do any of the following:

Become like them
Belong to them

Agree with them
Become a success as success was defined in your family
or in their families of origin (marry early, marry late,
have a great job out in the world, stay home and work
as a homemaker)?

Finally, did your parents ask you to compensate them for any
of the following:

An unhappy marriage
An unhappy childhood
Aborted career plans
Other children who were miscarried or who died
A divorce
Problems with in-laws?

Take some time to think and feel about your answers. If
your parents expected you to make them worthwhile in
some way, or to compensate them in some way, how did you
react to those expectations? How did your reactions affect
what you took in your toolbox to your new family?

---

## What We Need

All of us as children need a safe environment that can
contain us and contain our feelings. We need a sense that we
are being held, that we won't be dropped. In a sense, what
we need is something comparable to the resilient net you see
under high wire performers in a circus. We need to know
that if we trip or fall, we will not crash to the concrete floor
of life. Instead we will hit a parental net that will bounce and
hold us. Having a net gives us the freedom to grow, to risk
and to flourish.

We need our parents to be good enough. Please note that
I'm not saying we need our parents to be perfect or exem-
plary, merely adequate.

In part, adequacy requires that they be interested in us in
a particular way. We need them to be more attuned to our
needs than to their needs. The dilemma is that in order for
our parents to have in their toolbox the emotional empathy

required to put us first, they must have had parents who put them first.

Our parents need a sense of what is developmentally appropriate for us at different ages. For instance, if our parents are not attuned to the reality that we lack the physiological development to feed ourselves and be completely toilet-trained at nine months, they may ask something of us that we are both physiologically and psychologically incapable of. If, on the other hand, our parents are still attempting to feed us and are allowing us to soil when we're five years old, our built-in time clock for development is being interfered with by our parents' need to infantalize us. We need our parents to provide experiences and withhold experiences based on what will allow us to develop our strengths.

All of us, as children, need our parents' eyes, body language and behavior to show that we are seen and heard, that we matter, that we are being taken into account, that we are lovable, worthwhile, valuable and wanted. This loving attention is the bedrock of good self-esteem.

We need our parents to be people whom we can admire and people we want to be like when we grow up. We need desirable models we can move toward as we get older.

Because, as children, we are small and helpless in a world of giants, we need to feel protected by our parents in a very special way. We need to feel as if we can merge with them and borrow their size and competency temporarily.

We also need our parents to be what I call "benignly adversarial." We need our parents to establish limits that help mark safe from unsafe zones. When we are 18 months old and want to put a bobby pin in an electric outlet because we are curious, we need parents who can stop us and say, "No, you can't do that." Better yet, we need parents who will childproof the environment by putting safety covers on the electric outlets so there is no possibility that we can put a bobby pin in them. Limits say, "I'm not going to let you hurt yourself. I'm going to push back. I'll do it in a way that doesn't squash you and I'll do it in a way that respects your developing autonomy, but I'm going to push back so you learn how to internalize these limits for yourself."

Last, we need to feel we can have an effect on our parents. We need to feel powerful: We can get their attention, and we can make a difference.

We've been looking at some of the things that stood in the way of our parents' being attuned to us and seeing us for who we uniquely were. We needed them to be attuned to who we were so we could be emotionally complete and so we could learn how to be attuned to our own children. To the extent that they projected their unmet needs onto us, they were not attuned to us.

If these essentials were provided for us as children, we will then have the ability to give these same experiences to our own children. If they weren't provided for us, we will be lacking tools in our parental toolbox.

To the extent that our parents asked us to play a part in their drama, they got in the way of our being the separate and unique people we were born to be. We were born to develop our own unique sense of our selves and to play a part in our own dramas. To the degree that we were our parents' supporting actors, our own growth and development were compromised. We then were left with fewer tools in our toolbox to take into the process of building an intimate adult relationship and a parenting relationship.

# THE BIG PICTURE

# 8

# Our Family
# Time Line

W e are each reading this book in the hope of healing the wounds we feel in our relationship with our children. We are preparing ourselves to confront our regret and remorse and to be accountable for harm done as well as good done.

So far in our journey together, we have looked in our parental toolbox to see what we had available to us as we began our parental journey. In a subsequent section we will look at what we feel were/are our errors of omission and commission; we will look at our remorse and regrets; we will look at our wish that we had been better parents or had been better prepared to deal with our particular circumstances.

Before we do all that, however, we must become aware of one more context in order to understand more fully the parents we were and are. I call this context the big picture.

The big picture includes all of the circumstances and external events that were impinging upon us and upon our family as we were collecting tools for our parental toolbox and as we ourselves were parenting — cultural surroundings, specific historical events, normal life-cycle events for our family and for each individual in our family, particular losses, toxic events and major events our family experienced. All these affect the parenting tools we receive and the parenting we eventually do.

No event happens in a vacuum. When we were learning about who was "in" our family, the Great Depression was affecting our family as a whole. While we were learning whether we were allowed to cry or not, another sibling was born. While we were learning to play the role of family clown, our family moved to a new town. Events around us always affect what we learn. Cultural events, like the Depression; life-cycle events, like births; losses, like divorces; major events, like a new job; and toxic events, like incest, all affect the parenting we receive as children — and therefore affect what we learn about parenting.

Let me give you an example. Molly was born in 1939. Between the years 1939 and 1945, Molly's life was dramatically impacted by a number of external events, some cultural, some particular to Molly's family.

As you know, World War II began in 1939 and ended in 1945. Molly's birth in 1939 coincided with the beginning of WWII, a potent and dramatic shaper of the lives of all people in the United States and throughout the world for the next six years.

During the period from 1939 to 1945, Molly's parents separated, which altered Molly's father's draft status. Rather than be drafted, Molly's father joined the Marine Corps and went overseas, where he was killed in action. As a result of her marital separation, Molly's mother decided to relocate to California, where she and her children moved into a large house with her brother and several of her aunts.

A major cultural event, WWII, dramatically affected the course of Molly's life at the same time that losses (the loss of her father and home town) and a major event (moving into a new house with new people) were also affecting her life and the tools she would bring to her own parenting. In the first six years of her life she received modeling about intimacy both from her parents' separation and divorce and from the adults in the house she moved into. She learned who was in and who was out of her family — her father's family was out, and her mother's extended family was in, along with a number of nonrelated people the war brought into their household. The war, the divorce, her father's death and her mother's subsequent depression all affected Molly's sense of safety and security, potentially affecting the partner she would later select, her ideas about divorcing and staying married and the environment of safety and security she would try to provide for her own children.

In this section we are going to create a visual picture of the events that had an impact on our family of origin — and therefore on the parenting skills we learned — by drawing several time lines. Time lines take some thought and some work. You may be tempted to skip this work, but let me encourage you to make the necessary effort.

We parents tend either to hold ourselves totally accountable in a self-abusive way for all harm done to our children or, overwhelmed by remorse and regret, to defend ourselves against all information about harm done to our children. In both instances we operate as if we stood alone in time. The reality is that all of what happened in our family of origin and in the family we created happened in a cultural context and a context of personal life-cycle events, losses, and other major events.

Time lines can help us put our parental tools and our own parenting into perspective. Time lines can show us what our parental actions were anchored to and what they were in response to.

To do the work in the next few chapters, you will need five sheets of notebook paper and four pens of different colors: I will be using black, red, blue and green pens. Each sheet of paper will cover 15 years in time. You can adjust the years if these don't fit your particular circumstances, but 15 years to a page is a good guideline to use.

Let's begin our first sheet with the years 1920 to 1935. A sheet of paper has about 33 lines on it, so each year can take up two lines unless a particular year had a lot going on. Down the far left edge of the page, left of the margin line, number the lines from 20 to 35, skipping a line between each number. Down the left edge of the second page, number the lines from 36 to 50. Then number the third page from 51 to 65, the fourth page from 66 to 80, the fifth page from 81 to 95.

At the top of each of these five pages, to the right of the margin line write *Family of Origin*. You will list the events for your family of origin along the margin line. Draw three more lines on each page from top to bottom, leaving room at the right side of each line to make note of events we will discuss in this chapter. To the right of the first line, write *Extended Family*. To the right of the second line, write *Culture*. To the right of the third line, write *Myself*.

Now find the year that your parents married or partnered. Using the black pen, write *parents marry* or *parents partner* next to that date in the column labeled Family of Origin. Since we'll be using Molly's family as an example throughout this chapter, look at Molly's time line to guide you.

## Cultural Events

Before we add specific events to our family's time line, we need to document what was happening in the culture that affected our parents as they created their new family. Earlier in the book I said that our generation has seen social change at an unprecedented rate. All this change has affected our lives and our parenting.

Over the past hundred years, our family has had to deal with WWI, WWII, the Korean conflict and Vietnam. We have seen the overthrow of the Russian czar, the Bolshevik revolution, the rise of communism throughout eastern Europe and eventually China. We have seen the fall of the Berlin Wall, the dissolving of the Soviet empire and the opening of the People's Republic of China to outside commerce and influence. We've seen the democratization of the world through television, telephone, fax and photocopy. We've seen the rise of the civil rights and the individual rights movements, which include issues of gender and ethnicity.

| Year | Family of Origin | Extended Family | Culture | Myself |
|------|------------------|-----------------|---------|--------|
| 1920 | | | | |
| 21 | | | | |
| 22 | | | | |
| 23 | | | | |
| 24 | | | | |
| 25 | | | | |
| 26 | | | | |
| 27 | | | | |
| 28 | | | | |
| 29 | | | | |
| 30 | | | | |
| 31 | | | | |
| 32 | | | | |
| 33 | | | | |
| 34 | | | | |
| 35 | | | | |
| 36 | Parents marry | | | |
| 37 | | | | |
| 38 | | | | |
| 39 | | | | |
| 40 | | | | |
| 41 | | | | |
| 42 | | | | |
| 43 | | | | |
| 44 | | | | |
| 45 | | | | |
| 46 | | | | |
| 47 | | | | |
| 48 | | | | |
| 49 | Mom marries Stepdad | | | |

In a sense, all families are on the receiving end of two vectors that shape and influence their behavior. The first can be imagined as a vertical vector of values, expectations and unfinished emotional business coming from prior generations to impose upon our families and ourselves as developing children.

The horizontal vector is made up of a combination of individual life-cycle events, our family's life-cycle events and cultural events. We move through time on the horizontal vector, dealing with whatever family and cultural events presented themselves from year to year, all the while affected by the values and unfinished business pressing down on us from above. Let's look at the horizontal vector, starting with the cultural events on it.

| **Unfinished Business** | | | | **Expectations** | | **Values** | |
|---|---|---|---|---|---|---|---|
| | | | our family | | | | |
| 1940 | 1941 | 1942 | 1943 | 1944 | 1945 | 1946 | 1947 |
| marriage | birth | move | divorce | D-Day | ? | ? | ? |

Molly, for instance, was dramatically affected by living her early childhood in the shadow of World War II, the atomic bomb, the Cold War, the McCarthy era and the 1950s with their "return to normalcy."

Many of these events dramatically shaped decisions made by Molly's family. As we add more items to Molly's time line, we will see that her family moved frequently from the time Molly was 9 until she was 16. During that time Molly's family was living in Southern California. Her mother, having been terrified by the bombs dropped on Hiroshima and Nagasaki, was absolutely convinced that the Soviets would soon drop bombs on Southern California. She kept moving the family farther and farther away from major metropolitan areas, convinced that in doing so she was rendering her family safe.

Following is Molly's time line after she has included the cultural events that most affected her family between 1920 and 1957, the year she left home.

| Year | Family of Origin | Extended Family | Culture | Myself |
|------|------------------|-----------------|---------|--------|
| 1920 | | | | |
| 21 | | | | |
| 22 | | | | |
| 23 | | | | |
| 24 | | | | |
| 25 | | | | |
| 26 | | | | |
| 27 | | | | |
| 28 | | | | |
| 29 | | | Great Depression | |
| 30 | | | | |
| 31 | | | | |
| 32 | | | | |
| 33 | | | | |
| 34 | | | | |
| 35 | | | AA founded | |
| 36 | Parents marry | | | |
| 37 | | | | |
| 38 | | | | |
| 39 | | | WWII begins, Holocaust | |
| 40 | | | | |
| 41 | | | | |
| 42 | | | | |
| 43 | | | | |
| 44 | | | | |
| 45 | | | Atomic bomb, WWII ends | |
| 46 | | | | |
| 47 | | | | |
| 48 | | | | |
| 49 | Mom marries Stepdad | | | |
| 50 | | | Cold War, McCarthy Era | |
| 51 | | | Al-Anon founded | |
| 52 | | | *Man in Gray Flannel Suit* | |
| 53 | | | | |
| 54 | | | | |
| 55 | | | | |
| 56 | | | | |
| 57 | Molly leaves home | | Sputnik | |

Now it's your turn. Using the black pen, write on your time line in the Culture column the cultural events that you think most affected your family between the year your parents partnered and the year you left home. It may be important to include some cultural events that occurred before your parents partnered. WWII or the Depression may have postponed or speeded up your parents' marriage, or affected their feelings about money or security, for instance.

Also include on this list cultural events that affected your particular family. A drought or hurricane may have hit your local area. A particular strike or civil rights march may have had an impact on your family. An event within your religious or ethnic community may have affected your family. Take your time. Any thinking you do about this will take you back in time and loosen your memory banks for the rest of the exercises in this chapter.

Here is a time line of the major cultural events from 1918 through 1992 that can spark your thinking. Just reading through it, you can see the tremendous social change we and our families have lived through during these few years.

---

1918 WWI ends
1929 Great Depression begins
1931 From 4 to 5 million jobless
1932 FDR elected
1933 Prohibition ends
1934 Drought in Midwest, hobo camps
1935 AA founded
1937 Amelia Earhart disappears over South Pacific
1938 WWII begins; Hollywood, *The Wizard Of Oz* and *Gone With The Wind*
1941 Pearl Harbor, Japanese-Americans interred
1944 D-Day; FDR 4th term; General MacArthur, "I have returned."
1945 Atomic bombs on Hiroshima and Nagasaki, WWII ends, troops come home
1946 Nuremburg war trials, Dr. Benjamin Spock
1947 Television
1948 U.S. recognizes Israel, Kinsey sex report

1950 Cold War, McCarthy Era, world communism
1951 Al-Anon founded
1954 Brown v. Board of Education: "Separate but equal" is not okay
1955 Disneyland opens
1956 Elvis, Grace Kelly becomes princess
1957 Sputnik
1960 JFK elected, birth control pill
1961 Freedom Riders attacked in the South, Peace Corps
1962 Marilyn Monroe dies; John Glenn, Friendship 7
1963 JFK assassinated; Martin Luther King, Jr., "I have a dream . . ." Friedan, *The Feminine Mystique*
1964 Civil Rights Act, Beatles
1965 Watts, "Burn, Baby, Burn"; Medicare, U.S. escalates involvement in Vietnam
1966 Miranda Rule, Masters and Johnson
1967 San Francisco, the flower children
1968 Martin Luther King, Jr. killed, Robert Kennedy killed
1969 Mylai massacre, Woodstock, Armstrong/Aldren walked on the moon
1970 Kent State, Chicago Seven
1971 18-year-old vote, Attica prison riot
1973 Wounded Knee, Vietnam war ends
1974 Nixon, "I am not a crook," resigns
1976 Supreme Court okays death penalty
1977 ACoA movement begins
1978 Mayor Moscone and Harvey Milk killed
1979 Three Mile Island, inflation soars
1980 Mount St. Helens erupts, John Lennon killed, Reagan landslide
1981 AIDS virus identified
1982 Vietnam memorial dedicated, hope for ERA fades
1983 Grenada, Reagan calls the USSR "evil empire"
1984 Reagan re-elected, most U.S. bank failures since 1938
1985 Growing number of homeless, TWA hijacking
1986 Shuttle Challenger explodes, U.S. bombs Libya, Iran arms deal revealed
1987 Oliver North, stock market drops 508 points

1988  Reagan to USSR
1989  Berlin wall comes down
1991  Second Russian revolution
1992  Clinton elected, Hurricane Andrew, Ross Perot

## Baseline Givens

Before we add more items to our family time line, we are going to take a brief detour to list some of the important factors that were baseline givens at the time our parents partnered. This will provide an expanded context with which to make sense of our family of origin.

Here is the list of baseline givens in Molly's family when Molly's parents married.

|  | Mother | Father | Stepfather |
|---|---|---|---|
| Age at Marriage: | 18/30 | 26 | 43 |
| Locale: | Midwest | Midwest | Midwest |
| Setting: | Urban-small | Urban-small | Urban-large |
| Disabilities: | None | None | None |
| Illnesses: | None | None | None |
| Social Class: | Middle | Working | Working |
| Religion: | Methodist | Lutheran | Christian Science |
| Birthplace: | U.S.A. | U.S.A. | U.S.A. |
| Ethnicity: | English | Finnish | French |
| Language(s): | English | English | English |

**Mother's family position:** Last child of five, three brothers and one sister

**Father's family position:** Last child of four, three older sisters

**Stepdad's position:** Only child, born after the death of two siblings

**Mother's family at time of marriage:** Both parents and all siblings living, two grandmothers living

**Father's family at time of marriage:** Both parents and all siblings living, all grandparents living

**Stepdad's family at time of marriage:** One parent living, all grandparents dead

You'll notice that we included Molly's stepfather in the list. Since he entered her life in childhood and was a significant parent for her, we list what was given in his life when he partnered with Molly's mom.

When we look at this list of baseline givens, we are looking at a thumbnail sketch of some of the factors on the cassettes each of Molly's parents brought into their marriage. We can look at the differences on their cassettes and speculate how those differences might have created problems for this young couple. We also can see what kind of family Molly was born into.

There may have been religious conflict since Molly's mother's family was made up of rock-ribbed Methodists who were somewhat dogmatic, while her father's Lutheran family, although pious, were not doctrinaire or extreme. There may have been some problems because Molly's mother was so young when she married. We know from research today that the younger the marital partners are when they marry, the greater the likelihood that the union will not endure.

There was, in fact, conflict because of their differing ethnic backgrounds. Molly's father's parents never did approve of their son's marrying someone who was not from the same immigrant and ethnic background. Their son's wife always seemed too fragile and frivolous to them.

There were problems because of the class differences as well. Molly's father and stepfather both came from working-class backgrounds, in contrast to her mother's middle-class background. Today a working-class family in all probability would be classified as middle-class based on income, but at the time of Molly's birth, there was still a fairly clear distinction between blue collar and white collar work. Molly's mother's family, in fact, had definite expectations about who was "good enough" for Molly's mother to marry in terms of social class, and an ongoing stress in Molly's family was her grandparents' disapproval of her father and stepfather.

Fill out the following list of givens for your parents. As you write, you may find you have gaps in your knowledge about your parents. This is not unusual, especially if you grew up in a family with a "Don't talk" rule. If your parents did not talk about their younger years or their families as you were growing up, you might need to do some research now.

As you fill in these lists, remember that this is to be a picture of how things were when they first partnered. Include all significant parenting figures.

|  | Parent 1 | Parent 2 | Parent 3 |
|---|---|---|---|
| **Name:** | _____ | _____ | _____ |
| **Age at Marriage:** | _____ | _____ | _____ |
| **Locale:** | _____ | _____ | _____ |
| **Setting:** | _____ | _____ | _____ |
| **Disabilities:** | _____ | _____ | _____ |
| **Illnesses:** | _____ | _____ | _____ |
| **Social Class:** | _____ | _____ | _____ |
| **Religion:** | _____ | _____ | _____ |
| **Birthplace:** | _____ | _____ | _____ |
| **Ethnicity:** | _____ | _____ | _____ |
| **Language(s):** | _____ | _____ | _____ |

_____**'s family position:** _____

_____

_____**'s family position:** _____

_____

_____**'s family position:** _____

_____

_____**'s family at time of marriage:** _____

_____

_____**'s family at time of marriage:** _____

_____

_____**'s family at time of marriage:** _____

_____

As you look over this list of baseline givens, notice any differences that may have been sources of conflict. Notice also sources of commonality and strength. Notice potential conflict or compatibility based on each parent's birth order. Notice the lateral supports (or drains) that were present.

## Family Life-Cycle Events

Family life-cycle events are events that normally and predictably happen, not just in our personal family, but in nearly all families. Family life-cycle events and individual life-cycle events often interact with each other and with cultural events. We might see one child's birth at the same time the previous child starts school, for instance, which might affect the older child's experience of school and put on the younger child the expectation of "filling the empty nest." Both the family and the individual life-cycle events are the framework on which we will then hang the exceptional events that happened in our family.

Our family's life cycle is based around our family's tasks of partnering and rearing children:

Marriages/Partnerships
Births
Date each child started school (first and last children are most significant for the family as a whole)
Date each child left home
Parents' adjustment to childless home, renegotiation of relationship
Retirement
Marriages/Partnerships of children.

When we add family life-cycle events to Molly's time line, as follows, you will notice that her parents had children relatively quickly. Their first child was born when Molly's mother was 20, and the second when she was 21. As we add more things to the time line, we'll see what correlates with these family life-cycle events.

Again using black ink, write the significant family life-cycle events in your Family of Origin column and in your Extended Family column next to the year they occurred.

| Year | Family of Origin | Extended Family | Culture | Myself |
|------|------------------|-----------------|---------|--------|
| 1920 | | | | |
| 21 | | | | |
| 22 | | | | |
| 23 | | Stepdad's 1st marriage | | |
| 24 | | | | |
| 25 | | | | |
| 26 | | | | |
| 27 | | | | |
| 28 | | | | |
| 29 | | | Great Depression | |
| 30 | | | | |
| 31 | | | | |
| 32 | | | | |
| 33 | | | | |
| 34 | | Stepdad's son born | | |
| 35 | Mom finishes HS | | AA founded | |
| 36 | Parents marry | Stepdad's daughter born | | |
| 37 | | | | |
| 38 | 1st child born | | | |
| 39 | Molly born | | WWII, Holocaust | |
| 40 | | | | |
| 41 | | | | |
| 42 | | | | |
| 43 | 1st child enters school | | | |
| 44 | Molly enters school | | | |
| 45 | | | Atom bomb, WWII ends | |
| 46 | | | | |
| 47 | | | | |
| 48 | | | | |
| 49 | Mom marries Stepdad | | | |
| 50 | Last child born | | Cold War, McCarthy | |
| 51 | | | Al-Anon founded | |
| 52 | | | *Gray Flannel Suit* | |
| 53 | | | | |
| 54 | | | | |
| 55 | | | | |
| 56 | 1st child finishes HS, starts college | | | |
| 57 | Molly finishes HS, leaves home | | Sputnik | |

## Individual Life-Cycle Events

Now it's time to start filling in the Myself column. You will be using this column to plot the events of your individual life-cycle up to the time you moved away from home.

Common individual life-cycle events are these:

Birth
First word
First step
First day of preschool/daycare center
First day of grammar school
First day of junior high school
First day of high school
Last day of school
First friend
First period
First date
First girlfriend/boyfriend
First sex
First time driving a car
First job
Leaving home

You will see what Molly's time line looks like when she adds her individual life-cycle events as shown on the following page.

One of the things we might notice once we add Molly's individual life-cycle events is that Molly was just entering junior high school when her younger brother was born. She was also having her first period and developing breasts. She would be out pushing her baby brother in a carriage, and people would come up and ask her if he was her baby. As a 12-year-old just beginning to deal with her own sexuality, she would be mortified to be asked this question.

Using the black pen, fill in the individual life-cycle events that seem significant for you in the Myself column. If your first friend or first time driving a car weren't important to you, leave them out.

Life-cycle events don't end once you leave home, of course. We will look at the life-cycle events of our adulthood in another chapter.

| Year | Family of Origin | Extended Family | Culture | Myself |
|---|---|---|---|---|
| 1920 | | | | |
| 21 | | | | |
| 22 | | | | |
| 23 | | Stepdad's 1st marriage | | |
| 24 | | | | |
| 25 | | | | |
| 26 | | | | |
| 27 | | | | |
| 28 | | | | |
| 29 | | | Great Depression | |
| 30 | | | | |
| 31 | | | | |
| 32 | | | | |
| 33 | | | | |
| 34 | | Stepdad's son born | | |
| 35 | Mom finishes HS | | AA founded | |
| 36 | Parents marry | Stepdad's daughter born | | |
| 37 | | | | |
| 38 | 1st child born | | | |
| 39 | Molly born | | WWII, Holocaust | Born |
| 40 | | | | |
| 41 | | | | |
| 42 | | | | |
| 43 | 1st child enters school | | | |
| 44 | Molly enters school | | | Enter school |
| 45 | | | Atom Bomb WWII ends | |
| 46 | | | | 1st best friend |
| 47 | | | Television | |
| 48 | | | | |
| 49 | Mom marries Stepdad | | | |
| 50 | Last child born | | Cold War, McCarthy | Enter JHS Get period |
| 51 | | | Al-Anon founded | 1st boyfriend |
| 52 | | | *Gray Flannel Suit* | 1st kiss |

| 53 | | | |
| 54 | | | Drive car |
| 55 | | | 1st job |
| 56 | 1st child finishes HS, starts college | | |
| 57 | Molly finishes HS, leaves home | Sputnik | Finish HS 1st sex leaves home |

## Losses

Earlier, we looked at how our family dealt with loss and separation — how our family "did" endings. The ability to acknowledge and mourn a loss is part of being fully human. Families that are not able to acknowledge losses and facilitate grieving stack up unfinished business like cord wood in the backyard. The more losses there are that cannot be acknowledged and mourned, the more emotionally restricted our family becomes, and the more necessary it becomes for us to avoid those step-on-the-crack-and-you'll-break-your-mother's-back issues.

Even under the best of circumstances, even when perfectly mourned, loss exerts a tremendous strain on a family system and on a family's emotional resources. When we grieve, we must withdraw our energy from the person or the object we have lost. We must work out internally that the person or object we are still attached to inside no longer exists in external reality. The process is the same whether the loss is one of money, fame, person, pet or location.

In the process of mourning, we become less available to those around us. If a chief family member is lost, someone who was the hub of our family system, the people to whom we would normally turn to facilitate our mourning process are also bereaved and therefore less available to us. All of us are mourning the loss at the same time.

Even with a perfectly good grieving process, the more central the value of that which has been lost, the greater the degree of crisis and the greater the intensity and duration of the mourning process for the family.

Below I have listed some events that may have constituted losses for your family:

Accidents
Deaths (including those of pets)
Miscarriages
Disabilities (physical or mental)
Illnesses
Divorces
Desertions
Relocations
Departure of a family member
Ostracism of a family member
Relocation of significant others
Financial reverses (job loss, business loss, major investment loss, bankruptcy)
Religious disillusionment
Natural catastrophes (fire, flood, theft, drought, hurricane)

When Molly's losses are added to her time line it looks like this

| Year | Family of Origin | Extended Family | Culture | Myself |
|------|------------------|-----------------|---------|--------|
| 1920 | | | | |
| 21 | | | | |
| 22 | | | | |
| 23 | | Stepdad's 1st marriage | | |
| 24 | | | | |
| 25 | | | | |
| 26 | | | | |
| 27 | | | | |
| 28 | | | | |
| 29 | | | Great Depression | |
| 30 | | | | |
| 31 | | | | |
| 32 | | | | |
| 33 | | | | |
| 34 | | Stepdad's son born | | |
| 35 | Mother finishes HS | | AA founded | |
| 36 | Parents marry | Stepdad's daughter born | | |
| 37 | *Parents move* | | | |

| | | | | |
|---|---|---|---|---|
| **38** | 1st child born, *family moves* | | | |
| **39** | Molly born, *family moves* | | WWII, Holocaust | Born |
| **40** | *Family moves* | | | |
| **41** | *Family moves* | | | |
| **42** | | | | |
| **43** | 1st child enters school <br> *Parents separate, Dad joins* <br> *Marines, Mom and kids move* | | | |
| **44** | Molly enters school, *Dad killed* | *Loss of good will of Dad's family* | | Enter school |
| **45** | | | Atom Bomb <br> WWII ends | |
| **46** | | | | 1st best friend |
| **47** | | | Television | *Best friend moves* |
| **48** | | | | |
| **49** | Mom marries Stepdad, *move* | | | |
| **50** | Last child born <br> *Dog dies* | *Mom's sis dies* | Cold War, McCarthy | Enter JHS <br> Get period |
| **51** | *Family moves* | *Grandad dies* | Al-Anon founded | 1st boyfriend |
| **52** | *Family moves* | | *Gray Flannel Suit* | 1st kiss |
| **53** | *Family moves* | | | |
| **54** | *Family moves* | | | Drive car |
| **55** | *Family moves* | | | First job |
| **56** | 1st child finishes HS, starts college | | | |
| **57** | Molly finishes HS. <br> *Grandad dies* | | Sputnik | Finish HS <br> 1st sex <br> Leave home <br> *Auto accident* <br> *Break back* |

You will notice that some losses are family losses — the death of a pet, for instance — and go in the Family of Origin column. Some losses are particularly Molly's — when her best friend moves away — and go in her Myself column. Some losses occur in her extended family — grandfather dies — and go in her Extended Family column.

One of the first losses we see on Molly's family time line is the loss of location — the moving of Molly's parents to a neighboring state prior to the birth of their children. First events are always the most impactful on a family. The move to another state had tremendous implications for Molly's family, particularly for Molly's mother.

Generally speaking, a man has a ready-made social network that comes with his work. A woman who goes to a new location where her work is to be that of a wife and a mother does not have a ready-made social network. While her husband is plunged immediately into a group of peers with whom he has commonality, she has to go through the painful process of establishing a new network.

Such was the case with Molly's family. Molly's father loved his work, loved the terrain of the new state and loved the extensive travel away from home that his work afforded him. Molly's mother, on the other hand, felt marooned in a foreign environment miles away from her family of origin. Even though her family was hostile and rejecting of her, be it ever so miserable, there is no place like home.

You can imagine the strain that Molly's parents, as a young couple, experienced with their different attitudes toward being far, far from home. It was into this environment that Molly's brother and then Molly were born.

Now it's your turn. Take a red pen and add to your time lines the losses that you personally, your family and your extended family experienced. Speculate on how the losses may have affected the life-cycle events that occurred near the loss and how those losses may have affected what you learned about parenting and about "doing" endings.

This is also a good time to look at what lateral supports your family had available as shock absorbers while each loss was occurring. Remember that the degree to which our family of origin was able to parcel out to their lateral supports some of the stress associated with losses is the degree to which the loss was less toxic, more easily metabolized and less likely to create unfinished business. Loss resolution is a socially facilitated process.

## Toxic Events

There are other events beside losses that are difficult for a family. I call these difficult events "toxic events." Even though each of these toxic events also causes a loss in the family, they are not necessarily things we think of first and foremost as losses.

Here are some toxic events families experience:

Addictions:

alcohol
drug
food
spending
gambling
sex
work

Abuse:

incest
physical battering
emotional battering
neglect

Socially stigmatized events:

crime committed by family members
crime committed against family members
going to court
going to jail
infidelity
out-of-wedlock childbirth

Infertility
Relinquishment
Abortions
Eviction
Truancy/delinquency
A despised relative moves in.

When we add the toxic events in Molly's family onto her time line, it looks very different.

| Year | Family of Origin | Extended Family | Culture | Myself |
|------|------------------|-----------------|---------|--------|
| 1920 | | | | |
| 21 | | | | |
| 22 | | | | |
| 23 | | Stepdad's 1st marriage | | |
| 24 | | | | |
| 25 | | | | |
| 26 | | | | |
| 27 | | | | |
| 28 | | | | |
| 29 | | | Great Depression | |
| 30 | | | | |
| 31 | | | | |
| 32 | | | | |
| 33 | | | | |
| 34 | | Stepdad's son born | | |
| 35 | Mother finishes HS | | AA founded | |
| 36 | Parents marry | Stepdad's daughter born | | |
| 37 | Parents move | | | |
| 38 | 1st child born, family moves | | | |
| 39 | Molly born, family moves | | WWII, Holocaust | Born |
| 40 | Family moves | | | |
| 41 | Family moves | | | |
| 42 | | | | |
| 43 | 1st child enters school Parents separate, Dad joins Marines, Mom and kids move | | | *Molested* |
| 44 | 2nd child enters school Dad killed *Mom depressed* | Loss of good will of Dad's family | | Enter schl |
| 45 | | | Atom Bomb, WWII ends | |
| 46 | *Custody dispute — Mom v. Dad's family* | | | 1st best friend |
| 47 | | | *Television Best friend moves* | |
| 48 | | | | |
| 49 | Mom marries Stepdad, move | | | |

| 50 | Last child born | Mom's sis dies | Cold War, | Enter JHS |
|----|----------------|-----------------|-----------|-----------|
|    | Dog dies       |                 | McCarthy  | Get period |
| 51 | Family moves   | Pat. grandad dies | Al-Anon | 1st |
|    | *Mom's pseudo-illness* |         | founded   | boyfriend |
|    | *Mom's pill addiction begins* |  |           |           |
| 52 | Family moves   |                 | *Gray* | First kiss |
|    |                |                 | *Flannel Suit* | |
| 53 | Family moves   |                 |           |           |
| 54 | Family moves   |                 |           | Drive car |
| 55 | Family moves   |                 |           | 1st job |
| 56 | 1st child grads HS, starts college | | |       |
| 57 | Molly finishes HS |              | Sputnik   | Finish HS |
|    |                |                 |           | 1st sex |
|    |                |                 |           | Leave home |
|    |                |                 |           | Auto accident |
|    |                |                 |           | Break back |
|    |                |                 |           | *Alcoholism* |

You'll notice that toxic events often occur over a period of years. Molly's mother's pill addiction, for instance, began in 1951 and lasted until 1955. (I found it helpful to draw a vertical line from 1951 to 1955 to show that all the events in Molly's family between 1951 and 1955 were affected by her mom's addiction.)

When we look at Molly's time line to see what events correlate with these toxic events, we see that Molly's mother's sister died in 1950. To add to the trauma, the sister died of an unexpected illness at a relatively young age. Also in 1950 Molly's younger brother was born. Very often births and deaths are correlated on time lines.

It is not coincidental that Molly's mother's pill addiction began after the death of her sister. Molly's mother had a somewhat unresolved relationship with her sister, and her pill addiction is what I would call a "depressive equivalent" — an indicator that Molly's mother was both responding to her sister's death symptomatically and in all likelihood failing to fully mourn her sister's death.

It's your turn. Take your blue pen and write the toxic events of your childhood in the Family of Origin column, the Extended Family column and the Myself column. You may remember other toxic events I did not list. Maybe you had a horrible teacher or baby sitter in third grade who made a big impact on you. Anything you consider a toxic event can be included.

Then take some time to look for correlations. See if a toxic event stems from an earlier loss. Increased alcohol consumption, an affair or any acting-out behavior can be an indicator that the person is having difficulty mourning.

## Major Events

Now let's add the final category — major events — to our time lines. Just as you found in the last section that there are overlaps between the categories of losses and toxic events, you will find overlaps here.

Major events are events that we did not think of primarily as losses or as toxic events but that still had big impacts on our family and often had components of loss and toxicity. The list that follows is far from comprehensive, and you don't have to include all the suggestions. Trust your memory to let you know what was truly a major event for you or your family. If your family expected the end of the world to come in 1950 and it didn't, that was probably a major event for your family.

Adoption
People moving in (elderly parents, foster children, cousins)
New baby sitter, governess, nanny
Promotions or demotions
Major trips, vacations
New jobs, businesses
Confirmation
Bar or Bas mitzvah
Buying or selling property
Awards or achievements
Military draft
Returning from war
Significant new friends
Friends or family moving nearby
New cars
New pets
Switching religions, converting to a religion
Remembering incest or abuse

Entering addiction treatment, therapy
Becoming a feminist, communist, survivalist
Coming out to parents or friends or self as gay
New volunteer or political work
Joining a club, cult, church, social group
A significant class
Menopause
Operation
Midlife crisis
Braces
Helping family members into nursing homes.

When we add Molly's major events to her time lines, they look like this:

| Year | Family of Origin | Extended Family | Culture | Myself |
|------|------------------|-----------------|---------|--------|
| 1920 | | | | |
| 21 | | | | |
| 22 | | | | |
| 23 | | Stepdad's 1st marriage | | |
| 24 | | | | |
| 25 | | | | |
| 26 | | | | |
| 27 | | | | |
| 28 | | | | |
| 29 | | | Great Depression | |
| 30 | | | | |
| 31 | | | | |
| 32 | | | | |
| 33 | | | | |
| 34 | | Stepdad's son born | | |
| 35 | Mother finishes HS | | AA founded | |
| 36 | Parents marry | Stepdad's daughter born | | |
| 37 | Parents move | *Mom's dad returns after separation* | | |
| 38 | 1st child born, family moves | | | |
| 39 | Molly born, family moves | | WWII, Holocaust | Born |
| 40 | Family moves | | | |
| 41 | Family moves | | | |

| Age | Family events | | Historical | Molly |
|---|---|---|---|---|
| 42 | *Mom locates missing older brother* | | | |
| 43 | 1st child enters school parents separate, Dad joins Marines, Mom and kids move | | | Molested |
| 44 | 2nd child enters school Dad killed Mom depressed | Loss of good will of Dad's family | | Enters school |
| 45 | | | Atom Bomb, WWII ends | |
| 46 | Custody dispute — Mom v. Dad's family | | | 1st best friend |
| 47 | | | *Television* | Best friend moves |
| 48 | | | | |
| 49 | Marries Stepdad, moves | | | |
| 50 | Last child born Dog dies | Mom's sis dies | *Cold War, McCarthy* | Enters JHS Gets period |
| 51 | Family moves Mom's pseudo-illness Mom's pill addiction begins | Pat. grandad dies | *Al-Anon founded* | 1st boyfriend |
| 52 | Family moves | | *Gray Flannel Suit* | 1st kiss |
| 53 | Family moves | | | |
| 54 | Family moves | | | Drives car |
| 55 | Family moves *Mom is off pills, not sober Mom becomes fundamentalist* | | | 1st job *Become born-again Christian* |
| 56 | 1st child grads HS, starts college | | | |
| 57 | Molly grads HS, | | *Sputnik* | Grads HS 1st sex Leaves home Auto accident Breaks back Alcoholism *Begins college* |

You'll notice on Molly's time line that the major event of her Mom's conversion to a fundamentalist religion occurs simultaneously with her mom's becoming "dry." This had a big impact on Molly as a sophomore in high school, and she became a born-again Christian fundamentalist. Later on Molly will consider her mom's and her own entry into fundamentalism a toxic event, but at the age of 16 she would have considered it a major event. This is an example of an event that overlaps categories.

Now with a green pen, write the major events in your family under the Family of Origin, Extended Family, and Myself columns.

## Bird's-Eye View

We have created a picture — a bird's-eye view — of our family of origin, starting with the baseline givens. The baseline givens show us our parents' life circumstances at the point in time when they partnered. The givens show us what our parents brought to their new family on their cassettes and how ready or not ready they were to begin the process of parenting.

Some of our parents were like loaves of bread taken out of the oven too soon. Some of our parents faced the dilemma of having to finish baking and growing up at the same time they were trying to have an intimate relationship with their partner and parent us.

We added the family and individual life-cycle events to see what relatively predictable universal events occur in all families and in all individual lives. We can see from plotting the life-cycle events that even if there are no major losses or toxic events, families still have their hands full with the child-rearing and child-launching process.

We included cultural events — world, national, state, regional and community events — to see what impact those events had on our developing selves and on our families.

If we were living near Miami when a hurricane as destructive as Hurricane Andrew arrived, and at the same time one of our parents died and one of our siblings had a serious illness, we would clearly not only be bereft; we would have very little resiliency to deal with the demands put upon us as growing children by our circumstances.

In a similar fashion, large cultural events influenced the impact of some of our family life-cycle events. It was one thing to be born into an affluent, upper-middle-class family at the beginning of the roaring 20s; it was another thing to be born into an impoverished, itinerant, homeless, once-rural family in the middle of the Oklahoma dust bowl in 1936. The family resources that could be brought to bear on the children in each of these families was dramatically different because of class differences and the differences in the surrounding culture.

We have looked at the losses in our childhood history. Loss is part and parcel of both the human condition and the journey called life. However, some losses have a greater impact than others. A loss in childhood of a beloved parent will have an impact that continues to reverberate throughout the rest of a lifetime. We need to look at the losses on our time line to see how each loss affected our personal development and our family.

We have also looked at the toxic events in our families. In Molly's family two things were probably inherited: drug addiction and fundamentalism. Each functioned as a toxic event in the life histories of many of the people in Molly's life.

Finally, we added the major life events — those events that were not part of the expected life-cycle and were also not primarily toxic or a loss. These were the events that, although not "bad," had a big impact on our family.

As we look at our time lines, it is important to give close attention to certain time periods and events. When we look at our infancy, from 9 months to 36 months, we want to see if our environment was secure enough to leave us with a sense of trust in significant others and trust in the world.

This was the time period in which we began walking and talking. It included the terrible twos, or the terrific twos, depending upon whether our perspective was that of the adult or that of the child. This was the time we first began developing our sense of separateness and autonomy, when we first had a sense of our own emerging identity. It was very important during this time that we felt protected by our parents.

The time period from the ages of three to seven was important because it was the time in our own individual life-cycle the family atmosphere was pervaded by sexual energy. If we lost a parent, as Molly did, it could have far-reaching implications in terms of gender identity and sense of security in our identity as a male or as a female. It was when our conscience and our sense of right and wrong emerged. It was also the time our primitive rage could be either buried or acted out in destructive ways.

Between the ages of 7 and 12, we went out into the world and became full-fledged schoolchildren. Looking at this time period, we want to think about what was going on for us in terms of developing peer skills and our sense of competence. This was a particularly important time for us to put into our toolboxes the sense that we were "can do" people — people who were able to solve problems and be effective and competent in our environment. We were also people who could connect with others, form alliances and friendships and experience affection.

Last, of course, there was the period of adolescence merging into young adulthood. We will talk about this time period in more depth when we talk about how we left home, but, briefly, adolescence was the time when we tried to figure out who we were by trying on multiple identities, trying to discover who we were in terms of intimacy.

When we look at our time lines, it is important to notice individual or life-cycle events that are out of sequence. For instance, it is normal for us to lose our parents. But, in general, we don't lose our parents until we are in our forties or fifties. On Molly's time line, we see that Molly lost her father at the age of five. The impact of losing a parent at such a young age can be devastating for a child's development. So here we have the loss of a parent, an expectable loss if it occurs on time in midlife, but devastating when it occurs out of sequence. As you look at the family life-cycle events, individual life-cycle events and losses on your time line, notice whether things happened at their expectable times, or out of sequence, and speculate on the effects the out-of-sequence events had on you and on your toolbox.

Notice also those losses that were growth-promoting and those that were not growth-promoting. It is growth-promoting to lose your first tooth; it is not growth-promoting to lose a safe or stable environment in infancy or early childhood. It is growth-promoting, even though initially unsettling, to move from being a child in the neighborhood to being a child for the first time in a school setting. This loss and change makes greater demands on us and pushes us to develop new skills. However, it isn't growth-promoting if at the same time we move to a new town, leaving behind our secure base and everything that is familiar, and we lose a parent. All of these losses taken together impose a burden on us as developing children and weigh us down rather than free us up.

In an analogy developed by Claudia Black in her work with children of alcoholic parents, she talks about the unfinished emotional business of childhood as being like various-sized boxes that we have roped to us as we enter young adulthood. Picture yourself as a young adult getting ready to leave home, with boxes full of unresolved losses, perhaps the absence of a secure base in infancy, life-cycle events occurring out of sequence. The boxes are full of all the events you have not metabolized or worked through, and they will affect your adult intimate relationships and your parenting.

Now let's go back to the concept of resonance. When we become intimate and when we have children, two of our child selves are evoked. The first is the child self that remembers our experiences at two years of age when we have a two-year-old, who remembers our experiences at five years of age when we have a five-year-old.

The second child self evoked is our wounded child. When we look at our child of two, our wounded child of two feels wounded. It could be argued, by the way, that the pure fact of having a child evokes post-traumatic stress disorder in us as parents because having a child evokes the wounds from our childhood that have never been healed.

If we look at Molly's time line between the ages of three and seven, we see that, first, Molly lost her father through divorce; second, she lost her father to the service; third, she lost her father to death; and fourth, she lost her mother's attention because her mother became severely depressed in response to her father's death. One of the things we might wonder when Molly has a child between the ages of three and seven is how much of the wounding from Molly's years between three and seven will be unconsciously evoked? How much will Molly respond to her child as if her child were not the real child at the present time, but as if her child were little Molly between three and seven — fretful, bereft and feeling insecure and abandoned by her parents?

Molly may respond to her three- to seven-year-old by over-parenting and being oversolicitous, or she may become seriously depressed as her unmetabolized history is restimulated by her child's being the same age at which she experienced so many unhealed wounds.

We have taken our time lines up to the age we were when we left home. How and why and when we left home are crucial to understanding how we began our new family and how we parented.

# CHAPTER

# 9

# Our
# Springboard

Our family's job was to provide us with both roots and wings: roots to help us grow, develop and flourish; wings to help us leave home and develop a life and a family of our own. The mark of a mature adult is not necessarily marriage and children; mature adults are people who are able to form satisfying intimate relationships *outside* their family of origin.

When we look at the process of leaving home, we are partly looking at the extent to which our family was able to give us roots and wings, and we are partly looking to see if they gave us permission to leave. The loyalty code in some of our families said, "Don't separate." In other families the message was, "When you reach a certain age, we'll break your plate and burn your bed: you are a burden and are unwelcome here, so leave as soon as possible."

If we came from a family where there was a high degree of pain and/or dysfunction, that pain/dysfunction had a tremendous impact on the normal family life-cycle event called launching children — that is to say, launching us.

Serious family pain and dysfunction impedes normal developmental processes both for the family as a whole and for us individually as members of that family. Hence some of us may have come from families that never intended to say to us, "Be incomplete. Don't separate. Stay here forever." But the effect of familial pain and dysfunction on our growth process and on our family's growth process was such that we may have come to late adolescence with a feeling of not having received enough to feel complete and ready to separate from our family.

You'll recall the analogy of the loaf of bread that was taken out of the oven too soon. Sometimes, as part of our recovery process in adulthood, we needed to finish baking before we were complete enough to get on with our lives. The other analogy is the one in which we were hungry chiggers looking for someone's skin to get under. Both analogies describe instances in which we had too much unfinished emotional business and too much unfinished developmental business to feel complete enough to move into the world. Nevertheless, we were of an age when it was time to go, or the life circumstances in our family may have been such that, no matter how incomplete we were, we had to leave.

These are examples of our springboard — the platform from which we were launched and from which we launched ourselves into the world of intimacy, work and parenting. How we left home, the circumstances under which we left home, the extent to which our family, particularly our parents, could function as lateral supports for us in the leaving process and in the postemancipation period of early adulthood had a great deal to do with whether or not we faltered as young adults, young intimates and young parents.

## When

If our father was a rageaholic, physically and verbally abusive, and we were a young male of 15, it may have no longer been safe for us to stay at home. The potential violence between us and Dad mounted with each passing day, particularly when Dad directed his violence toward Mom or one of our younger siblings. We may have left home prematurely in order to head off a confrontation with Dad and in order to go out into the world and no longer experience our impotence in the face of Dad's power and rage.

Leaving home at such a young age and under such circumstances had enormous implications for us as we moved forward in time. In a sense we were that loaf of bread that was not able to stay in the oven long enough to be fully done. Some of our finishing process had to occur in our early intimate relationships and in our early parenting endeavors.

For instance, maybe we felt competitive with our own children for our partner's attention. Maybe the hungry, yearning little boy in us still longed for completion. Seeing that the family we created had only limited supplies of nurturing, we may have fought to get our share.

In this example, our leaving home was an out-of-sequence life-cycle event. It was expectable that we would leave home in late adolescence. It was not expectable that we would leave home at the age of 15.

The opposite case can also be true. Rather than leaving home prematurely, perhaps what we did, in effect, was to stay too long at the fair. At 30 years of age we may have still been home with Mommy and Daddy, working independently in a job away from home, but emotionally tied to our parents and incapable of forming an intimate alliance with an adult in our generation.

Perhaps we framed the issue as one of fear: I'm afraid to go it alone, and I'm afraid to be in the world by myself. But, in fact, we may have been playing out our loyalty to Mom and Dad, completely unaware that loyalty was the real issue for us. Or perhaps we were unaware that the real issue was comfort. Mom and Dad had made it so comfortable for us to stay home that we had very little impetus to emancipate. At some level, we need our parents' help in getting launched. We need the message from them to be, "It's time to go."

## Why

Let's look at another factor on our springboard: why we left when we did. Part of the reason for leaving home was the normal pressure of our individual life-cycle and our family's life-cycle, and part was of cultural expectations.

For instance, in this culture the pressure to emancipate begins in adolescence. By the time we were in our twenties, the culture expected us to be standing on our own two feet, struggling with our own intimacy issues and settling into our occupation. The cultural expectation, though perhaps not that we "marry," was that we would form an intimate alliance outside our family and begin bearing and rearing children.

If we had not begun doing this by our thirties, there was some degree of concern from the adults around us that something was amiss. It was feared/assumed that we might never find a suitable partner, settle down or produce grandchildren.

Being single in our thirties would not raise such concern nowadays because there is a trend toward leaving home and starting a family later in life. Particularly in the past 30 years, greater and greater amounts of education and professional achievement have combined with later ages of marrying, the absence of the necessity of marriage for committed unions and child-bearing and the entrance of more and more women into the ranks of higher education, professions and occupations.

All of this is to say that why we left when we did was culturally influenced. That is only part of the picture, however. Why we left may have had a great deal to do with what was going on at home. If we came from a family where the message was, "I'll break your plate and burn your bed," that was a clear indicator that if we did not leave, things would get bad.

I think of the woman who was left at home after all of her older siblings had emancipated. Her parents had separated, and her mother's expectation was that she was to leave as soon as possible. As the last born, and unwanted, she was seen as a burden. The *why* of leaving home for this particular woman was to escape the abusive relationship with her mother.

There are a multitude of ways to leave home. One is to leave by choice in a timely manner when we are ready and well prepared to go. Another way to leave home is to be extruded from our family, either subtly or not so subtly.

We may have been extruded from our family for a whole host of reasons. Perhaps one of our parents was seriously ill, and we didn't know about the illness. It may have been for that reason that we were catapulted unexpectedly into the adult world, given premature permission to marry at a very early age, for instance. Our parents' may have hoped that we would be settled and well taken care of before our ill parent died. We may wish, in retrospect, that our parents had not granted permission. It may appear that our parents did not establish an appropriate boundary for us.

Let's say we left home because we had a sense that our family was disintegrating because of dysfunction. We thought that if we did not get out, we too would become subject to the family's disintegration. Or maybe we left home because we had a sense that our family's ties were truly the ties that bind. We knew those ties were fastened with Super Glue and that if we didn't take the first chance we had to get out, we would never be able to leave.

If, in our leaving home, we were making a decision to be a survivor — that is to say, we were escaping the pain, the chaos, the Super Glue, the disintegration — we may subsequently suffer survivor guilt. We may feel that our healthy, normal need to emancipate from our family was at the expense of our parents or younger siblings who experienced our emancipation as desertion. In such circumstances we may struggle with a lifetime of guilt about the life trajectory of a younger sibling who did not do well, whose life course appeared to have been blighted by familial dysfunction.

This was particularly apt to be true, by the way, if we were the parentified child in our family of origin and had functioned as a surrogate parent to this sibling. Our dilemma was that we were not this child's parent although we functioned as if we were. Our need to separate and have a life of our own seemed to be at the expense of a sibling we could not take with us and who seemed imperiled by our leaving.

Molly experienced just such a dilemma. When Molly was 22, her brother, 10 years younger than she, begged her to let him come and live with her. At the age of 22, Molly was actively alcoholic and barely launched into adulthood. She was not able to take on the responsibility for her younger brother. In subsequent years he would say to her, "I'm not blaming you for not taking me in, but my life would be very different today if you had said yes."

## EXERCISE

Take a moment to think back to the time you left home. At what age did you leave home? What was going on at home when you left? Why did you leave home?

Does it seem to you that when and why you left home gave you a good start on your adult life? How might the when and why have affected your first intimate relationships and your parenting?

## Resonance Again

Let's look at how resonance affected our springboard. When we think back to our adolescence, it's important to remember that our parents' child selves were resonating when we moved into the developmental time period when it was appropriate for us to begin experimenting with intimacy, transferring some of our allegiance from our parents to our peers, looking at what we would do with our lives occupationally and preparing to leave home.

All parents have two inner child selves restimulated based on what their children are doing. When we were 14, our parents' unconscious experience of being 14 was evoked, and our parents responded to this bank of experience often totally out of conscious awareness. Second, our parents' wounded or traumatized 14-year-olds were evoked. Our parents may have experienced post-traumatic stress disorder when we were 14 because of the restimulating of their wounded 14-year-olds of the past whose feelings they had never been able to address and metabolize in a conscious way with support.

With the emergence of our adolescent sexuality, they may have remembered for the first time some occluded memory of abuse in their own adolescence. They then had to deal with all the feelings around that memory at the same time they were confronting their future without us.

How our parents left home when they were adolescents was also restimulated when we began the process of leaving home. Any feelings that were unresolved for our parents about their leaving process may have intruded into our leaving process.

Molly's mother, for instance, had forfeited the opportunity for a college education when the family's resources were diverted so that her youngest brother could go to college. She spent a lifetime feeling inadequate because of a lack of education. Even if nothing else had complicated Molly's emancipation process, her mom's unprocessed feelings about her own leaving home would have made her mom ambivalent about watching Molly go off to college.

## The "Nevers"

Family turbulence was also generated by our parents' unconscious sadness about what I call the "nevers." Our parents confronted in us that they would never again be 14 or 16 or 18. When we became adolescents, the house was not only full of our racing hormones and emerging sexual energy; the house was also full of hope and of the promise of things to come. Our parents began confronting their own life histories through us when we entered this stage in our lives.

If our parents' marriage had been relatively fulfilling, and if their fulfillment had come through channeling their energy into us, they may have looked at marital bankruptcy and emptiness when they envisioned a home without us. They might have inadvertently got in the way of our leaving in order to forestall confronting a marriage that needed either to end or to be worked over dramatically in order for it to be a viable vehicle to take them into the next stage of their lives together.

As the house became filled with sexual energy and the promise of things to come for us, our parents measured the reality of their lives against what they had hoped their lives would become. On some level, they mourned. They mourned for the 14-year-olds they had been and for the 14-year-olds they did not get the opportunity to be. They mourned for whatever dreams they had had at 14 that they had not been able to fulfill.

---

### EXERCISE

Look back at the time lines you created in the previous chapter. What was going on at the time your parents left home and partnered? What stories have you heard about their adolescence and their leaving-home process? Do you see any parallels between their experiences and yours? What do you imagine might have been resonating for them?

Do you know what adolescent dreams your parents had for their lives? Do you know if they had any regrets as they grew older? How do you imagine their unfulfilled dreams might have affected your teen years and leaving process?

---

## Mourning

One of the problems we and our parents had was that the culture did not give us permission to mourn. They were supposed to be glad we were going. The song says, "Thank God and Greyhound she's gone." The feelings of sadness and excitement that overlapped, both for our parents and for us, may not have been articulated or understood either by us or by our parents.

We were supposed to want to emancipate and be excited about what was to come. Having been sheltered to some degree, we were given little help in articulating our fear of what it might be like to stand unsheltered in the world.

## Lateral Supports

If we had been a parent surrogate to our parents, we may have feared that if we left home, our parents would fall apart. When we did leave home and our parents did fall apart, we may have felt punished for needing to have a life of our own. This is one of the reasons the concept of lateral supports has been emphasized throughout this book.

Appropriate lateral supports for our parents are other adults of their generation. If our parents had been getting their needs met with one another, with their extended family and with their peers, they would have been less likely to reach down one generation to us to draft us into inappropriate roles, such as surrogate spouse or surrogate parent, which were detrimental to our emancipation process.

---

## EXERCISE

Did you and your family feel free to express all your emotions about your leaving home: fear, excitement, sadness?

Did you and your family have lateral supports that helped you with the process?

---

## Intimacy

During adolescence we began developing our sense of identity, part of which included our gender identity and a view of ourselves as sexual beings. Some of us were late bloomers, kids who were still climbing trees and were more interested in latency-age issues in adolescence than our peers were.

Others of us were race horses who were bursting out of the gate. At the very early age of 11 or 12, we were sexually curious, sexually preoccupied, physically well-developed and ready for and interested in sexual exploration.

Recently I got together with an old friend from high school. I reminded her that all of us girls who ran around together had elected her, at the age of 15, to be the emissary for our group. She was to go to her mother and ask her mother on behalf of all of us what sex was like. At 15 we had either little or no sexual experience.

Now, bear in mind that I am of the generation of good girls/bad girls. Good girls "didn't do it" and didn't pierce their ears; bad girls "did it" and did pierce their ears. Because I grew up in that era, it would have been impossible for any of us to acknowledge if we were in fact having sexual experiences. The assumption was that we were good girls and, therefore, not "doing it."

In our curiosity about sex, we wanted to know from her mother what sex was like and, in particular, what intercourse was like. When I reminded my friend of this conversation, she laughed and asked why it was that her mother had been chosen. I told her that none of the rest of us had mothers with whom we could even begin to be so bold as to ask such a question. When she had asked her mother, even her mother said nothing more than, "You'll cross that bridge when you come to it."

Now compare that example with the sexuality part of the springboard for the contemporary generation. The contemporary generation is likely to be sexually active at a very early age, on the pill, using condoms because of AIDS and seen as "out of it" if they are not sexually active.

When we look at our first adolescent and young adult experiences with intimacy, we must put those experiences into a context. First, we must put them into a cultural context. What was the cultural expectation about sexuality when we were adolescents and young adults? Were we expected or not expected to be sexual? Were we expected or not expected to talk about what we were experiencing?

If we were male, the expectations about sexual experience were far different for us than they were if we were female. Was our first intimate experience by choice, or was it an experience of disempowerment?

For instance, the socialization for males, and perhaps some of the drive provided by testosterone, encouraged males to push and push and push until they could push no more. For an adolescent male, "No" or "Stop" may not have meant "No" or "Stop." It may have meant, "Push until you can get your partner to yield no further."

As young adolescent females, many of us may have had early sexual experiences more by default or ignorance than by choice or out of a genuine expression of our own sexual desire. Our early sexual experiences may have been an outgrowth of our socialization to be nurturing, cooperative and pleasing; not to be angry; and to take care of other people's feelings.

Many of us females had our first intercourse without having consented. Many of us were not fully aware of the potential of becoming pregnant. Some of us ended up with an unwanted pregnancy and no full awareness of how we became pregnant.

If, by the time we came into adolescence, our life experience included a history of sexual abuse by a parent, a parent surrogate, a sibling or someone outside the family system, much of our sexuality had been preempted. We did not come into adolescence with excitement about our emerging sexuality and a sense of ownership about our own bodies. We came into our earliest experiences with a sense of shame and defilement that dramatically affected our early intimate history.

---

## EXERCISE

Take a few minutes to think back to your adolescence and young adulthood. When did you become aware of your sexual feelings? When did you begin acting on those feelings?

When you first became intimate, was it by choice or by default? Was it pleasant or unpleasant? Was it frightening or exhilarating?

Did you feel as if you were in charge of your own body? Were you in charge of how you were touched, by whom you were touched, who you touched and how you touched?

Did you come from a sexually permissive or a sexually repressive environment? Was the home environment highly charged sexually and loaded with the expectancy that you would be sexual? Might you have acted out some of your parents' unmetabolized sexual energy and sexual aspiration?

---

### Our First Partner

We've talked about how we left home and how we became intimate. Let's talk now about how we picked the person with whom we became intimate and formed a sufficient union to begin the process of becoming a parent.

We've talked about the unfinished emotional business we bring from our childhood into young adulthood. Both too much of a good thing and too little of a good thing from our parents was not helpful to us as children.

Let's say we were over-parented by our parents — that is to say, our weaknesses rather than our strengths were reinforced, and our dependency rather than our autonomy was responded to. When we left home, we were likely to have been attracted to, and to have left home for, someone who held out the promise of taking care of us in the way our parents did.

The opposite may also have been the case. We may have left home with many of our developmental needs not met because of our family's inability to provide for our emotional needs appropriately. We then went out into the world as the hungry chigger looking for what we had not received.

In either instance, we looked at potential partners as people who would either love us the way we'd been loved in childhood or love us in the way we'd never been loved. Both of these possibilities made for a very large fantasy component when we began the process of partnering.

It has often been said that falling in love is a form of temporary insanity. Falling in love is the projection of all of our unfulfilled wishes and desires onto another person. We fail to see that person for who they are, but instead see them through lenses that are clouded and complicated by who we need them to be.

The state of "falling in love" doesn't last throughout the entire course of a relationship, of course. When we attempted to "stand" in love, that period of time after we quit falling, we could finally see the real person with whom we partnered.

We then began experiencing the restimulation of all the hopes and fears of all the years that would not be met. With that came a primitive rage and a primitive hurt felt by us in our child selves.

Honeymoons are notorious for the fights we have as they end. There is an end to the fantasy of being in love and the fantasy of who this person is going to be. The reality of day-to-day life with another real person sets in and we begin to see how well-matched we are.

| EXERCISE |

Take a moment to think about the partner(s) you became intimate with. With the power of 20/20 hindsight, can you see what childhood needs or adolescent fantasies you hoped each partner might fulfill? What happened when the real person emerged?

## Children

I don't have space to cover in depth all of the ways in which partnered and marital relationships can become disappointing and go sour, but let me say they are legion. And it is within the context of this relationship, whether a fulfilling or a terribly disappointing one, that the issue of having children arises.

In looking back at ourselves as young parents, I would like us to look back on whether we became parents by choice or by default. We may have become parents by default because of some expectation that we did not feel we had a right to question.

The expectation might have been cultural. Only the last generation or two has felt it had the right to talk about having children by choice. All prior generations had children because it was the socially expected thing to do.

The expectation might have been familial. Perhaps we were the child who felt as if we were glue for our parents' personalities and our parents' lives. If we got a strong message that we were to have children to fulfill and complete our parents' lives, most likely we never considered not having children.

Let's take an example where the expectation was both cultural and familial. Let's say we are Jewish and part of a religiously and culturally observant large extended family. At all family get-togethers when we were growing up, tremendous emphasis was placed on the preciousness of the children born to all members of our family. Family get-togethers, in fact, were often in honor of new family members as they were born.

As we sat at a family dinner with 25 or 30 adults and children of our extended family, we may have silently questioned whether we were capable of adequately parenting a child, but we were faced visually with our only possible answer: having children was the only option for us. We could look forward in time and see that in order to have a fully respected place in this family, we needed to bring babies and toddlers and adolescents and young adults to this dinner table in years to come.

How did our children come to be? Did they come to be by choice? Did we and our partners mutually decide that we wanted to have children? Was it a well-informed decision? Were we financially and emotionally prepared to have children?

At the other end of the spectrum, we might have decided that we wanted to have children, but we were uneducated, unemployed and had little adult capacity. We brought our girlfriend home to live with our parents; she was pregnant because the two of us wanted to have a child.

That is a scenario far different from the one in which we were launched, emancipated and had a job and the financial wherewithal to provide for a family. We both wanted children, felt emotionally prepared to have a family and decided it was time.

In many cases, one of us wanted children and the other didn't. Maybe since one spouse clearly did not want to have children, we agreed to forfeit children as part of our joint life journey prior to our union. But once the union was in progress, one of us changed our mind and made the continuation of the relationship contingent upon the bearing of children. Needless to say, the consequences for the marriage, for the family and for the children were considerable.

If we were the one who did not want children and were put in the position of either losing our spouse or having children we did not want in order to keep our spouse, it's likely that the resentment between us and our spouse continued to grow and our ability to attach to, prize and really embrace our children was dramatically impaired.

---

## EXERCISE

Think for a moment about how your children came to be. How did you answer the "children" questions:

- Should I have children?
- How many children should I have?
- When in my marital history and occupational history should I have children?

Who influenced those decisions? How heavily was each influence weighted by your family of origin, the culture, the church, your partner and your siblings?

---

## Looking Back

Before we make time lines for the family we created, this is the time to stop and review what was going on for us as we began our adult life.

First, how did we leave home? Were we moving away from someone or something, or toward someone or something?

Second, how did we become intimate? Was it by choice? What was the meaning of sexual intimacy to us? What was the meaning of emotional intimacy to us?

Third, when we began a partnered relationship, how much unfinished business did we bring from our own childhood? Who was the fantasy person toward whom we were moving? What was the childhood wish we were trying to complete — to duplicate what we got in childhood or to get what we hadn't received in childhood?

Finally, how did we decide to have children? Was it a choice or did it happen by default? Was it a unilateral decision or a bilateral decision? Whose choice was it? How much was the decision influenced by culture and family?

## Baseline Givens

Now that we have looked at the springboard from which we launched ourselves or were launched, let's look at the baseline givens we and our partners brought into our new family. You will recognize this list from the last chapter. Remember, this is a picture of how things were when you first partnered. Include all significant parenting figures.

|  | Myself | Parent 1 | Parent 2 |
|---|---|---|---|
| Name: | _____ | _____ | _____ |
| Age at Marriage: | _____ | _____ | _____ |
| Locale: | _____ | _____ | _____ |
| Setting: | _____ | _____ | _____ |
| Disabilities: | _____ | _____ | _____ |
| Illnesses: | _____ | _____ | _____ |
| Social Class: | _____ | _____ | _____ |
| Religion: | _____ | _____ | _____ |
| Birthplace: | _____ | _____ | _____ |
| Ethnicity: | _____ | _____ | _____ |
| Language(s): | _____ | _____ | _____ |

My family position: _____

_____

_____ 's family position: _____

_____

_____ 's family position: _____

_____

My family at time of marriage: _____

_____

_____ 's family at time of marriage: _____

_____

_____ 's family at time of marriage: _____

_____

As you look over this list of baseline givens, notice any differences that may have been sources of conflict. Notice also any sources of commonality and strength. Notice potential conflict or compatibility based on each parent's birth order. Notice the lateral supports (or drains) that were present. Take a moment to think about how these baseline givens might have affected your intimate relationships and your parenting.

## Cultural Events

Pull out the time lines you started in the last chapter. This time we are going to create a visual picture of your new family so that you can see all the different influences on you, on your intimate relationships, on your parenting and on significant events in your life.

Once again, start by listing the cultural events that most affected you, your intimate relationships and your new family. You can refer to the list of cultural events in the last chapter for ideas.

## Family Life-Cycle Events

Now add the life-cycle events for the family you created. Since all the events for you as an individual, as well as for your new family, will be listed in the Myself column, you may find you need to use more sheets of paper just for the Myself column. In that case, simply number the years along the left-hand side of the new sheets so they match the sheets you've already numbered and keep the sheets side by side. That way you can still read all the events that happened in one year straight across.

Write "I marry" or "I partner" in the Myself column next to each date you married or partnered. Notice what cultural events were happening at those times that might have affected your partnering.

Since you now have your spouse and your spouse's family in your life, you will be adding significant events in their lives to your time lines when they seem important as well. You can put the events for your spouse's family in the Extended Family column. The events for your spouse and your children will go into the Myself column, because whatever affects a member of your new family affects you as well. Once partners have become ex-partners, if certain events in their lives affect you and/or your children, put them into the Extended Family column. They are now part of your extended family as supports or drains.

Add the family life-cycle events to your time lines in black ink. You will be adding events to your Myself column for the family you created, to the Family of Origin column for your parents and siblings, and to the Extended Family column for your spouse's family or other extended family.

Remember from the last chapter that our family's life-cycle is based around our family's tasks of partnering and rearing children:

Marriages/Partnerships
Births
Date each child started school (first and last children are most significant for the family as a whole)
Date each child left home
Parents' adjustment to childless home, renegotiation of relationship
Retirement
Marriages/Partnerships of children

## Individual Life-Cycle Events

In the previous chapter, you plotted the individual life-cycle events for yourself as a child and adolescent in your Myself column. This time, using black ink, write the significant life-cycle events for each of your children in the Myself column. You don't need to include all of these events, just the ones you see as significant. As you enter them, you are again looking for ways in which cultural events, family life-cycle events and events in your extended family and family of origin might have affected your children or your parenting during these important individual life-cycle events.

Here is the list of common individual life-cycle events:

Birth
First word
First step
First day of preschool/day-care center
First day of grammar school
First day of junior high school
First day of high school
Last day of school
First friend

First period
First date
First girlfriend/boyfriend
First sex
First time driving a car
First job
Leaving home

## Losses

As mentioned in the previous chapter, losses cause a strain on a family. If the loss was central to you, it made you less available to your children while you mourned. If the loss was central to the whole family, your whole family went through an upheaval.

Using a red pen, write the losses you and your family experienced in the Myself column. Write the losses your family of origin and your extended family experienced in the appropriate columns.

Below are listed some of the losses your family may have experienced:

Accidents
Deaths (including those of pets)
Miscarriages
Disabilities (physical or mental)
Illnesses
Divorces
Desertions
Relocations
Departure of family member
A family member is disowned
Relocations of significant others
Financial reverses
Religious disillusionment
Natural catastrophes (fire, flood, theft, drought,
    hurricane)

Once you have listed the losses, look at the events near each loss that were probably affected. Also think about what lateral supports you and your family members had available as shock absorbers while each loss was occurring.

## Toxic Events

In the last chapter I defined toxic events as "other events besides losses that are difficult for a family." Take a blue pen and write, in the appropriate columns, the toxic events that affected your family. Make a vertical line next to all the years each toxic event was present. Your workaholism, for example, may have lasted ten years; your partner's physical battering may have lasted three years.

As you enter each toxic event, notice what life-cycle events that toxic event is affecting for your family and for each of your children. Also notice what losses the toxic event comes after. Do you see any correlations between losses and nearby toxic events?

Here are some toxic events families experience:

Addictions:
  alcohol
  drug
  food
  spending
  gambling
  sex
  work
Abuse:
  incest
  physical battering
  emotional battering
  neglect
Socially stigmatized events:
  crime committed by family members
  crime committed against family members
  going to court
  going to jail
  infidelity
  out-of-wedlock childbirth
Infertility
Relinquishment
Abortions
Eviction
Truancy/delinquency
A despised relative moves in

## Major Events

Now add the final category — major events — to your time lines. You may recall that these are events that were not primarily losses or toxic events, but still had big impacts on your family.

Use the green pen to enter major events into your columns, and as you do, again notice the other events listed nearby to see how they may have interacted to affect you, your partnership, your children or your parenting.

The list that follows is far from comprehensive, and you don't have to include all of these. Trust your memory to let you know what was truly a major event for you or your family.

Adoption
People moving in (elderly parents, foster children, cousins)
New baby-sitter, governess, nanny
Promotions or demotions
Major trips, vacations
New jobs, businesses
Confirmation
Bar or bas mitzvah
Buying or selling property
Awards or achievements
Military draft
Returning from war
Significant new friends
Friends or family moving nearby
New cars
New pets
Switching religions, converting to a religion
Remembering incest or abuse
Entering addiction treatment, therapy
Becoming a feminist, communist, survivalist
Coming out to parents, friends or self as gay
New volunteer or political work
Joining a club, cult, church, social group
A significant class
Menopause
Operation
Midlife crisis

Braces
Helping family members into nursing homes

## Molly

Let's use Molly as an example again so we can see some of the things you might notice as you think about your own time lines.

| Year | Family of Origin | Extended Family | Culture | Myself |
|------|-----------------|-----------------|---------|--------|
| 1955 | Family moves<br>Mom is off pills, not sober,<br>Mom becomes fundamentalist | | | 1st job<br>Born-again<br>Christian |
| 56 | 1st child finishes HS, starts college | | | |
| 57 | Molly finishes HS | | Sputnik | Finishes HS,<br>First sex<br>Leave home<br>Auto accident,<br>Back broken<br>Alcoholism<br>Begin college |
| 58 | Family moves | | | Spiritual crisis<br>Loss of faith |
| 59 | | | | |
| 60 | 1st child marries<br>Dog dies | | JFK,<br>birth control | |
| 61 | | | | Begin to flunk |
| 62 | | | | Quit school,<br>New job |
| 63 | Family bankrupt<br>Family moves<br>Mom's pill addiction reactivates | | JFK killed<br>Civil Rights<br>Feminism | |
| 64 | Divorce, Mom moves | | | Start school,<br>Quit |
| 65 | | | | |
| 66 | Mom's menopause | | | Start school<br>Quit |
| 67 | Family moves | Mat. grandmother<br>dies | | Marry<br>Alcoholism<br>Rcvy thru AA |

| Year | Family of Origin | Extended Family | Culture | Myself |
|------|------------------|-----------------|---------|--------|
| 68 | Last child finishes HS | | MLK killed | |
| 69 | | | Woodstock | Finish college, Move, begin grad school |
| 70 | | Husb's parents lose business | | |
| 71 | | | | Pregnancy Move, divorce New job |
| 72 | | | Watergate | Daughter born |
| 73 | Mom remarries | Ex-husb remarries becomes alcoholic | Vietnam War ends | Major depress. Therapy thru '78 |
| 74 | | | Nixon resigns | |
| 75 | Mom sober w/AA | | | Move |
| 76 | | Pat. aunt dies | | Cut-off between self and Stepdad |
| 77 | | | ACoA movement begins | Buy house Start self-employment |
| 78 | Mom's emotional breakdown | Mat. uncle dies (Mom's fav) | | Child begins school |
| 79 | | | | 16-yr dog dies |
| 80 | Mom loses financial stability Mom divorces | Ex-husb heart attack | Reagan elected | Remarry Acquire teen stepchildren |
| 81 | Mom's business fails | | AIDS identified | |
| 82 | | | | |
| 83 | Mom repeated psych hospitaliz thru '90 | | | |
| 84 | | | | Sell house, buy house |
| 85 | | Ex-husband alcohol recovery | | Remodel house |
| 86 | | Fav uncle dies | | Rcvy thru AA |

| Year | Family of Origin | Extended Family | Culture | Myself |
|------|-----------------|-----------------|---------|--------|
| 87 | Mom major surgery | | | I reconcile with Stepdad |
| 88 | | | | Stepchildren Finish HS and leave home Sell house, buy house |
| 89 | | | Berlin wall falls | Menopause |
| 90 | Mom to nursing home | | | Divorce Child finishes HS, begins college Therapy to '92 |
| 91 | | 1st ex-husb dies Fav aunt dies 2nd ex-husb remarries | | Leave bus. partnership Sell house, buy house |
| 92 | | | Clinton elec | Ill, to hospital |

Molly left home "on time," that is, at the age of 18. Although it looks as if she should have had an easy launching since no traumas were currently going on in her family of origin, she was actually too immature to be out in the world. As a result, she was in and out of college for 12 years and struggling with her loyalty to her family of origin.

Her leaving home felt to her almost like an act of disloyalty to her mother and her younger sibling. She had been a pseudoparent for both of them and was leaving them in a deteriorating situation.

During Molly's twenties, her family of origin sustained a number of losses. While she was struggling with her issues of intimacy, emancipation and occupation, she had the additional strain of helping her family deal with their losses and of watching her mother's pill addiction reactivate.

We can see that Molly's mother probably returned to pills in response to the number of losses she was experiencing, including the loss of her children, who were growing up and leaving home. Since her own adolescence, departure from home and first marriage had been very painful for her, we can imagine that these experiences were resonating for her as her children reached adolescence and left home.

We can also see that Molly didn't have much support for her first marriage when she was in her twenties. Her family moved away shortly after she was married, and her husband's family was in financial trouble. Molly's family of origin had already gone bankrupt.

Molly's daughter, Janet, was born at a turbulent time. Molly had moved, divorced and started a new job just before Janet's birth. Shortly after Janet's birth, Molly went through a major depression, not unlike the depression her own mother had gone through after her divorce and move when Molly was three. The fact that Janet's father remarried shortly thereafter didn't make life any more stable for her, since she from then on would also have to deal with the tension between Molly and her new stepmother.

While Molly had had few lateral supports available to her during her first marriage, during her second marriage in her forties she had an abundance of support from the family of her second husband. She was also, however, at midlife and part of the sandwich generation. She was dealing with an ailing mother, a new marriage complete with the challenges of a blended family, struggles with her siblings over the care of her mother and the need to look at her own mortality. She needed to complete any business she had with the older generation, make peace with her siblings as the generation that would go with her into the last third of her life and learn about stepparenting.

It's interesting to note that Janet acquired a stepfather when she was eight years old. Molly had acquired a stepfather when she was nine. Molly can see from the parallels between her springboard time line and her family of origin time line that she was most likely filled with resonance and unfinished emotional business during this time period. History does in fact repeat itself.

By the time Molly's second marriage ended in 1990, all three of her stepchildren had left home, and her daughter had started college away from home. Molly had the same feeling that her family was falling apart that she had experienced as a young adult when she left home and began her own life while her family sustained losses and her mother's pill addiction reactivated.

The difference in 1990 for Molly and her daughter was that Molly's addiction did not reactivate. The generational legacy had been broken in Molly's family with her recovery and her having sought excellent psychological help.

When we look for parallels, we can see some similarities and some differences between the family Molly created and her family of origin. Both Molly and her mother had first marriages of short duration and second marriages that ended when they were in midlife. Molly, however, had more lateral supports during her second marriage, which made both her and her daughter's lives easier.

Molly received better parenting than either of her parents had received. In turn, her daughter received better parenting than she had received.

Molly had the advantage of growing up during the cultural time period when there has been an emphasis on recovery and an encouragement to seek lateral supports above and beyond those available in the family's extended network. While her daughter did have to go through Molly's depression, just as Molly had gone through her mother's depression, Molly had already recovered from alcoholism and could use therapy to grow from her depression instead of spiraling downward. Molly's recovery and the shock-absorbing benefits of more lateral supports had a big impact on making her daughter's life better.

If we imagine Molly looking over her time line, we would hope she would get a broad picture of the context in which she was operating as a young adult, a young married person and a young parent. We would want her to notice the difficulties her daughter may have experienced because of some of the external events out of Molly's control. And we would want Molly to become more forgiving of herself and more aware of the multiple stresses both she and her husbands were juggling.

Hopefully you have had a similar experience as you have looked over your time line. If you can see your life in terms of the big picture — the context in which you parented — as well as look at the tools and unfinished emotional business you brought to parenting, you can develop compassion both for your children and for yourself as the parent who survived and grew through it all.

## Moving On

Up to this point, we have been on a long and sometimes very arduous journey together. Some of what we've done has been painful and difficult. We have taken a journey back into our own families of origin, opened our toolboxes and become aware of what we did or did not have available to us as we began our journey as young intimates and young parents. Hopefully, we can now look back at ourselves as young parents and realistically appraise (1) who we were, (2) what tools we had available to us, (3) what lateral supports or drains were present or absent for us and (4) what the givens and events were over which we had no control.

My hope is that having taken this part of the journey, we now have more compassion for ourselves and for the young parents we once were. Compassion means really knowing in our bones that we couldn't know what we didn't know and we couldn't give what we didn't get. We did the best we could with what we had at the time.

Please remember that this is not a journey for sissies. Pause for a moment and commend yourself for having had the courage to pick up this book and to come this far.

We are now ready to take the next leg of our journey. This leg takes us through healing and accountability.

In the self-help group Alcoholics Anonymous, one of the recommended ways to heal regret and remorse about harm done is to talk about what we were like, who we were, what happened and what we are like now. We have just completed looking at what we were like and how we came to be who we were.

During the healing and accountability leg of the journey, we will be looking together at what we did and what we didn't do about which we have remorse and regret. Our companion as we travel must always be our compassion for the young adult we were.

This next leg of the journey is not about self-flagellation. It is about healing. It is a time to own what we did well, what we did poorly and what we deeply wish, with our 20/20 hindsight and our current maturity, we could have done better. It is a chance to heal our regret and our remorse in order to have a better relationship with ourselves, our partners and our children.

Up to this point, we have been living in the problem. In this next section, we will begin living in the solution.

# SECTION

## III

# OUR HEALING JOURNEY

# CHAPTER

# 10

# Getting Ready: Preparation For The Healing Journey

### by Constance B. Huey

Before we parents plunge down the path that can both heal our relationships with our adult children and allow us to lay down our burden of parental guilt, we need to get ready for the journey. Most of the time we are unconscious of our own preparations.

Every once in a while, we have a moment of wonderful communication with our children that gives us hope for a better relationship with them: we are suddenly aware of some pain in our children's lives caused by our parenting, a life-threatening event urges us to get moving or a memory of parenting surfaces unbidden. I call these occurrences Magical Moments, Rumbles,

Alarms and Memories. They randomly punctuate our lives, rising like bubbles from the compost at the bottom of a lake, popping in without invitation.

We can ignore these events, even see them as unwelcome intrusions, or we can use them to help us prepare for our healing journey. Some people leave for a trip by just walking out the door with the clothes on their backs; others spend weeks packing. The "bubbles" that pop into our lives are like personal valets that tap us on the shoulder and say, "You'll be going soon. Here's a map; here's a first aid kit. It will be easier if you pack a little now."

Recognize and value these moments. Use them to get ready for your journey.

## Magical Moments Of Communication

The first Magical Moment of Communication I can remember happened eight years ago. My 14-year-old daughter, Jennifer, and I were having a rip-roaring argument over some earth-shattering subject such as whether or not she had to clean the bathroom before she could go out with her friends. An outsider seeing us, toe-to-toe, screaming and flailing our arms, would have had difficulty ascertaining who was the parent and who was the child. (As I look back, I realize Jennifer was being the parent.)

In the midst of our shouting match, Jennifer suddenly thrust her hand in front of my face like a cop stopping traffic. I immediately became mute and curious. She then took two "Mother-May-I" jumps to the side, away from my toes, and said, "Mommy, have you forgotten that I am a teenager? I won't always be a teenager, but right now this is how you and I are supposed to behave. So, don't worry about it too much, but please keep up your part. You do 'mad' very well! Get it?"

I replied, "Got it!" She jumped back into character, and we were back to our screaming fight.

When Jennifer stepped out of the fight and we had that Magic Moment of Communication, I felt something click inside me: hope. After that I knew —

    1. Jennifer and I could begin again as mother and daughter, making a joint effort to communicate differently.

2. I would have to come to terms with my guilt and shame over whatever real or imagined harm I had done to her as a parent if we were going to be genuine with each other and be in our appropriate roles.
3. I would have to go to any lengths to learn how to become an honest, loving and self-forgiving parent. Then when Jennifer had children of her own, she could take a better image of a parent and better communication skills into her own parenting, and she could be confident that what she gave her children was good enough.

Particularly ripe and poignant Magical Moments of Communication occur in the lives of all recovering parents, when the possibility of developing a healthy new relationship with our children suddenly becomes evident. I say *possibility* because for some parents, even recognizing a Magical Moment is difficult, let alone knowing what to do when it occurs. Yet when you and I, as recovering parents, are able and willing to embrace these moments — these opportunities — and when our children are receptive at the same time, we set an entire process in motion. We begin a journey that will ultimately lead to a greater sense of purpose and fulfillment, as well as to a greater experience of belonging, than we have ever known.

Sometimes the healing and/or forgiveness work we have done with our own parents can help us embrace the Magical Moments with our children. I'm not saying this is a necessary part of the process, but the healing between ourselves and our children will be much more complete if there is an intergenerational wholeness. Also we can use what we learn with our parents when we work with our own children.

A few years ago Jean, a woman I worked with, told me of the abuse she had suffered from her alcoholic parents. Her mother had beaten her on several occasions. In one incident Jean, at age 12, was taking a bath on a winter afternoon. Her mother came raging at her, hitting Jean with her fists and telling her she was not to take a bath until she had finished her chores. She chased Jean, who was naked, out of the house into the freezing weather just as a neighbor boy her age was walking past. The mother locked Jean out. Jean just crouched on the front porch, hiding her head in shame. This was one of many abusive experiences Jean related about her mother.

Her father was sexually abusive with Jean on at least two occasions. Both parents, Jean would discover later, had abused her out of their anger with each other. Both believed the other was having an extramarital affair when, in fact, neither was.

Jean inherited both the genetic disposition toward alcoholism and the emotional scars of being a child of alcoholic parents, resulting in Jean's becoming an alcoholic herself. Susan, her only child, was neglected until Jean got into recovery for her alcoholism. Jean suffered tremendous loneliness both from her own childhood abandonment and from her inability to connect with her daughter on any meaningful level until after she had confronted both of her parents.

What made it possible for Susan and Jean to begin their Magical Moment was that Jean was able to talk with both of her parents individually before they died. Once each parent had validated that her memory was accurate and asked her for forgiveness, Jean was ready for the next Moment to communicate with her daughter when it happened. Jean's openness in forgiving and accepting her parents allowed her to hear her own daughter when Susan complained about Jean's lack of attention. Jean responded to Susan warmly and told her, simply, she loved her. This honest response was the first step in their healing process.

When experiences such as the one I had with Jennifer, or Jean had with her daughter, occur and we know they are occurring, we become open, vulnerable and risk-taking with our children. It's as if we have had scales over our eyes and now we can finally see. An internal shift takes place in us and we are ready for whatever lies ahead. We begin to have more and more Magical Moments of Communication with our children, which, in turn, provide more impetus and energy to continue Getting Ready.

## The Getting Ready Process

Lessons in life are like the seasons: they occur predictably over and over again, a little differently each time. If we look carefully at the trees or the grass or any other part of nature, we see that growth takes place over time — that each year, for instance, a rhododendron knows what its role is in winter (its roots go deeper) and in spring (new blossoms appear). This growth and change is never finished; it is repetitive and predictable, and that's just how life works on this planet. I believe the rhythm of our emotional and spiritual growth is no different. We take risks, grow, change, pull back, contemplate, rest and begin again, over and over.

Additionally, I believe we get every opportunity we need to move toward health and away from pain. For some of us, it takes many, many Magical Moments before we are able to embrace the Getting Ready process wholeheartedly. It may then take many, many experiences within the preparation process before we are able to move into the heart of recovery work itself. Eventually, however, the recovery process will lead us to a feeling of peace and, hopefully, a healing of our relationships with our children.

It's important to remember that while we control the direction we take and the methods we use, the outcome is out of our hands. We can only have faith that hard work and love will bring us both things we seek: peace and a new relationship with our children.

## EXERCISE

1. At least twice each day, close your eyes and put two or three fingers on your pulse (e.g., wrist, neck). Do not count the beats, just feel them. Feel the life flowing through you; say thank you to life with each beat.

2. Using headphones, lie on your bed or on the floor and, with your eyes closed, listen to a favorite piece of soft and melodic background music. Pretend your forehead is a screen. Have everyone you have ever loved walk across the screen from left to right, stopping halfway across to smile at you.

3. Either make or buy an "I love you" card for yourself and read it every day for a week. Then make or buy a new one to read daily. Do this weekly until you are convinced.

4. List every Magical Moment and positive experience you have had with your children.

5. List every quality in yourself and in your children that will aid this process.
6. List every outside support you can pull on.
7. Finish the following sentence:
   I feel hopeful because . . .

---

## The Rumbles

Most parents reading this book are in the midst of recovering from some form of dysfunction (e.g., workaholism, co-dependency, alcoholism, gambling, drug addiction, bipolar depression) that prevented us from parenting as well as we wanted to. At one time or another in this recovery process, we realize we are carrying around some guilt and shame about our past parenting. This is typically obvious to us when The Rumbles strike and we observe that —

1. Our children are in some emotional pain.
2. Our children are behaving in ways that could only reflect coming from a dysfunctional family.
3. We and our children cannot seem to talk with each other without shouting.
4. We do a Fourth Step in an Anonymous program and in the process of our searching and fearless inventory we realize our parental failings.
5. Our children are vocal about our inadequacies as parents.
6. We see our children repeating with their children what we did with them.

The primary feeling when the Rumbles strike is shame. We realize our children know our parental failings when we thought we had hidden them so well. We feel exposed. We feel "bad."

Fortunately, the Magical Moments of Communication pop in from time to time to give us hope or the Rumbles would paralyze us with guilt. Although it is tempting to feel guilty when our adult children are describing our sins one by one, hope allows us to depersonalize the criticisms and deactivate our defenses. It allows us to say, "Yes, I did those things" or "I don't remember doing what you are describing, but I want us to work out whatever we need to work out." Rumbles are like squeaky wheels that warn us something is wrong. If we pay attention to the noise instead of ignoring it, we can fix the problem before something terrible happens.

The Rumbles are contagious. The best way to get them is to talk with another recovering parent about our regretful experiences while raising our children. Once our own awarenesses arise, coupled with the criticisms from our children, we will feel shame. We need to keep talking. If we can share with at least one other recovering parent how foolish we feel now that our earlier behavior is being exposed, the shame will slowly dissolve.

I worked with a woman whose adult child was dying from bone cancer. One day the mother arrived at her session just after visiting the hospital where her son had been blaming her for the fact that he had become sick. He believed that because he was the oldest child and had taken care of the single parent family of four children while he was still a child, he had had no childhood, had become depressed and got cancer as a young adult.

The mother was appalled at this accusation. She could not assess the accuracy of his analysis, of course, but that didn't matter. What mattered was that she had very little time to work through the results of her alcoholism in order to heal their relationship. Time was of the essence. We set to work acknowledging regrets, reducing shame and developing hope. As her guilt and shame emerged, any denial about the effects of her drinking disappeared.

The young man lived another seven months. After six months he and his mother had resolved their conflicts enough to help him die knowing he was loved. The loud Rumble of his accusations had spurred her to action.

In this seven-month period, the mother had gone through the Getting Ready process and the first stages of the grief process. After he died, she still had to go through more grieving and move into the healing process. But she did it! By so doing, she began the rest of her life with more peace and acceptance than she had ever known.

For me, the Rumbles began when Jennifer was 20 years old. We were having another, now familiar, toe-to-toe argument. She was pleading with me to stop treating her like a child. When I asked what she meant, she couldn't believe I didn't know all the things I had been saying and doing for years that caused her to feel inept.

The shame of not knowing what I had been doing arose immediately in me, and I wanted to run away. I asked her to tell me specifically what I had been saying and doing. It would have been better if I had asked for, and limited her to, just a few examples. Maybe then I would not have become so defensive. Maybe then I could have heard her. As it was, it took me a long time to regain some hope.

Slowly I realized that I really had been unaware of her abilities to take care of herself. I also realized that I needed to get at what lay beneath her accusations, and that I had better look for opportunities to do so. There would be fewer and fewer chances as she grew older and grew away from me. Jennifer and I were fortunate that more situations presented themselves to us while we still lived near each other.

## EXERCISE

1. List things your children have said they didn't like about your parenting.

2. Finish the following sentence: When I think about my parenting, I feel shame for . . . Feel free to add to your list over the weeks ahead as you recognize shame arising.

3. With one other person, preferably another parent, talk about as many accomplishments in your life as you can think of. They can be as miniscule as you want, and they do not have to be what you think others would say. Just being a parent is one, even if you feel like a failure right now.

4. Find or draw a baby picture of yourself and look at the child with tender love. Tell the child you love him/her even if you don't feel the love right now. Put this picture where you can see it every day. Realize that your children need to blame you right now and reassure your inner child that you are going to protect her/him from this blame while you go through the Rumbles.

5. Make a list of all the people you blame and what you blame them for.

Sample: I blame _____ for _____.

DO NOT READ BELOW THIS LINE UNTIL YOU HAVE MADE YOUR LIST.

6. Cross out the word blame for each person on your list and replace it with one of the following:

    a. Forgive

    b. Want to Forgive

---

## Alarms

Alarms are single events or insights that let us know something has to change *now*. They scream at us, "Pay attention. Time is running out!" An alarm happens when you pass an accident on the freeway with your still-squeaky wheel.

The feeling after an alarm is urgency, a need to make things right again, or maybe for the first time. We reel and we feel queasy as we contemplate our need to change who we are, to become who we want to be and to try to rectify our errors, all as quickly as possible.

We're aware that the opportunities to be with our children are slipping away. We worry that our capacities to make the needed changes are limited. At some point we may become aware that we are wanting an unconditional acceptance from our children (now that we are finally learning how to love them unconditionally) that we didn't get from our own parents. So then we also take on the task of trying to make up for our parents' poor parenting as well as our own. What an ordeal!

Alarms are the kinds of experiences that bring practicing alcoholics to their knees. In fact, the similarity between hitting bottom as an alcoholic and being hit by an alarm is striking.

I once worked with a woman who had just finished an alcohol inpatient program. When I asked her what had caused her to enter the program, she said that specific events had occurred over the past few years she just couldn't ignore.

First, a male friend had called her on the phone one morning to ask her not to call him again at night, as she evidently had the night before. He would not say what my client had said, and she had no memory of the call. She was in a blackout. Needless to say, she was humiliated and felt out of control.

Another time she showed up drunk at an open house at her son's school, where she had taught years before. Many of her colleagues were still teaching there and were obviously appalled at her behavior. This experience also stuck with her.

The third event, though the least dramatic in nature, had the most profound effect. She and her husband owned a wine shop, and she made certain that after each wine-tasting party, they brought home the remaining bottles of very expensive wine. She would line them up in the refrigerator and drink them by herself, day after day.

One evening her husband came home with an inexpensive jug of wine from the grocery store and said, "Here. If you're going to drink so much, drink this junk, not our expensive wines." Her internal response was a jolt of alarm through her whole body and an internal voice that said, "Oh, he's noticed."

These events, plus several others, finally resulted in my client hitting bottom and she signed herself in for treatment. You will notice that an alarm doesn't have any particular level of danger or drama or a specific content; you recognize it simply by the feeling of urgency that sweeps over you.

Alarms will hit us parents of adult children in the same way.

Last spring a friend of mine told me he had heard a song on the radio that served as a wake up call. As a result of listening to that song, he really knew that he had to settle his grievances with his dad before it was too late — before his dad died. Suddenly I thought about Jennifer's father and wondered how long it would be before I was Jennifer's only parent. The impact of that thought shook me to my bones.

Shortly thereafter, Lorie Dwinell asked me to read a poem entitled "Brand New" by Linda Shelton for our first workshop. Again, I was shaken. It made me aware that I still had healing work to do as a parent and that I'd better get moving on it.

This event was followed by a phone call from Jennifer, who was a student at the University of Oregon. She was trying to make a decision about where to work for the summer. She had been hired as camp director for American children on a Navy base in Korea. She was reluctant to go because her father's health was worsening rapidly. (He had been suffering from heart disease for 12 years.)

One day shortly thereafter, her father called me to make sure Jennifer would take the job in Korea. He also wanted to make sure that my life was a good one. (We had been divorced for many years but were still very close friends.)

Each of these diverse experiences left me with a sense of urgency that said, "You might be a single parent very soon. You'd better become as emotionally and spiritually ready as you can, as strong and available to Jennifer as you can — *now*." I realized that when Donn died, I would have my own grieving as well as Jennifer's to deal with and would have to face all the weaknesses I had had in the parental role. Fortunately, I paid attention to these alarms and got a head start in preparing for the trauma and grief ahead.

---

## EXERCISE

1. Take three minutes to finish each sentence:

I feel an urgency to heal my relationships with my children because . . .

I feel an urgency to stop feeling guilty about my past parenting because . .

2. List experiences that have sparked this feeling of urgency.

3. Finish this sentence: The single, most important thing I would say to my children today if I could is . . .

---

## Memories

As we progress further into our recovery as parents, memories of our own childhoods emerge. Undoubtedly we have some memories that are painful and some that we realize, sadly, we have visited on our own children. We are sandwiched between the two generations. We feel like a child, with demanding parents coming at us from both sides. Our greatest wish has been not to be like our own mothers or fathers in certain ways, and yet here we are, repeating some of their patterns, including the ones we like the least.

I think the main purpose of memories like these is to remind us that our lives do have continuity. Our childhood has affected our parenting. Remembering what we did and didn't receive from our parents can help us understand why and how we became dysfunctional. Though the understanding itself will not change the past or heal our wounds, it will give us an appreciation of the enormous task we are undertaking.

Painful memories of our own parenting will arise as well, and while they can remind us to get on with the healing process, pleasant memories are just as essential. Like life jackets in a stormy sea, pleasant memories keep us from feeling overwhelmed and hopeless. They can help us remember that the process will be worth it.

## EXERCISE

1. On the left side of a piece of paper, list the numbers from 1 to your current age in a column. Then after each age, write at least one memory you have of that year, beginning as early as you can. Notice where the blanks are. On another piece of paper write about the year before and the year after any blank year, then see if that will help you remember the blank one. Don't worry that there are blank spots; we all have some.

2. Keep a journal to jot down memories that surface. Divide it into four sections:
   a. Positive memories about your childhood
   b. Negative memories about your childhood
   c. Positive memories about your parenting
   d. Negative memories about your parenting.

3. Carry a small pad and pen with you at all times to jot down memories whenever they come up. Just carrying the pad will give your unconscious the message that you are willing to remember.

4. Find a pleasing photo of yourself as a child. Also find one of you with a favorite adult. Put them both where you can see them often.

5. Find a pleasing picture of you and your children. Put it alongside your childhood pictures.

## New Beliefs

As we get ready for the healing process, certain new beliefs emerge that most parents find helpful. The first is the belief that we are accomplishing something very important, even critical, by going through this process. We need to trust that there will be a reward and that our efforts are worth it.

Some of us do not have a choice. By this I mean that as human beings, we move in the direction of the least pain. Thus, the pain of having a horrible relationship with our children can become greater than doing whatever we need to do to heal this relationship. The reward we believe in may be nothing more than the reward of less pain.

Is it worth it? Recently three separate women, all in their forties and all on the same day, told me that they were individuating from their mothers, as they supposed most people do in their teens. First I assured them they were not alone in being "late;" then I asked them why they thought it had taken until now.

All three gave essentially the same answer: "My mom was too dysfunctional when I was a teenager. Since I was the parent, there was no one to separate from. Since Mom has become healthy, I have been able to relate to her as 'my mother.' Now it is time to become my separate self and my own mom, so that we can relate as two adults." Their mothers, all in recovery, had gone though incredible changes, which in turn gave the daughters incentive to change.

Over the years in my work with dysfunctional and then recovering parents, I have discovered five more beliefs held by parents who become the most peaceful — beliefs often expressed at our meetings by parents who are already part of 12-Step programs and have a head start.

First, we realize we can *let go of the need to be perfect*, a need most of us have had since childhood. We have the right to be adequate instead of the best. Usually we come to this awareness after having tried for a long time to "do perfection" and having discovered each time that it doesn't really make a difference in the quality of our lives. Not only is being perfect impossible; trying to be perfect doesn't make us happier.

Second, we recovering parents begin to *simplify our lives*. We become aware of the need to reorder our priorities and to eliminate whatever keeps our lives in constant turmoil. The idea of living peacefully rather than in crisis becomes much more appealing. It also creates the time and energy needed to do the healing work.

Third, as we get older, we begin to accept the fact that *we really have very little control over what happens in life*. We like to think we are in control of our lives, but there is a difference between taking charge of our lives to the degree that it is possible and fighting a reality we can't change just because we don't like it. (Parents familiar with 12-Step programs will recognize this belief in the serenity prayer.)

If giving up the illusion of control is difficult, it's helpful to realize that, although we are limited as to what actions we can take, we are fully responsible for our reactions. To say "I choose" rather than "I have to," when that is realistic, is empowering.

Fourth, *all we have is right now*. We might logically predict that we'll be alive tomorrow just as we are today, but there is no guarantee of that. To learn to live in the present moment, and in so doing to relinquish the guilt of the past or the fear of the future, is a tremendous accomplishment.

When we first begin to understand and actualize this concept, we can do it only for a few minutes. With practice we can learn to bring ourselves back to the present many, many times during a given day.

Now that I am over 50, I have given myself permission to do what I want to do and to not do what I don't want to do much more often than I did before I was 50. I often say to myself (and sometimes to others as well), "Oh well, now that I am over 50, I can _____" and feel absolutely no guilt about whatever fills in that blank. Living in the now is quite a bit like that. I could as easily say, "Now is all I have, so . . ."

I'm not suggesting we ought not have goals for the future. Nor am I saying we are not responsible for our actions in the past. I *am* saying, though, that this moment is all I have, and I can choose to make it work for me.

The fifth belief is that *nothing in life stays the same.* The bad news about this is that we can count on very few constants; the good news is that if our relationships with our children have not been good, they can change and become wonderful.

Recovering parents who are establishing good relationships with their children struggle with these concepts. And many become quite mournful when they realize how helpful these beliefs would have been when their children were younger. Remember, 12-Step programs teaching these beliefs are everywhere now, and our adult children can learn them there. When both parents and adult children hold these pivotal beliefs, the prognosis for family healing is very good.

---

## EXERCISE

1. Ask other recovering parents what makes it worth going through this process.

2. Make a list of all the things, people, places, ideas, books, etc. that you have liked or loved in your lifetime. Do this in one sitting and don't write what you think you were supposed to like, or what you were told you liked, if you really didn't.

3. Now make a list of the things and people you have disliked or hated. Be honest!

4. Write each of the following beliefs on a card:
   • Recovery is important; there is a reward waiting.
   • Be adequate, not perfect.
   • Simplify: live in peace, not turmoil.
   • There is much in my life I cannot control.
   • All I have is right now.
   • Nothing in life stays the same.

Carry one card each day and read it several times.

On the day you read the card, take five minutes to imagine what your life would be like if you really believed what it says. Then take another five minutes to imagine what each of your children's lives would be like if they believed what the card says.

5. With a partner, take turns completing the sentence: "I believe . . ." Do this for three minutes. If there are any beliefs you told your partner or heard from your partner that you think will help you in this process, put each one on a card and read one each day.

6. Ask each of your children to tell you an important value they have (e.g., honesty). Share one of yours with them.

---

## Changes

One day when Jennifer was 16 years old, I was driving her to school on my way to conduct a training session for the counselors of a treatment center. Anyone who knows me well knows that I struggle with public speaking and say no to engagements more often than I say yes. Jennifer also knew this and, as we sat in the car together on the first morning of the seminar, she said:

"Do you want me to come with you?

"You always do a good job, so I know you'll be just fine.

"Here's my worry rock; you may take it with you.

"In 20 years you'll look back and see how relatively unimportant this presentation is.

"If you need me, I'll be in French, Room 104, during first period; History, Room 209, during second period, . . ."

I thought to myself, "Jennifer is an excellent parent."

Just five years later I was planning another seminar. Jennifer was now 21 and was packing to be gone for the summer. When I mentioned one more time that I was anxious about this presentation, she was no longer co-dependent. This time she said:

"I'm sure glad I'm never going to be a therapist.

"When are you ever going to stop being nervous about these presentations?

"Thank God, I'll be in Korea this summer — you're on your own!"

Five years before, I might have felt abandoned, but on this day I chose to feel gratitude that Jennifer did not need to take care of me. I had learned to deal with my own abandonment issues, and Jennifer had become her own person. We had both changed. Now we had a chance to learn to talk with each other in a new way, sometimes with brutal honesty.

I knew, however, that I still had work to do before we could be accomplished communicators. It had taken time for us to get that far. It would take more time before we were healed.

Besides changes occurring in behavior, those of us who are Getting Ready have a series of predictable feelings we must go through before we plunge into the healing process. I have diagrammed the most significant ones on the Feelings in Grief Readiness chart (Figure 10.1).

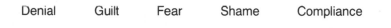

Denial        Guilt        Fear        Shame        Compliance

Anger
(Rebellion)

Grief

**Figure 10.1 Feelings in Grief Readiness**

People often follow the order I have drawn, beginning with Denial and proceeding around the circle through Anger and back to Denial again. But this is not necessary. Each of us has our own individual process.

First of all, each of us has an emotion of choice, just as we may each have had a drug of choice. When something is threatening or confusing, we may always feel anger first, or fear, or guilt. We land on that emotion, and we may remain stuck there because it is familiar, and familiarity holds out the illusion of safety.

Once we are willing to let go of our emotion of choice, we may go around the circle of other feelings several times before we finally leap into the center of the healing process. Let me illustrate how this happened for me.

Earlier I alluded to Jennifer's father's illness. He did indeed die while Jennifer was in Korea. I suddenly became her only parent, and even though she was 22, I found myself thinking of her as a young child who needed early childhood parenting. This thought frightened me, so I tried to push my fears away with some affirmations:

"I'm doing the best I can.

"She's lucky to have me in her life.

"I can be her mother and her father and do a good job."

Using affirmations is not a bad idea. But in this case, I was using them to stay in *denial*. By repeating these phrases I thought I could become a supermom and keep at bay my memories of the times when Jennifer was young and I felt inadequate as a mother. I also was attempting to avoid my own feelings of loss over Donn and the loss I had never fully mourned when my father died.

All this guilt, fear and grief had little to do with Jennifer's needs. She needed mostly space to deal with her father's death in her own way. My role as her mother was relatively unimportant in her process, and there was going to be no way I could compensate for the past by attempting to be both parents to her now.

While I was willing to deal with my grief over Donn and my father, I was not yet ready to face the pain of what I had done and hadn't done as Jennifer's parent when she was younger. I could not yet accept my imperfection.

However, about three weeks after Donn's death, Jennifer and I had another one of those Magical Moments of Communication that led me out of denial and through the rest of the feelings on the diagram.

I was driving us to Green Lake because we had agreed to take a walk together. She began the conversation by telling me I always drive too close to the cars in front of me. This was followed by, "How come you don't ever send me packages at school like everybody else's mom does? In my four years there you have only sent me a few packages." Next she said she did not like my Chevrolet Cavalier, and that her VW Jetta got much better gas mileage.

So far I had not responded verbally, but inside I felt terribly *guilty*. I was hearing that I did not measure up as a driver, a mother or a buyer of cars. She concluded her statements with, "And are you ever going to let me grow up?"

At this point I asked, with irritation in my voice, "What are you talking about? Why does this topic keep coming up? How do I not let you grow up?"

She responded with three or four examples and concluded with, "Take me home. I don't want to walk around the lake with you, and I don't want to ride in your car any more."

I plummeted into *fear*. I was afraid she was going to divorce me as her mom, that I would never be redeemed in her mind. I did a great job of overreacting. But it didn't show. Behaviorally, my adult stayed in charge while my feelings moved from fear into *shame*, the predictable next step.

For the next few minutes I was sure I was the worst mom that had ever existed. I felt horribly exposed and discovered. It was as if she could see beyond my exterior into my soul where she and I agreed, momentarily, that I was bad. I was expecting that at any moment she would launch into an account of all the ways I had been inadequate throughout her life. I anticipated her asking, "Why did you have me if you weren't going to do a better job?" Of course, she said none of this. I was clearly on my own trip.

From shame I moved into what I call *compliance;* others have called it bargaining. I said, "I'm so sorry I haven't sent packages. What would you like me to send? I can imagine how it must feel to be the only girl in your sorority who doesn't receive packages from home. And about my driving, I'll practice not tailgating. You're absolutely right; I drive too close to the cars in front of me."

I was becoming nauseating, and the only good thing that came from it was that my compliance suddenly turned into *anger*. (Whenever we comply, we will rebel in some way at some time.) I continued talking as my anger built. "And by the way, my Chevrolet is just as good as your VW, probably even better."

Jennifer argued with me about that for a while and then again asked me to take her home. This time, I pulled the car over and turned off the motor. The following conversation then occurred:

*Connie:* Jennifer, what we are arguing about is not what we are really angry about. I'd like to work this through.

*Jennifer:* Then you work it through, but take me home.

*Connie:* I can't resolve this without you.

*Jennifer:* But you'll act like a therapist if we try to talk.

*Connie:* How do you want me to talk?

*Jennifer:* Like a person, like an adult, like my mother.

*Connie:* What does "mother" mean to you at this point? (This was my best line of the day!)

*Jennifer:* That we are two adults who do not get in each other's way. That you don't see me as a little girl you have to take care of. That you give me credit for being able to do most things for myself. That you know that I know that you were not a perfect mom as I was growing up. And that you know that sometimes I'm angry with you for that and sometimes I'm not. I don't want you to be my friend, and I don't want you to baby me.

*Connie:* Is there anything else?

*Jennifer:* Yes. Could we walk around the lake now?

*Connie:* You bet.

*Jennifer:* I'm glad you're my mother.

*Connie:* Me too!

---

## EXERCISE

1. What is your emotion of choice? Write a letter to it, telling it why it has been important to you. Tell it why you are afraid to let it go. Discuss this with a friend or counselor.

2. What have been the five most significant events in your life? How have they changed you? Discuss these with a friend or a counselor.

3. List or tell a friend the changes you have made since you started thinking about healing your relationship with your children.

4. List or tell a friend the changes you've seen between yourself and your children since you started thinking about this issue.

## The Leap Of Faith

When I pulled the car over and asked Jennifer to talk with me about the *real* issue, I took a Leap of Faith. I was saying to both Jennifer and myself, "Okay, I'm ready to deal with this now." If I hadn't done my preparation, if her honesty had not blessed us with a Magical Moment of Communication, I would have missed a golden opportunity to move out of the circle of emotions into a real grieving stage. As it happened, I was ready, and we were blessed. So I moved on to the grieving and healing work that will be outlined in the following chapters.

As I see it, the processes of Getting Ready are not linear; they are circular. Hopefully we get as many chances as we need to begin again.

We parents do have a chance to heal our relationships with our children, to let go of the guilt and to become the people we want to be.

# 11

# Grief Work: The Next Step On The Healing Journey

## by Patsy Burnett Carter

Doing grief work means feeling the feelings, thinking through the difficult issues and taking the actions put before us by the loss of a good relationship with our children and with ourselves. We are now "in the soup," for this is a messy, untidy process.

Let's say our children are not speaking to us. We need to feel the anger, pain and loneliness that the loss of contact brings up. We need to think through the reasons behind our children's decision. We need to take specific actions — talk to a family friend, write our children a letter or make an amend to them.

Sometimes the current loss triggers old losses we never mourned. Then, in addition, we need to feel the feelings, think through the issues and take the actions we should have felt, thought and taken at the time the original loss or painful event occurred. No matter how small the current loss seems to be, we need to know that this grief deserves full attention — time every day. Grief is a valid set of feelings about real losses.

Did we yell or cry when our partner beat our children and we lost our children's trust? Did we think through what it meant for us to lose trust in our partner or ourselves? Did we act in the face of our loss — apologize to our children and do what was necessary to keep them and ourselves safe? If not, what we have left undone is in the way of our relationship with our children — waiting to be addressed.

## Either Grief Work Or Crisis

"Grief doesn't sound like any fun," you may say. "Isn't there some other choice?"

Yes. Unfortunately, our other choice is to go into crisis. If we don't allow ourselves to feel the feelings of grief and to resolve whatever issues have come up because of our loss, the feelings and issues fester, make us irritable or depressed, sap our strength and leave us feeling overwhelmed. We are less able to handle life's ups and downs. Eventually we end up in crisis.

When I first worked in an emergency room, I always asked patients who had been brought in after bar fights, "Have you had any major losses in the past year? Perhaps the death of a parent, the death of a best friend, an automobile accident, a shooting?" I could almost always find a major loss that had not been mourned. Some event had remained untouched and unprocessed, creating the tension and blocked feelings that became fertile ground for the next crisis.

Some of us reading this book may be in crisis right now, having ignored the Rumbles and Alarms and gone around the circle of feelings too many times. Perhaps we stayed silent while our son began drinking too much: Now he has lost his job and wants to move back in with us. Perhaps we changed the subject every time our daughter tried to say anything angry about her father: Now her husband has been jailed for sexually assaulting our grand-daughter, and our daughter has accused us of never having protected her from her incestuous father.

We have slipped into crisis. Let me say a little about how crisis operates and how to get out of it before I talk specifically about grief work.

| | | |
|---|---|---|
| Precipitating | | Anger |
| Event | | Denial |
| | | Guilt |
| Higher | | Fear |
| Functioning | | Shame |
| | | Compliance |
| Repetitive | | |
| Feelings | Crisis | Anger/Guilt |
| | | Numbness |
| Change | | Paralysis |
| | | "Stuck" |
| Precipitating | | Disoriented |
| Event | | |
| | | Help |
| Chronic | | Learning |
| Crisis | | Choice |
| | | Reframing |

**Figure 11.1. Crisis Time Line**

Take a look at the Crisis Time Line (Figure 11.1). As Constance Huey mentioned, it all starts with a *precipitating event* — an Alarm or a Rumble. We may have weathered many smaller Rumbles or Alarms, but this particular event is the final straw.

Next, we are thrown onto the circle of feelings, which I have called, on the time line, *repetitive feelings.* When we first hit the circle of feelings, we may be able to convince ourselves that these feelings will pass of their own accord, that we can force ourselves to live, essentially, in our normal pattern. As time goes by and the feelings do not abate, we must decide whether to make the Leap of Faith into the healing journey or to keep trying to ignore our feelings and, therefore, slip into a crisis. Remember, if we decide to do our grief work soon enough, we may be able to circumvent the crisis phase and go directly to the change phase.

As we can see on the Crisis Time Line, once we slip into *Crisis*, we experience even more feelings that are intense, painful and confusing. We feel *angry* and *guilty* that we didn't handle the event differently, or that other people prevented us from handling it differently. This angry guilt is not a helpless feeling, it is a powerful feeling.

At any time of the day, *numbness* can strike us. We may be pushing our shopping cart past the crackers and suddenly feel wrapped in cotton. We know that on the other side of that cotton is terrible pain. Remember the old advertisement for toothpaste that put an invisible shield between the tooth and tooth decay? Decay could pound and pound on that shield, and it would never break. Numbness is like that shield.

When we shift from the circle of ordinary feelings into the realm of crisis feelings, we often feel *paralyzed*. There are times we physically just can't move our bodies. We can't do anything at all.

We also feel stuck emotionally. We can't move forward or backward; we can't get into this grief process and we can't get out of it. We can't get our work done or have fun. Time seems to stand still.

Finally, we feel *disoriented*, almost as though we were intoxicated. There are times we don't know what time it is; can't remember what day it is. If we are admitted to a hospital at this point, the intake worker will ask us questions that would sound silly ordinarily. "Who is the President? What day is it?" When we are deeply in crisis, we can't answer those questions.

All this sounds pretty frightening and depressing, I know, but if you are in crisis right now, don't be discouraged. Crisis is not all bad. Crisis brings with it a glorious window of opportunity for *Change.* Only pain, and often only pain at the crisis level, can convince us to change some of our deepest habits. As long as we can remain comfortable, there's not a reason in the world why we should change.

Religion probably won't make us change. Persuasion probably won't make us change. Unless the circle of feelings we drop into after the precipitating event makes us uncomfortable enough, it probably won't make us change. Even this section of the book warning us to change before we go into crisis may not motivate us. Only the pain and the disabling of our lives that crisis brings may convince us to face our biggest fears and change our deepest patterns.

The word for *crisis* in many languages is synonymous with the word for change or for opportunity for change. Once crisis has occurred, there will be change. We cannot stay, unchanging, in a state of crisis forever, because when we are in crisis, we lose the ability to function.

So here we sit, facing the need to heal ourselves and our relationship with our children — facing change. Whether we have come directly from the circle of feelings or had to go through crisis first, we will need *help*. If we are in crisis, we will need help to get unstuck. If we are not in crisis, we will need help to do our grief work. We may have to ask for help, or it may be forced upon us. Sometimes that help comes from a book like this, sometimes from a person.

Change gives us an opportunity to learn and, in fact, insists that we learn. What we learn determines whether we graduate to a higher level of functioning or sink into a state of chronic crisis; so it's important to take learning seriously.

Even though we may feel paralyzed when we're in crisis, we still have choice. The choice not to change is a choice. The choice to change opens up a lot of other choices.

Finally, in the process of change, we usually have to reframe some of our experiences. *To reframe* simply means to consider an idea from a different point of view. Much of the information and many of the exercises in this book are helping us reframe our parenting. Looking at our parental toolbox, for instance, may have allowed us to reframe some of our parental actions from "good or bad things I did" to "good or bad things I was taught to do."

If the help we get, the learning we do, the choices we make and the reframing we do during the change phase are helpful, we will face the next difficult situations with a *Higher* level of *Functioning*. If, however, we don't get good help, if we learn hurtful rather than helpful things, if we make bad choices or choose not to try to change, or if we find harmful ways to reframe our experiences, the next difficult situation may become the *precipitating event* that throws us into a state of *Chronic Crisis*.

Grief work is the first step in healing and the first step toward change. We can take one of two positions in relation to grief work. We can lean into our pain: seek out the pain, push at it, try to push through it. Or we can try to lean away from our pain and shield ourselves from it.

Imagine pain as a strong wind. If we lean into it, we can end up standing upright, ready to face our lives with even more strength. If we lean away from it, we may find safety by huddling in a simple shelter, but we will not come out stronger and will not learn how to deal with wind.

When we do our grief work effectively, we will move to a higher level of functioning. No matter what happens in our lives — and I guarantee that people will die, lightning will strike and jobs will be lost — our functioning, our ability to cope with those misfortunes, will be better than it was the last time. We may never need to go through crisis again. We may go onto the circle of feelings again, but the next time we may be able to use our new skills to deal with those feelings before they become crises.

## Grief Work

Let me start by countering any training we may have received in our childhood about feelings. Doing grief work means feeling our feelings, and if we are like many other people, we were raised not to feel. "Big boys and girls don't cry." "Don't feel that way." Some of us may have used an addiction to help us numb our feelings. Well, let me offer some new "rules":

- We are entitled to feel whatever we are feeling, including grief.
- We are entitled to release our grief through mourning.
- We are entitled to act on our remorse.

What has happened in our lives is truly a cause for bereavement. We must mourn the lost opportunities. We have lost the opportunity to be a dependable parent for our young children. We have lost the opportunity to have our young children know that we will never bail out on them, that we will never turn into a different person in the middle of some transaction with them. That opportunity is lost.

We must mourn the death of possibilities. It is not possible to do what was not done, and it is not possible to undo what was done.

We must grieve over the finality of what is lost to us. What's gone is lost, not temporarily, but forever.

It may help to recognize we are not alone in our loss. Our children have suffered loss, and perhaps a co-parent has also. It may help to know we don't have to do all our grief work alone.

Nevertheless, we must do the grief work ourselves, with or without company. Only we can do it.

## Grief Work Preparation

The following three assignments lay the foundation for the entire process of grief work, indeed, for the entire healing journey.

### 1. Budget your time

Recognize grief work as real work. I often think of grief work as a part-time job. You may allow four hours a day for it, as you would for a half-time job; you may only be able to budget two hours a day. But you must budget some time for it to take place deliberately, or it will sneak up on you and insist upon your time when you don't want it to. It will interrupt other things you are trying to do. It will demand its time the same way an unruly child who has not been given enough attention will demand your time.

### 2. Get help

Use counseling or crisis intervention; use professional and non-professional help. Choose it, use it, regard it as a tool. You would not try to build a house without a tool; you would not try to do any kind of work without a tool. Counseling is your tool.

When I was grieving heavily, a colleague of mine suggested I might want to use a therapist as a person who would monitor my recovery. She said, "You're already doing most of the work. You shouldn't also have to be burdened with supervising the work."

When I engaged a therapist with that in mind, it took a huge load off me. It was as though I had delegated part of the work to someone who could do that part better than I could, leaving me with more energy to pay attention to myself.

### 3. Access your spiritual support

You must access some power beyond the simple strength of your own muscles and your own brain. Get in touch with whatever you believe in or whatever you would like to believe in.

If you have been out of touch with your spirituality, you may start by searching through the experiences of your life for what has touched you spiritually. You may want to return to the church of your childhood.

A few years ago I went back to my childhood church and found that it no longer provided the kind of emotional closeness I remembered as a child. The principles of that church, however, are still important to me. I've needed to come to an agreement with myself to allow my spirituality to be a fairly private matter which I share with the God of my childhood.

My own definition of spirituality is "that which we allow ourselves to do cognitively with the unknown." We have to do something with whatever is unknown in our lives. (What is unknown may change from day to day, because people keep coming up with explanations for things!) We may explain the unknown by saying it's God's will, or by calling it karma, predestination or luck. We need to seek access to a spirituality that fits our deepest biases, our deepest beliefs and our deepest, maybe even corniest, definitions of truth.

## Grief Work Exercises

Grief work entails both nurturing ourselves and challenging ourselves. We need to get support, stay in touch with ourselves, keep our balance and take care of ourselves while we experience and release our grief.

## Get Support

### 1. Identify a mentor

A mentor is someone who has more experience than you do. It could be a therapist, a pastor, a teacher, or it could be somebody who grieved about their parenting 25 years ago and has a lot of experience at it. It doesn't have to be a professional. It simply has to be someone you can look up to and who is willing to help you.

### 2. Identify lateral supports and allies

You remember the concept of lateral supports. This is the time to identify all the lateral support people you might be able to call on for small favors or major aid. Lateral support people might be friends, family members, neighbors, co-workers or members of any church or group you attend.

An ally is a particular kind of lateral support. An ally is someone who is at about the same level in the recovery process you are. Your ally may be a co-parent — someone who had the same experience you did or someone who was with you and didn't have the same experience. Your ally could be another parent who is having similar experiences now or someone who is grieving over a different kind of loss entirely. You want to find allies who are able to be empathetic and who can share the whole process with you.

### 3. Use your allies as coaches

Ask your allies to help you monitor your progress. They might say, "You know, you've been talking about that same thing now for about six weeks. Are you sure you're not just overdoing that? What's the next thing you ought to be thinking about?" They can prompt you to take new risks. They can push you just a little bit. And you can do that for them as well.

## Stay In Touch With Yourself

### 1. Keep a journal of your changing perceptions

Any of you who have been in a recovery program have been told to keep a journal a million times, but I'm asking you to focus on something very specific. Don't write what happens during your day; just write your perceptions and your feelings.

Get in touch with whatever you feel at the very moment you sit down in front of your journal. On Tuesday you might write, "I'm furious at my children for asking me to pay for their therapy. They have no right to do that." You might write a page and a half about how angry you are. And on Thursday you might sit down at the same journal at the same desk and write, "This is depressing. This doesn't seem to be getting me anywhere. I don't know if I even want to write in this journal."

The fact that you have such different feelings on different days does not mean you are losing ground. It just means that your feelings are all over the place. Later, when you look back at your journal, you'll see how many feelings you went through. You will respect and appreciate the work you did in this grief process.

Don't try to stay consistent. You'll be tempted to try to stay consistent too quickly, and to try to find patterns too quickly. I think there's a mandate in our society to have feelings that remain predictable — in the absence of power over our feelings, we'll settle for predictability. That is not productive for this kind of journal work.

### 2. Let your state of mind change

If your state of mind changes all of a sudden, you don't need to force it back to where it was in order to stay orderly. That impulsive change may give you access to a change you need to make. Trust yourself. When your impulses carry you to a new state of mind, it may mean you're ready to move.

When I found myself moved to throw away my mother's cards and letters, at first I recoiled from the idea. I didn't want to lose touch with her ways of expressing herself.

Then I began to pay more attention to my own speaking and writing style and realized I didn't need her letters. I had internalized some of her language and expressions and made them my own.

When a widowed client found herself moved to sell the house her husband had built at the start of their marriage, she discovered she didn't need that structure as a memorial to their good years together. She had integrated those memories into her values and personal choices, into the fabric of her everyday life.

### 3. Think whatever you want

Again don't try to be consistent. You are entitled to have any thoughts that occur to you — they may be pleasant thoughts, or they may be unpleasant thoughts.

Well-meaning friends and family may tell you not to think about certain things. You may even tell yourself not to think about certain things. You may say, "Ugh, the more I think about this, the more miserable I get."

In one workshop, a woman walked past me, talking more to herself than to me, and said, "I don't know why I keep having to pay people enormous amounts of money to make me this miserable." She was thinking it; she was saying it. Even though she knew she was leaning into her grief, she had misgivings about it. All of that is okay. She allowed herself to think whatever she wished to think.

## Keep Your Balance

### 1. Remind yourself that grief is a process

Frequently, happily, in any way that you wish, remind yourself that your grief is a process and not a steady state. Any time you feel stuck, any time you feel overwhelmed, simply find a way to remind yourself that there is a process going on.

You might refer to your journal and notice that what you wrote six weeks ago is different from what you wrote yesterday. You might take some time to remember how you felt when you first fell into the grief soup. It will help you recognize how far you've come.

When I am counseling, I encourage people to make a record of how they feel at their worst. If they write, make a tape recording or draw pictures when they are in their deepest despair, they will recognize their changes later. They will learn that no matter how bad they feel at any given moment, it will change.

### 2. Learn to set limits

You must stop at the end of the time you have allotted for grief work. You might fear grieving because you are afraid your feelings will take over your whole life. Learning ways to end on time and to put a lid back on your feelings will ease those fears. Time limits can be difficult to respect when you're in a state of intense feeling, so you need to set up a system in advance.

The easiest way to set a limit is to change the sensory context. You might play a music tape during your grief work time. When the tape is over, your grieving time is up. After your grief work time is up, you might move to a different room, change the temperature, change the light level. You might call a friend and talk about something entirely different.

You could set up a special place for doing grief work. When you are in that place with that light level and that sound system, you are grieving. When you don't have those particular sensory inputs, you are playing, relating to someone or working.

### 3. Budget time for intense grieving

If you get fully into the grief work, you will experience some intense grief. Don't be surprised if you need to scream, shout or cry loudly. Find a place to do that where people won't try to stop you. As a last resort, you may be able to do it in your car on the freeway, particularly if you're in a traffic jam and you don't need to focus on your driving.

## Encourage Your Grief To Emerge

### 1. Allow a flood of memories

Allow a flood of memories to occur from time to time, but set limits on that experience. One of the reasons people don't allow a flood of memories is that they're afraid they're going to get swallowed up in them and not be able to get separate from them again. If you say you're only going to allow a flood of memories to occur for an hour or 20 minutes, you can set a limit by changing the sensory context, as I've already described, and by promising yourself you will allow another flood at another time.

Find a safe place and time when no one will interrupt you. Make yourself comfortable and let yourself think about specific events. Re-create the motion picture of what happened. Let yourself hear the conversations, see the faces.

Use sensory cues to bring back memories and feelings. The senses of taste and smell are deeply anchored neurologically, and they will sometimes help you access memories that would not be available in the higher levels of your brain. Smelling certain foods or perfumes or even certain household cleaners may bring back memories you thought you had lost.

When I was going through my mother's things after she died, I found a tape that wasn't labeled. When I played the tape, there was my mother's voice talking about her trip to the Grand Canyon. Enormous waves of intense feelings washed over me.

Photographs and videotapes are evocative. Watching home movies of times when you were parenting your children or watching videotapes that show some of the things you wish you had done differently will help you to access feelings.

### 2. Make rituals

Make rituals that will help you access your feelings. Go to that ocean beach where you punished your children when they didn't deserve to be punished, to the mountains where you had an awful camping trip because you got drunk. Take your adult children with you, or take a friend, and experience something wonderful there. Overlay the old memory with a new memory.

Go to the shopping mall where you made a scene and embarrassed your children in front of their friends because you couldn't stand all the demands being made on you. Allow yourself to sit down and imagine how you would handle that situation in your present state of mind.

### 3. Write a letter

Write an impulsive letter of apology to your children. Write the letter that says, "I'm sorry for what I did; I'm sorry for what I didn't do; I'm sorry for how I failed you." This letter will not be sent to them, and it will not be carefully composed; it will simply give you an opportunity to let your own feelings flow out uncensored.

### 4. Write another letter

At some other moment, write the letter you should get from someone who didn't help you parent well. It might be from a spouse, a co-parent, a counselor, a schoolteacher or your own parents. Again, this is not a letter to send to anyone, but sit down and write it impulsively with all the feeling you can muster.

### 5. Confirm past reality

If you were addicted while you were parenting, your addiction probably blocked some of your memories and feelings. Even if you weren't addicted, almost invariably your memories will have changed over time, and they will be different from the memories of your children. So when the accusations come, it's hard to remember what really happened.

It's important to confirm as much reality as you can, because however bad the reality was, your imagination of it is usually worse. You have the right to look up school records and hospital records. You can read old personal letters and look at old photographs. You can talk to people who were present at the time. Do whatever you can to get concrete evidence of what happened in the past.

### 6. Spend time with your memory caches

Most of us have memory caches — a place, a box of belongings, certain photographs — that hold memories we can't access any other way. For myself, it's my mother's kitchen gadgets. I look at those gadgets; I touch them and they give me memories. I don't put them in a place where I'll never see them. I put them in my gadget drawer and use them every day.

Memories you access from objects are often very detailed. A side benefit you derive from retrieving these detailed memories is that your shame — or your embarrassment — is usually tied up in details. Once you have the details and the parameters of your shame, once you can define your shame very precisely, you can work through it. You can't exorcise it unless you know it clearly.

## Take Care Of Yourself

### 1. Put some comfort foods into your nutritional plan

You can eat for comfort and, at the same time, eat in a disciplined way. There are foods that comfort you. They may not be absolutely excellent for your health, but you can let yourself have some comfort food. Then you need to use discipline so comfort foods don't take over your entire nutritional program. Discipline prevents comfort from becoming an addiction in and of itself.

### 2. Stay balanced about physical exercise

I'm sure you've heard by now that physical exercise is the core of our chemical/emotional wellbeing. Exercise can affect our metabolism and our energy level and produce endorphins that elevate mood.

I had a friend who, when she was so depressed she could barely function, would force herself to walk outdoors for 15 minutes every day. After that 15 minutes she would have a window of time during which she felt good enough to do her most important chores.

Physical exercise sounds like a virtue, right? Well, I'm beginning to see people who are addicted to physical exercise, who are not using discipline to balance physical exercise in their lives. So go swimming frequently if you love swimming and it gives you comfort; just stay balanced about it.

Try to make your physical time a pleasurable time and a playful time as well. Being outdoors may be more fun for you than being in a gym. Looking at a lake or a mountain may be as important as the length of your run.

### 3. Pay attention to pain

Many of you who are in recovery programs may think you need to bear pain, even grin and bear it. But pain carries a message. It tells us there is too much of something going on or too little of something going on. Pay attention to it; see if you can figure out what the message is. It comes from a place inside yourself which is nonverbal, maybe even preverbal, and can almost always be trusted.

Now some of you may ask, "If I pay attention to the pain, am I not just engaging in self-pity?" Self-pity is its own form of pain. If you're engaging in self-pity, it means that not enough other people are feeling sorry about what's happening to you. Not enough empathy is coming your way, so you're having to provide some of it yourself. The message is, "Beef up your lateral supports and get more empathy from someone."

### 4. Spend positive time alone

Some of you who were only children may have learned to spend time alone pretty well many years ago. I find to my surprise that lots of people don't know how to spend time alone comfortably. People who are twins or triplets or who grew up in large families with lots of close siblings may not know how to spend positive time alone.

My personal theory is that there is a whole generation of you called "baby boomers" who had entirely too much company for everything you did, all the time. There were mobs of you. I saw you coming up right behind me in school. I don't think you were ever alone. I don't think there was room for you to be alone. And you may not have learned the skills needed to be alone in a positive way. Being alone may feel like deprivation. You may need to teach yourself how to enjoy being alone.

### 5. Use your support people

Once you have identified your lateral support people, use them. This means asking them to do things with you and for you.

A few years ago my fiance died suddenly. When all of the people came to say, "Let me know if I can do anything to help you," I discovered I needed to start saying what they could do right away.

I started giving instructions. I said, "Please take Thursday off and go with me to the funeral home. I do not want to do that by myself. I need your company." Another time I said, "I need to scatter some ashes over water. Can you help me figure out how to get an airplane lined up to do that?" I asked my five or six closest friends, "Please take me and my fiance's family to dinner. I don't think I can do it alone."

I needed to give instructions and I found, to my pleasant surprise, that my dearest friends needed to have instructions. They genuinely did not know what to do and were massively relieved to be told.

### 6. Use counseling

Identify some kind of professional help. You can use it any way you want. You can use it every day if you can afford it. You can use it every week; weekly is a common experience. You may do it any way you wish. You may make any kind of agreement with your therapist you wish. You are the customer. You are always right about how you want to use professional counseling help. You call the shots. If you find a counselor who tells you that you can't do that, you probably need to find another counselor.

### 7. Give yourself the opportunity to hold, to touch and to be touched in a loving way

There's something especially helpful about physical contact, about simple physical nurturing, about the acceptance of your body as a part of you that also needs comfort, about easy access to giving and getting hugs. Explore ways to restore, enhance or make yourself open to that kind of loving relationship.

Ask a trusted massage therapist, an old friend or a new friend for back rubs. Revitalize your marriage. Start a sweet, juicy romantic love of long or short duration. These may be sexual relationships or not; they may be temporary or forever. Whatever the context, given that it is responsible and caring, you need to receive and express physical affection.

## Grief Work Energy Levels

Many of us are already familiar with the stages of grieving identified by Elisabeth Kubler-Ross in her first book, *On Death And Dying.* She has since said that she wishes she had never labeled them as stages because people have assumed you have to go through them in the right order or you haven't grieved correctly. Instead of thinking of them as orderly stages, it's been productive for me to think of them as mind states, all of which are necessary somewhere in the grief process.

It's easiest to remember the mind states in their classical order since it makes a nice acronym, DABDA: Denial, Anger, Bargaining, Depression and Acceptance. But that's not the order in which they always occur in people's grieving. Many people start in anger, and others start in depression.

Anger

Bargaining

Individual Normal ——————————————————— Acceptance

Denial

Depression

**Figure 11.2. Grief Energy**

Look at the Grief Energy chart (Figure 11.2). Here I've deliberately left the mind states out of their classical order. Notice that each mind state carries a different level of energy. The broken line on the Grief Energy chart represents the normal level of energy for each of us. Some of us were probably called lazy by our parents because we had low energy, some of us were always thought of as high-energy people. What I've indicated on the Grief Energy chart is the relative difference in energy we may expect in each of the mind states.

We want to respect the variable energy levels we have available in these different mind states when they hit us. When we're in *anger*, our energy level rises. That's a good time to do things that require a lot of energy — make phone calls, make lists, burn things.

*Denial* tends to take us to an energy level a little below our normal one. The energy we use to avoid looking at what's obvious becomes unavailable to use for other things.

*Bargaining* is my personal favorite. Bargaining is when we try to make tradeoffs with our Higher Power, with the universe, with the other players in our lives. "If you will forgive me for what you believe I have done to you, I will try to be a better parent from here on out: I will try to make it up to you. If you will stop your addiction, I will give you all the things I didn't give you when you were a child."

Sometimes we bargain with God. When I was 39 years old and grieving over my mother's terminal illness, I marched up and down the hallways of the hospital in which she was dying and said to the God of my childhood, "If You will save her, I will truly be a better person. And, furthermore, if You don't save her, I'm going to be the worst backslidden Christian You ever tried to deal with in Your existence."

As you can see, bargaining uses a high level of energy because "hope springs eternal." We do believe that if we can just reach the right tradeoff, we can make the pain go away.

*Depression* has a bad reputation among many health-care professionals. Counselors don't like people to be depressed. It is my personal belief that that depression is a necessary mind state for resting. We use depression as an opportunity to stop struggling for a little while — to sleep more than anybody wants us to sleep, to slow down all of our metabolic processes. That may mean eating less; it may mean hiding out from social events. We may need to experience depression more than once during the grief process, just to rest up from the work that's involved.

Toward the end of our grief work there is some kind of *acceptance.* I won't promise that our energy level will be back to where it always was, and I can't promise there will be perfect peace. But I can promise some restoration of our ordinary energy level, some sense that if we need energy, it will be there for us.

The tricky part of all this is that we will bounce back and forth between these mind states. We will have peace and acceptance intermittently during the grieving process, not just at the end. At any moment we may find ourselves back in anger or engaging in denial because we've just been given news a little bit worse than we thought there was.

We won't stay in a nice clean line with these mind states, but the energy access is somewhat predictable; so we need to take our emotional temperature and use our energy appropriately. We don't need to make ourselves carry out a list of tasks when we're in depression, and we can make ourselves accomplish things when we're in anger.

## Traps To Avoid

The grief process can be seductive because grief generates intense feelings. For those of us who habitually have not been able to access intense feelings, trying to avoid these feelings or basking in them may trap us.

## Don't Be Seduced By Guilt

Guilt is sneaky because it has a hidden payoff. I know this is hard for many people to take, but I don't believe we can feel guilty without feeling an intense sense of personal power. "I could have done it better. I'm smart enough to have done it better." We can get stuck in guilt as the easiest source of empowerment. Guilt and power so nicely balance each other off that we don't even have to feel conceited about the power.

## Don't Let Well-Meaning Friends Slow You Down

We can't let well-meaning friends and family drive us back into denial or drive us away from the work. We will recover, ourselves. We will be able to construct new relationships where the old ones are being dismantled.

People who want to protect us will say, "Oh, don't think about those things; that's just unnecessary pain for you. Try not to get so heavily into this. You're just making trouble for yourself."

In my family we called it borrowing trouble. When I would get into my feelings, someone would inevitably say, "You're just borrowing trouble. Think about something else for a while."

We can't let people do that to us. All they're going to do is slow down the process. We don't have to chastise them for it. They really do hope to protect us. But we can resist their influence.

## Don't Get Stuck At Any Stage Of Recovery

I borrowed the Steps in Recovery graph (Figure 11.3) from Sidney and Suzanne Simon when I attended their workshop on The Dynamics of Forgiveness a couple years ago. The graph is deceptively simple because it appears that we can just start at the bottom in *denial* and end up well integrated at the top. However, it is possible, even tempting, to get stuck on one of these steps.

Obviously it's very easy to get stuck on the bottom step of denial, but that's not really the seductive part. When the Rumble or the Alarm occurs and we're thrown onto the circle of feelings, there's an element of *self-blame,* an element of *mea culpa, mea culpa, mea maxima culpa.* This step is so powerful that some religions have even made a ritual of it. They recognize there is something rewarding about being able to say, "Yes, indeed, it is all my fault. Yes, indeed, I need to punish myself."

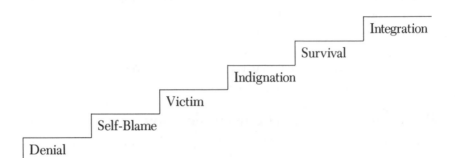

**Figure 11.3. Steps In Recovery**

From there, it's an easy step to thinking of ourselves as *victims.* First of all, we're victims of the blame that we're piling on ourselves. Second, we may suddenly remember that we too were victimized by parents who didn't do a better job of it than we did. This memory is truly seductive because it not only explains our own dysfunction but also gives us a way to externalize the blame. Feeling like a victim of prior generations is a place where we can get stuck for a long time.

Feeling like a victim leads very easily into *indignation.* My personal favorite is righteous indignation. I love to feel righteously indignant. If I'm sure of my ground and feel righteously indignant, I can go in and make speeches. I can insist upon social change. I can advocate the rights of people whose rights have been abridged. It gives me power. For me, then, indignation can be a very seductive place to get stuck. I have to discipline myself to take a good look at what I'm doing from time to time, to make sure I'm not coming just from my own personal stuff.

As indignant people, it's easy to think of ourselves proudly as *survivors.* These things have happened to us. We have had this or that misfortune. And we have survived. We are intact. We are competent. Look how powerful we're getting. We are advocates for others.

We're entitled to feel like survivors. It's a glorious feeling. But we must not get stuck there. We must be able to discipline ourselves to include that survivorship in our total personal self-image.

Yes, we are survivors, but we are not just survivors. We are not just indignant people. And please, we are not just victims. No matter what's happened to us, we are not just victims. We participate in the victimization of others either willingly or unwillingly; wittingly or unwittingly. Every time we pay our taxes, we may be paying somebody to do something bad.

We cannot see ourselves in just one of these roles on one of these steps all the time. Eventually, we need to *integrate* all of our experiences into the wholeness of ourselves.

The easiest places for most people to get lost is either in victim identification or in indignation. There are organizations geared to provide support to survivors of crime victimization. These organizations intend to provide support throughout the apprehension, trial and imprisonment of the assailants, but may end up helping people stay in that place between victimization and indignation. I'm almost positive that no one can move off those steps until the courtroom saga is over and litigation is completed.

## The Payoff

If we get stuck in one of the seductive traps of the grief process, we deny ourselves the ultimate payoff. The ultimate payoff comes when we can finally accept what has occurred and use the misfortune in our lives as material with which to grow to a higher level of functioning.

If we do this right, each generation gets a little bit more insight than the previous one had. If we grieve appropriately, if we take the whole healing journey, we can pass on what we've learned, and the whole human race benefits.

# CHAPTER

## 12

# Taking Stock

**W**ell, here we are. We have finally arrived at the most frightening and most difficult chapter in the book. In this chapter we face the formidable task of making an inventory — taking stock — of the pluses and the minuses in our history as parents.

Before we begin, I'd like to give you a couple of warnings. First, I'd like to suggest that you do this stock-taking in bits and pieces. Bite off small bits to chew. Process each bite with one of your lateral support people — with another parent in recovery or with your therapist or with your sponsor in a self-help group, such as

Al-Anon or Co-dependents Anonymous, or with a sibling who is on a similar leg of their journey as a parent. Most importantly, do not sit down and read this chapter from beginning to end and do all of the exercises in one fell swoop without telling anyone what you're doing.

Healing is a process, not an event. This chapter is part of the process. It needs to be digested a little at a time and shared with at least one other person who will not shame you, invalidate you or redefine you in some way that gets in your way as a healing parent. You are now a healing parent.

The second warning I would like to ask you to remember repeatedly throughout this chapter is that your parental journey was not about intention. As you look at your regrets and your remorse, your errors of omission and commission, please remember that you did not set out to do harm. Like most parents, you probably began your parenting journey with feelings of excitement and anticipation for what you hoped would be a gratifying and fulfilling endeavor.

As you read this chapter, remember from time to time what your vision was for yourself as an adult person, as a parent and as a spouse or a partner. Remember also what your vision was for the family you created. You had hopes and dreams and aspirations, some of which have been realized and some of which have not.

You may pause from time to time to ponder how you got off track, where you lost your way. Notice the places where you feel you were able to rekindle your vision, to get back on track and to find your way again. For some of us, it will only be now, as we do this emotional healing work, that we have a sense that getting back on track is a possibility.

Also, as you read this chapter, you will find yourself wondering what you would have changed if you had known then what you know now.

The fact that you are reading this book says to me that you are willing to be accountable. My hope is that you will give yourself credit for having come this far in what is a ferociously frightening journey. It is much easier to hold others accountable for harm done than it is to hold ourselves accountable.

In having come this far in the journey, we are in the process of realizing our greatest fear — the fear of being found lacking, the fear that we did our best and it wasn't good enough. For many of us, our children could never blame us as harshly as we blame ourselves. Please pause for a moment and give yourself credit for having faced your fear.

I am reminded of how lions hunt their prey. The lionesses are the hunters and are positioned at one end of the valley. The old male is positioned at the other end of the valley with the herd of prey between him and the lionesses. The male roars ferociously. The prey, in the wish not to be eaten, turn and run from the roar into the jaws of the waiting lionesses. The irony is that if the prey were to turn and face the roar, that is, to turn and face their fear, they would not be eaten.

We, as parents, are in the process of turning and facing the roar. The real danger — the danger that is often as silent as the lionesses — is the continued deterioration of our relationships with our children and ourselves. To the extent that we run from our fear, we co-create this wreckage. To the extent that we stop and turn and face the roar, we contribute to our own healing and to the potential healing of our relationship with our children.

Now let's begin taking stock. Throughout this chapter we will be referring to work we have done earlier in the book, so many of the exercises will be familiar.

## Model For Relatedness

Think back for a moment to the first few years you were parenting. What adjectives would you use to describe the quality of relatedness you created in your new family? Here is the list from Chapter 2 of some of the ways in which people organize their need for relatedness. Put a small *m* for "myself" next to the adjectives that fit the style of your early parenting years. Then put a capital *M* next to those that describe your style now. Add any other adjectives that come to mind.

close/distant
open/closed
communicative/silent
warm/cold

public/private
pleasant/civil/rude
sensitive/insensitive
sexual/asexual
friendly/apathetic/hostile
physically demonstrative/standoffish, rigid, withholding
calm/chaotic
affectionate/cold
lively/dead
respectful/abusive
including/excluding
connected/isolated
committed/indifferent
engulfed/separate
family is primary source of intimacy/secondary source
clinging/detached
uncontained/contained
direct/indirect
trusting/mistrustful

Notice any changes you have made over time. Then look back at this same list in Chapter 2, where you marked the style of the family in which you grew up. Notice any similarities or differences between your style and your family-of-origin's style.

Now put a plus by any items on this list you feel proud of and a minus by any items you feel remorse about. You may feel proud that you changed some bad patterns over time, or that you improved on the models your parents gave you. You may simply feel proud of some of the choices you made.

Our model for relatedness will define our children's unconscious comfort zone just as our family defined ours. Think about your adult children's lives now. What similarities and differences do you see between their style of relating to their partners/families and the style of relating they grew up with in your family?

## Model For Parenting

The list that follows was also in Chapter 2. It contains some of the styles you had to choose from when you developed your own parenting methods.

As you look at the list, remember that you and each of the people who parented your children may have had different styles. First go through the list and put a small *m* for "myself" next to each word that fits your parenting style as it was when you began raising your children. Then go back over the list and put a capital *M* next to any words that describe your style now.

permissive/strict
democratic/authoritarian/anarchistic
laissez-faire/highly structured
unprotective/protective/abusive
overprotective/appropriately involved/uninvolved
    (smothering)                          (detached)
intrusive/respectful of boundaries
over-giving/under-giving
    (martyr)     (scrooge)
over-receiving/under-receiving
(expects to be taken care of)/(you can never pay them back)
consistent/inconsistent
cooperative with you/competitive with you
cooperative with other parent/competitive with other parent
unilateral/bilateral
(one does all the parenting, / (both give input and share
other gives no input)        responsibility)
present/absent

oscillating presence
(drug addiction, mental illness, criminal arrests)
one present/one absent
both absent/(surrogate parent figure(s) present, e.g.,
    grandparent, aunt, sibling, orphanage)
passive/assertive/aggressive
critical/accepting
controlling/doormat
responsible/irresponsible

Notice the changes you made over time. Then turn back to the list of parenting styles in Chapter 2, and notice how different or similar your style was from that of your parents.

Now go through this list once for each significant parenting figure in your children's lives and put each parent's initials next to the words that fit their styles. You may need to use small letters and capital letters for them as well if they changed over time. Remember to include the nontraditional people who parented your children — grandparents, oldest child who was the parent in your absence, ex-husband's wife, etc.

When all the letters are on the list, you will have a snapshot of the parenting styles that were modeled for your children. Notice any differences between parenting styles that your children had to cope with.

Now put a plus by those items you feel proud of and a minus by those you feel remorse about.

If your children are parents now, mark their styles on this list as well. What do you notice about what they may have learned from you and your partner(s)? Did they do a 180-degree pendulum swing on anything?

## What Winds Our Springs?

You will remember from Chapter 3 that there are three interpersonal needs that wind our springs as human beings:

- Who's in and who's out (inclusion)?
- Who's on the top and who's on the bottom (control)?
- Who's near and who's far, how near and how far (closeness)?

Let's look at each of these interpersonal needs in terms of the family we created.

### Inclusion

Take a moment to think about the family you created. Did you include lots of people (global) or few (narrow)? Was the boundary rigid, or was your family chaotic and nearly unbounded? Was the boundary guarded? Who guarded the boundary and decided which people were allowed in and which were not? Did they guard the boundary ferociously, or were they flexible about how people were to come and go?

First plot the family you created on the lines below as it was when you began parenting by marking a small *f* for family. Then add any changes over time by marking a capital *F.*

Global                                                      Narrow

Chaotic, Unbounded                            Rigid

Unguarded                          Ferociously Guarded

Who was the guard? _____

List the people included in your family:

_____     _____

_____     _____

_____     _____

_____     _____

_____     _____

What changes do you notice over time?

Look back to the exercise you filled out in Chapter 3 on your own family of origin. What similarities and differences do you notice?

Most families have a predominant style of inclusion, which you just charted. But there can still be disagreements or different styles between the parents. My Swedish, Lutheran friend's family, for instance, basically followed the father's rules, except when he wasn't home.

Think for a moment about each person who parented your children. Plot yourself first and then each of the other parents on the following lines. How did each of you define who was in your family? Again, use initials to represent different people as we did in the Parenting Styles exercise.

Global                                                      Narrow

| Unbounded | Rigid |
|---|---|

| Unguarded | Ferociously Guarded |
|---|---|

Once you have completed these three scales, notice the discrepancies, if there are any, between the cassettes of the parents in your children's lives. How did your parents resolve these discrepancies? What messages did your children get about inclusion because of these discrepancies?

As we discussed in Chapter 3, each interpersonal need has two dimensions — what we do (expressed) and what we want (wanted). On the lines below, plot yourself on the two dimensions of Expressed and Wanted inclusion. How much did you *do* to get yourself included and to include others? How much did you *want* to be included and to include others? Feel free to turn back to Chapter 3 if you need to refresh your memory about inclusion.

Again, use a small *m* for how you were when you first began parenting, and a capital *M* for how you are now.

*MYSELF*

**EXPRESSED**

| Never | Sometimes | Always |
|---|---|---|

**WANTED**

| Never | Sometimes | Always |
|---|---|---|

Have you changed over time?

Turn back to this exercise in Chapter 3, and compare your lines with those of your parents. What do you notice?

Are there differences between what you wanted and what you expressed? How do you imagine your children experienced these differences?

Next plot the people who were significant parenting figures for your children on these lines. Again, use their initials, and if they changed over time, use small letters for early years and capital letters for now.

*PARENT 1*
**EXPRESSED**

---

Never                    Sometimes                    Always

WANTED

---

Never                    Sometimes                    Always

*PARENT 2*
**EXPRESSED**

---

Never                    Sometimes                    Always

**WANTED**

---

Never                    Sometimes                    Always

How did you and your partner(s) work out your different needs for inclusion? How did these differences affect your children?

Think about each of your children in turn and plot them on the following lines.

*CHILD 1*
**EXPRESSED**

---

Never                    Sometimes                    Always

**WANTED**

---

Never                    Sometimes                    Always

*CHILD 2*
**EXPRESSED**

---

Never                    Sometimes                    Always

**WANTED**

---

Never                    Sometimes                    Always

Who is each child most like? What do you notice about the "match" between you and each child? How did you and each child work out any differences?

The category of inclusion is also about exclusion. Identify the people who were excluded from your family. When did you exclude them? Why did you exclude them? How did you exclude them?

What might your children have learned about how and why to exclude someone?

Mark a plus beside anything in this inclusion section you feel proud of and a minus beside anything you feel remorse about. There may be specific people you wish you hadn't included in your family, or others you wish you had, for example. Or you may wish you had made the boundary more rigid or less rigid.

## Control

Inclusion is the first interpersonal need a new family must satisfy. You and your spouse/partner, as young parents, had to decide who was in your family and who was not. Once the family group was formed, your next questions were about control. Who makes the decisions in the family? Who has the control? How much structure does each of us want?

Whether we use the word *control*, or perhaps *structure* or *dominance*, there are two dimensions to consider — expressed and wanted — just as there were with inclusion.

Remember that expressed control has to do with *behavior*. How often did you take over being responsible, structuring? High expressed means you took over all the time. Low expressed means you never took over — even if your children were hurt.

Wanted control means how much did you *want* someone else to provide structure and control? Maybe you wanted your partner to make all the decisions, or maybe you never wanted anyone ever to tell you what to do.

Take a moment to think about yourself as a young parent. Plot yourself on the following lines, using a small *m* for "myself" when you first began parenting and a capital *M* for "Myself" as you are now.

*MYSELF*
**EXPRESSED**

| Never | Sometimes | Always |
|---|---|---|

**WANTED**

| Never | Sometimes | Always |
|---|---|---|

Have you changed over time?

Turn back to the chart you filled out on your parents in the Control section of Chapter 3. What similarities and differences do you notice? Are you like one parent or the other? Are your control needs a reaction to how they dealt with control? How did your control needs match or not match those of each of your parents?

Now plot the other parents who influenced your children on the following lines.

*PARENT 1*
**EXPRESSED**

| Never | Sometimes | Always |
|---|---|---|

**WANTED**

| Never | Sometimes | Always |
|---|---|---|

*PARENT 2*
**EXPRESSED**

| Never | Sometimes | Always |
|---|---|---|

**WANTED**

| Never | Sometimes | Always |
|---|---|---|

Notice whether or not you, as parents, were willing to give your family structure or set limits. If not, did one of the children end up having to be a parent? If all of you wanted control, how did you resolve the ensuing conflict? Do you think you provided your children enough structure? Too much? Too little?

Plot your children on the following lines.

*CHILD 1*
**EXPRESSED**

---

Never                     Sometimes                     Always

**WANTED**

---

Never                     Sometimes                     Always

*CHILD 2*
**EXPRESSED**

---

Never                     Sometimes                     Always

**WANTED**

---

Never                     Sometimes                     Always

Are any of your children like you? How did the control needs of each of them match with yours? Have any of them changed over time?

What do you imagine your children learned about control from watching you? What might they have learned about how to resolve conflicts about control?

Mark a plus by anything you feel proud of in this control section — it may be something you feel you did better than your own parents did, or it may be something you improved over time. Mark a minus by anything you feel remorse about. Write notes in the margins about anything you feel proud of or sorry for on the issue of control.

## Closeness

Think back to the time you were just beginning your own family. How much closeness, intimacy and affection did you want in your new family? How much did you express? Plot yourself on the following lines, again using an *m* for "myself" at the age you began your new family and using an *M* for "Myself" as you are now.

## *MYSELF*
## EXPRESSED

| Never | Sometimes | Always |
|---|---|---|

## WANTED

| Never | Sometimes | Always |
|---|---|---|

Did you change over time?

Were you consistent in what you expressed and what you wanted? If you gave mixed messages, how did your children deal with the discrepancies?

Look at the lines you filled out on your parents in Chapter 3. Are you similar to either of them? How well did your closeness needs match with theirs?

Now plot the other parents that raised your children, using their initials in small letters for the past and capital letters for now.

## *PARENT 1*
## EXPRESSED

| Never | Sometimes | Always |
|---|---|---|

## WANTED

| Never | Sometimes | Always |
|---|---|---|

## *PARENT 2*
## EXPRESSED

| Never | Sometimes | Always |
|---|---|---|

## WANTED

| Never | Sometimes | Always |
|---|---|---|

How did each parent's needs match with yours? Were the other parents consistent in what they expressed and what they wanted? If not, how did you and your children deal with the inconsistencies?

Think for a moment about how you and your new family let each other know when you wanted closeness or when you had had enough closeness. Were you able to express your needs directly without resorting to indirect methods like getting sick? Were you able to move in and out of closeness as your needs changed?

Now plot each of your children on the same lines.

**CHILD 1**
**EXPRESSED**

| Never | Sometimes | Always |
|---|---|---|

**WANTED**

| Never | Sometimes | Always |
|---|---|---|

**CHILD 2**
**EXPRESSED**

| Never | Sometimes | Always |
|---|---|---|

**WANTED**

| Never | Sometimes | Always |
|---|---|---|

How did each of your children match with you? How did you and each child work out the differences between you? How did they match with the other parents who raised them?

What do you imagine your children learned about closeness from watching you and your spouse(s)/partner(s)? What do you imagine they learned from reacting to your needs?

Put a plus by anything you feel proud of in this closeness section. Put a minus by anything you feel remorse about. Write notes in the margin if anything else occurs to you about how your closeness style or closeness needs affected your children.

## Communication

Look back at the communication in your family when your children were young. Plot the communication style of your family on the line below. Note anything that changed over time by writing the years the changes happened. Maybe communication was indirect during your active drinking years, 1960-67, and more direct as your years of recovery grew. You might put 1960-67 at the indirect end of the scale, 1968-70 toward the middle of the scale and 1971 to present near the direct end of the scale.

Direct                                                            Indirect

Did your family have a switchboard operator? Who was it?

Did your family have other triangles or other ways to communicate indirectly?

Now plot your family on the quantity-of-communication line that follows. Again, note any changes that happened over time.

Sparse                                              Overly Abundant

Were you comfortable with the amount of communication in your family? How did each of your children react to the amount of communication? Did one become silent, another join in and another try to fill the silences?

What topics were not allowed in your family?

In your family, was everyone allowed to finish their thoughts (responsive) or were people interrupted or talked over (reactive)? Were there topics that were like hidden mines — topics that blew up if your children said the wrong thing (reactive)? Or could you and your children bring up even sensitive topics and discuss them openly (responsive)?

Plot your family on the reactive/responsive continuum that follows.

---

Reactive                                                    Responsive

Now turn back to your answers to the questions on communication in Chapter 4. How similar was the communication style in your new family to the one in your family of origin? Did you have the same forbidden topics?

When you listen to your children communicating with their partners and children, do you see any similarities?

Mark a plus by anything in this communication section you feel proud of; mark a minus by anything you feel remorse about. Some things may have both a plus and a minus if you feel proud of the changes you made but still feel regret that those changes were not enough.

## Enforcement

As you were raising your children, you and your partner(s) had to figure out what enforcement methods you would use to enforce your family's rules. When you couldn't agree, each of you may have used different methods, or one of you may have reluctantly used the other person's methods.

Think back to times when you personally corrected or punished your children. What methods did you use?

---

Remember some of the methods we mentioned in Chapter 4: silence, comparisons, physical abuse, name-calling. Mark a minus by the methods you used that were shaming (attacking the child's self). Mark a plus by the methods that were not shaming (attacking only the child's behavior).

Did you use different methods for different children?

Now list the methods your partner(s) used to enforce the family rules.

---

---

Again, mark a minus by those that were shaming and a plus by those that were not shaming. Even though the shaming methods your partner(s) used were not your fault, you may feel regret for not stopping them.

Now turn back to the Enforcement section of Chapter 4. How similar or different were the methods used by you and your partner(s) from those used in your family of origin?

What enforcement methods do your children use with their children?

## Conflict

Think back to some specific conflicts in your family as your children were growing up. Think about conflicts in the first five years of child-raising, the second five years, the third five years, etc. Did the conflicts and your handling of them change over time?

When you think about those conflicts, who was allowed to be angry? What indirect methods did people use to express their anger? List the members of your family in the first column below. In the Anger column write *yes* or *no* to indicate whether or not this family member was allowed to express anger openly. Since we know that anger that is not expressed openly will still come out somehow, in the Indirect Methods column write the ways each person's anger came out indirectly. Include yourself as you were when your children were young and write down anything you changed over time.

| Name | Anger | Indirect Methods |
| --- | --- | --- |
|  |  |  |
|  |  |  |
|  |  |  |
|  |  |  |
|  |  |  |
|  |  |  |
|  |  |  |
|  |  |  |

How would you describe your family's method of conflict resolution?

_____

What did your family consider "unresolvable" conflicts?

_____

What did your family do about these conflicts?

_____

If you have trouble identifying specific "unresolvable" conflicts, think back to any addictions, cutoffs, abuse, acting out or scapegoating you remember in your family. Then ask yourself, "What might have been the underlying issue when we used cutoffs or scapegoating?"

Did you directly or indirectly ask your children to play a role in "unresolvable" conflicts between you and your partner(s)?

Did you call in outside support to help with the most difficult conflicts?

Did you encourage empathy, good listening, validating the other's point of view and experimenting with various solutions?

Turn for a moment to the Conflict section of Chapter 4. Compare what you just wrote about the family you created to what you wrote in Chapter 4 about your family of origin.

Now think about how your children handle anger and conflict in their current relationships. Do you see anything they learned from you?

Put pluses on the things you feel proud of and minuses on the things you feel remorse and regret about in this conflict section.

## Mistakes And Human Fallibility

When you created your new family, did you expect your children to make about the same number of mistakes all humans make? Another way of saying this is: how realistic or unrealistic were you and the other parents of your children in what you expected of them as they were growing up? Did you expect perfection (expectations too high), or did you expect failure or nothing (expectations too low)? Plot yourself and each of the other parents on the following scale. Remember to include any nontraditional people who parented your children — Uncle Jim, Bess who lived next door and so on.

Since your expectations may have been different for different children, mark a different line for each child. Use a small *m* for "myself" during that child's early years and, if you changed over time, a capital *M* for "Myself" now.

**CHILD 1**

_____

Too high                                            Too low

**CHILD 2**

_____

Too high                                            Too low

What did you do when each child made a mistake? What did the other parent(s) do? Again, you may have responded differently to different children.

_____

_____

What did you and the other parent(s) do when each child asked for help?

_____

_____

How did you and the other parent(s) react when each child had an illness, an addiction, a disability?

_____

_____

How would you describe your attitude toward human beings? Would you say humans are basically good and trustworthy or basically bad and untrustworthy? Plot yourself and each person who parented your children on the line that follows.

_____

Basically good                                  Basically bad

Now turn back to the section on mistakes and human fallibility in Chapter 4, and look at what you wrote about your own parents on these issues. How are you similar to or different from them?

Think about how your adult children now handle mistakes and disabilities. Can they ask for help? Do they offer help? Are they realistic about what they expect from their own children?

Mark a plus by anything in this section you feel proud of; mark a minus by anything you feel remorse about. Remember, some things may have both a plus and a minus.

## Loss

Think back to your children's first experiences with loss. How did you and the other parent(s) help your children understand the losses?

_____

Did you comfort them and allow them to express their feelings and thoughts?

_____

How did you explain death to your children?

_____

How did you and each of the other parents deal with losses that happened to you? What might your children have learned from watching you deal with your own losses?

_____

Did you change over time in how you dealt with your own losses and in how you helped your children deal with theirs?

Were there "unspeakable" losses in your family? What were they?

_____

Turn back to the section on losses in Chapter 4, and compare your answers here with those you gave when you described your family of origin.

Think about your children as they are now. How do they deal with loss?

Mark a plus by anything in this section you feel proud of; mark a minus by anything you feel remorse about.

## Difference And Autonomy

In the family you created, was it all right for your children to be unique, to be different from you and from the other family members, to be separate? Did you respect differences, or did you ridicule, shame or punish differences?

First, let's look at your family's attitudes about differences in general. In general, did you expect your children to be different from you, from the other parent(s) and from their siblings? Plot your attitudes and each of the other parents' attitudes on the following line. Again, use a small *m* for "myself" in the early days of childrearing and a capital *M* for "Myself" today if you have changed over time. Use small letters and capital letters for the other parent(s) as well.

---

Different          Same

You may have had different attitudes toward different children. If you are a man, perhaps you expected a son to be like you but not a daughter. Perhaps one child had an appearance, talents or a temperament that led you to want that child to be like you. Plot your attitude toward each child on the lines below.

*CHILD 1*

---

Different          Same

*CHILD 2*

---

Different          Same

Were there particular differences you had strong reactions to? What were they?

---

Do you know why you reacted so strongly to those differences?

Were your children allowed to have a different relationship with each parent?

Do you remember apologizing or admitting mistakes to your children? Do you remember making amends?

Do you remember blaming?

How much autonomy were your children allowed to have?

When and how did you expect your children to leave home?

Turn back to the sections about differences and autonomy in Chapter 4, and compare what you said about your family of origin to what you just wrote here. Notice differences and similarities.

Take a moment to think about your children as they are now. In what ways are they different from you? How do they communicate to you the ways in which they are different from you?

Are your children now able to admit mistakes? Apologize? Make amends? Are they more likely to blame?

Mark a plus by anything in this section you feel proud of; mark a minus by anything you feel remorse for.

## Role, Gender, Birth Order

List each of your children's names in the Name column in the order in which they were born. Put your firstborn next to the number 1, your secondborn next to the number 2, etc.

Think back to when each child was young and identify the roles that child played in your family. Note any that changed over time.

If you need to refresh your memory, roles are explained in Chapter 5. The basic roles are (1) the clown/distracter/pleaser; (2) the hero/caretaker/responsible one; (3) the adjuster/lost child; and (4) the scapegoat/acting-out child.

**Name**                    **Role(s)**

1. _____    _____

2. _____    _____

3. _____    _____

4. _____    _____

5. _____    _____

Next to each name, write an F for female or an M for male.

How did gender affect the roles your children played?

How did gender affect your way of relating to them? Were males and females treated differently in your family? How did you react to each child's style of being male or female?

How did birth order affect your way of relating to them?

How did the combination of gender and birth order affect your way of relating? Did you relate differently to the oldest male and the youngest male, for instance?

Take a moment to turn back to your answers in Chapter 5. What similarities and differences do you notice between the attitudes your parents had toward you and your siblings and the attitudes you had toward your own children in terms of role, gender and birth order?

Which of your children played the same role you did?

When you think about your children in their current lives, can you see any patterns that may relate to their birth other? What role(s) do they play in their current relationships? Are they playing the same role(s) they played in your family when they were children?

Put a plus by anything in this section you feel proud of; put a minus by anything you feel remorse or regret about.

## Family Size And Composition

Did your children grow up in a little family or a big family? Was there enough time and attention for each child? Did they have siblings to learn from and to practice sharing and teasing with? How did the size of your family affect your children?

Did you have a large or a small lateral support system? Was there enough lateral support to help you? To help your children?

Was your extended family — parents, grandparents, siblings — accessible to you and your children? Were relatives helpful or detrimental? If they were detrimental, did you protect your children from them?

Was your family gender-skewed? That is to say, were there mostly people of one gender in your family? If so, how do you think that affected your children's attitudes about their own gender? About the opposite gender?

Feel free to refer back to Chapter 5 where some of the effects family size and composition can have on children were explained.

Now, put a plus by anything in this section you feel proud of; put a minus by anything you feel remorse about.

## Personal Characteristics

In the columns below, list each child's name in the Name column; list the person each child looked like, if anyone, in the Looks column; list the person each child was named for in the Named For column. Finally, write what your relationship was with each of the people in the Looks or Named For columns in the column labeled Relationship. Did you like or dislike each of them? Did you have easy or difficult relationships with them?

| Name | Looks | Named For | Relationship |
|------|-------|-----------|--------------|
| _____ | _____ | _____ | _____ |
| _____ | _____ | _____ | _____ |
| _____ | _____ | _____ | _____ |
| _____ | _____ | _____ | _____ |

Take a moment to think about how each child's appearance and name may have affected the way you treated him or her, the expectations you had for him or her.

Now list each child in the following Name column. Briefly describe each one's temperament in the Temperament column. Note any traits that worried you or made you think that child might have inherited a family disability (physical, mental; obesity, addictions) in the Traits column.

| Name | Temperament | Traits |
|------|-------------|--------|
| _____ | _____ | _____ |
| _____ | _____ | _____ |
| _____ | _____ | _____ |
| _____ | _____ | _____ |

How did each child's temperament match yours? Did any child's temperament remind you of someone in your past or present?

How might each child's temperament or traits have played a role in the way you treated him or her? The expectations you had for him or her?

Now list each child in birth order in the Name column. Put your firstborn next to number 1, your secondborn next to number 2, etc. Then list yourself and your siblings in birth order in the Myself column. Finally, list your partner(s) and siblings in their birth orders.

| Name | Myself | Partner 1 | Partner 2 |
|------|--------|-----------|-----------|
| 1. _____ | _____ | _____ | _____ |
| 2. _____ | _____ | _____ | _____ |
| 3. _____ | _____ | _____ | _____ |
| 4. _____ | _____ | _____ | _____ |
| 5. _____ | _____ | _____ | _____ |
| 6. _____ | _____ | _____ | _____ |

Take some time to consider each of your children in turn. How did you feel about your sibling who was in the birth-order position of each child? How was that sibling treated in your family of origin? What role did he or she play?

Which child is in the same birth-order position you are in? Your favorite sibling is in? Your least favorite sibling is in? Do you notice any similarities between your feelings toward each sibling and your feelings toward, or expectations of, the child in that sibling's birth-order position?

Consider the same questions about each child and your partner(s) and their siblings.

Look back over this section. Mark a plus by anything you feel proud of; mark a minus by anything you feel remorse or regret about.

## Unmet Needs

We may have unconsciously or consciously expected our children to meet our unmet childhood needs and the needs we couldn't fill in our adult lives, making it hard for us to see our children's unique selves and unique needs. Whenever our pent-up demands clashed with the needs of our children, whenever we asked our children to forego a normal task of childhood to fill a need of ours, we may have created a knot of guilt inside ourselves and an empty space or a knot of pain in our children.

In Chapter 7 we looked at how our parents' unfinished business from their childhoods may have affected what they expected of us. Now I am going to ask the same question of you: How did your unfinished business affect what you expected of your children? Think of each of your children in turn as the following questions are posed.

Did you hope this child would take the place of a "missing person" in your childhood? Put the child's name next to the role you hoped that child would play.

A sibling
A playmate
A friend
A parent
A cuddly teddy bear
A victim who let you be the powerful one this time
An outlet for your anger/revenge

Did you hope your children would fill in your lacks? Put the child's name next to any of the following that apply.

Carried the anger you weren't allowed to have.
Carried any other feeling you weren't allowed to have.
Was assertive/said No for you.
Was your social network.
Was a pseudo-adult/parent, competent where you were not.
Was the scapegoat/took the blame for family pain and problems.

Did you ask your children to protect you from any of the following:

Seeing feelings that might trigger your own feelings (sadness, anger)
Seeing behaviors (teasing, etc.) that might trigger old feelings for you

"Upsetting" you

"Upsetting" a partner or grandparent

Feeling powerless (they should not bring unresolvable problems to you).

There are many ways we can triangulate our children, asking them to play roles that have nothing to do with who they are and what they need. The following questions will help you inventory possible triangles in the family you created.

Did you hope any of your children would be the glue child that could hold your marriage/relationship together?

Did you directly or indirectly ask any of your children to be your spokesperson or ally in conflicts with your partner?

Did any of your children stimulate memories of an old triangle you were in as a child?

Did you have any of your children for a third party — the church, your parents, your in-laws — or in competition with a sibling?

Before our children were even born, most of us had an idea of what our children would be like if we were successful parents. We may have also been aware of our parents' ideas about what good grandchildren would be like. In order that you might feel successful, did you ask your children to do any of the following:

Become like you

Belong to you

Agree with you

Become a success as success was defined in your family or your family of origin (marry early, marry late, have a great job out in the world, stay home and work as a homemaker).

Finally, did you ask any of your children to compensate you for —

An unhappy marriage.

An unhappy childhood.

Aborted career plans.

Other children who were miscarried or who died.

A divorce.

Problems with in-laws.

Take some time to go back over this section, and mark a plus by anything you feel proud about; mark a minus by anything you feel remorse or regret about. Give yourself the time you need to really think about these questions. They are hard ones.

Even though the list of things you feel remorse about may feel overwhelming at this point, it's important to take the time to consider *all the ways you did not hurt your children.* If you were abused as a child and did not repeat that pattern with your own children, take some credit for that. If you had an unhappy marriage and did not make your children feel they had to pay you back for staying in it "for their sakes," give yourself a plus. Those are things to feel proud of.

If you tend to do black/white thinking, if you tend to be very hard on yourself or if it's difficult for you to acknowledge anything you did well when you feel bad about what you did poorly, you must make a contract to come back and let yourself own what you feel good about. Your inventory is not complete until you accept the positive as well as the negative.

## Your Time Lines

Turn now to the papers you filled out with your personal time lines. You will use these time lines to complete your inventory.

## Losses

Look at the losses you noted during the years you were raising your children. List on the lines below the losses you feel remorse about — either because you caused the painful loss or because you handled the loss poorly with your children. Then list the losses you feel proud of — losses you handled well with your children — and losses of things you were pleased to leave behind.

You may find that some losses have parts you feel proud of and parts you feel remorseful about. In those cases, list each component of the loss in the appropriate column. The move to Chicago, for instance, might have been a brave and economically sound thing to do, but you may have been drunk when you told your children about it. Or you may have handled it well with one of your children and not the other.

**Proud**

**Remorseful**

_____   _____

_____   _____

_____   _____

_____   _____

_____   _____

_____   _____

_____   _____

## Toxic Events

Now look at your time line again and list in the Remorseful column below any toxic events you feel remorse about causing or not preventing in your children's lives. In the Proud column, list the toxic events you are proud you stopped or handled well with your children.

**Proud**

**Remorseful**

_____   _____

_____   _____

_____   _____

_____   _____

_____   _____

## Major Events

Again, look at your time line, and this time pick out any of the major events that you feel remorse about or are proud of and list them below. Remember that parts of some events may be listed in both columns because there are things you feel both proud of and remorse about. You may also have handled an event differently with different children.

**Proud**                          **Remorseful**

_____          _____
_____          _____
_____          _____
_____          _____
_____          _____
_____          _____

## Life Cycle

Now look at the individual and family life-cycle events on the time line. List below any that you feel you handled particularly well with your children in the Proud column and any you feel you handled particularly poorly in the Remorseful column.

**Proud**                          **Remorseful**

_____          _____
_____          _____
_____          _____
_____          _____

## Cultural Events

Finally, look at the column of cultural events on your time line. Even though you didn't cause these cultural events, you did help or not help or hinder your children in understanding and dealing with them. There may be some you feel you could have protected them from by moving or counseling them differently. If there are any you feel you handled particularly well with your children, list them in the Proud column. If there are any you feel you handled particularly poorly, list them in the Remorseful column.

**Proud**                          **Remorseful**

_____          _____
_____          _____
_____          _____
_____          _____

# The Roar

Those of you who are actively involved in 12-Step programs are intimately aware of the function of the fourth, fifth, eighth and ninth steps whereby you make a fearless inventory of your behavior and become willing to make amends. I hope that doing the inventory in this chapter has not only helped you to be accountable for things about which you feel remorse or regret but also helped you to have compassion for yourself and to give yourself credit for things which you did well.

Remember, for example, Molly's time line at the end of Chapter 9. Molly had recovered enough from her alcoholism not to return to it when her second divorce occurred. This is a change in the generational legacy of her family — Molly's mother's pill addiction had been reactivated in Molly's mother's forties and had, in all likelihood, led to the end of her own marriage and the creation of tremendous pain for her family.

Were Molly to be completing this chapter, it would be important that she write on her list of assets the breaking of several generational legacies. She interrupted the legacy of alcoholism and the legacy of fundamentalist sobriety, i.e., sobriety achieved with white knuckles and willpower and a fundamentalist anti-alcohol stance. Instead, Molly had sought therapy and ongoing involvement in a 12-Step group to support her sobriety and her growth.

As we continue our healing journey, it might be useful to remind ourselves of the "12 Steps To Healing The Hurt" developed by Rosalie Jesse in *Healing The Hurt* and modified slightly for our purposes here:

1. We admitted that we were powerless over our children's hurts as a result of our chemical dependency/other life dysfunction and that their lives and ours had become unmanageable.
2. We came to believe that a power greater than ourselves could restore our children's mental health and the parent-child relationship.
3. We made a decision to turn the life of our child over to the care of the God of our understanding, relying

only on knowledge of divine will for our relationship with our child and power to carry it out.

4. We made a searching and fearless inventory of our parenting.
5. We admitted to God, to ourselves and to another human being the exact nature of our wrongs with our child.
6. We were entirely ready to have God remove all of these defects of character.
7. We humbly asked God to remove our shortcomings.
8. We made a list of the hurts that we had brought to the lives of our children, and we became willing to make amends to them all.
9. We made direct amends to our children wherever possible, except when to do so would injure them or others.
10. We continued to take personal inventory; and when we were wrong in our parenting, we promptly admitted it to ourselves and to our children.
11. We sought through prayer and meditation to improve our conscious contact with the God of our understanding, praying only for knowledge of God's will for us and the power to carry that out.
12. Having had a spiritual awakening as a result of these steps, we tried to carry this message to other parents in recovery and to practice these principles in all of our affairs.

As these 12 Steps show, taking stock is an ongoing process. You have taken the biggest step, however, by completing this chapter. Give yourself some heartfelt appreciation and respect. You have faced your worst fears; you have faced the roar.

# CHAPTER

---

# 13

# Self-Forgiveness

## Are We Willing To Forgive Ourselves?

The journey we have just completed in Chapter 12 is possibly one of the most arduous journeys we will ever make. From time to time it has been said that this parent's journey is not a journey for sissies. We have amply discovered the truth of that statement in the very difficult work we have just completed.

Many of us are now facing both the "nevers" mentioned in Chapter 11 and what I call the "evers." The "nevers" tell us that we will never be able to go back and undo the past. The past is the past. In thinking of the "evers," we ask whether we will ever be able to forgive ourselves and whether we will ever be worthy of our children's forgiveness.

We make of ourselves a harsh judge and jury, and so we must face not only the roar of our fears but also the roar of our own self-condemnation and self-hate. The enemy is our lack of compassion for ourselves and our feeling that our self should be punished.

Eventually, if we are to heal, we must become willing to forgive ourselves and do what members of Alcoholics Anonymous call dropping the rock. That is, we must drop the heavy rock of resentments against ourselves and give up our demand for punishment.

## Six Steps To Self-Forgiveness

Nancy Whitaker-Emrich, in her work on compassion and self-forgiveness, has delineated six steps in forgiving the self. I have found these steps to be useful both in my own self-forgiveness and in my work with clients over the years.

1. *We acknowledge that we are unforgiving with ourselves.* We need to take responsibility for the fact that we are unwilling, or have been unwilling up to this point, to forgive ourselves. We have been unable or unwilling to let go of our self-hate and self-punitiveness.

2. *We grieve.* When we fully encounter our lack of willingness to forgive ourselves, and when we fully confront the many manifestations of our self-hate and self-punishment, we will feel tremendous sadness. Hopefully, a sense of compassion for ourselves will be born from this sadness.

3. *We share our grief with the God or Higher Power of our understanding and with at least one other human being.* In order to heal this grief, we must acknowledge the reality of the loss, feel the feelings associated with the loss and then share the loss. In this step we confess our anger with ourselves and our unwillingness to forgive ourselves. We openly acknowledge out loud, not just privately, to a Higher Power and to one other human being the exact nature of our wrongs.

**4. We acknowledge what is valuable about ourselves as people.** In Chapter 12 we included what we did well as parents in our assessment. In this step, we do a more general assessment of our good qualities. Are we giving and forgiving toward other people, even though we are not giving and forgiving with ourselves? Are we kind to animals?

For many of us, it will seem quite foreign to make an assessment of our good qualities. Even if we have difficulty with this step, we should not move through the rest of the steps until we can complete this step adequately. If necessary, we can ask our friends and family members what they like about us. How might they describe our good qualities? We can then include those good qualities on our list.

**5. We make amends to ourselves.** A good way to begin making amends to ourselves is to write ourselves a letter like this:

---

*Dear Self:*

*I have been too hard on you. I have held you too responsible for too many things, and I want to make amends for having been so hard on you.*

*These are some of the things I have been hard on you about:*

*a. I have expected you to be infallible and too perfect.*

*b. I have cut you no slack when you have failed to meet unrealistic standards.*

*c. I have punished you to a far greater degree than anyone you have ever harmed could have punished you.*

*d. I have given you indeterminate sentences for what I consider to be your flaws, and I have refused to commute your sentences or to find some way to discharge your responsibility for the harm you've done.*

*I deeply and truly regret having done this to you, and I would like to ask for forgiveness. I pledge to you that I will actively work at being aware of my self-hate and my lack of self-forgiveness. When I find myself punishing you, I will promptly admit the exact nature of my wrong to you and will cease self-hating behavior.*

*Sincerely, Self*

---

This letter might be a first draft. As it stands, it includes only general amends. However, as Whitaker-Emrich says, our shame is hidden in the details. So in order for the fifth step in this process to be effective, we will need to include examples of what we have not forgiven ourselves for. For instance, under the category of indeterminate sentences, I might add something specific: I have beaten up on you repeatedly because you were too strict and too rigid with the children. I wish you could have been more democratic and less authoritarian, but you can't change the past. In the present, you are actively working on changing your authoritarianism, your need for control, your rigidity and your tendency to see things in black-and-white terms. I make an amend to you for having continued to punish you for not being more flexible when the children were teenagers.

**6. We write what we have learned about ourselves in this process.** To consolidate our learning, we must not only silently review what we have learned; we must write it down. Writing it makes it concrete and takes the healing to a deeper level.

One of the themes in this book is that healing is a process, not an event. We will need to come back to this exercise repeatedly. As we become aware of feelings of regret or remorse or self-hate, we can use those feelings as cues to repeat these six steps immediately and take another self-forgiveness inventory.

---

## EXERCISE

See if you can begin Step 1 right now. Pull out a piece of paper and write down, "I have been unforgiving of myself and punitive toward myself."

Take some time to breathe and to notice how you feel as you read this statement a few times. This is the first step in acknowledging your unforgiving stance and becoming willing to let it go.

Write any thoughts or feelings you have about this statement.

---

## Forgiving Our Parents

We are simultaneously on several journeys at once. We may be on the journey of recovering from a primary addiction or dysfunction. We are on our parental journey, looking back at what we were like as parents. We are also on our own inner child journey: discovering, honoring, grieving and healing the wounds we experienced in childhood.

While it is true that authentically forgiving our parents will help us forgive ourselves, let me issue a caution here. We cannot cut short our inner child's journey. We cannot simply decide to forgive our parents because forgiving them will help us forgive ourselves. We must take each step as it comes, feel all the feelings as they come and let the healing occur in its own time.

Some of us are now in the middle of our child's journey. We are feeling the grief and rage. We are hoping our parents will step up to the plate and acknowledge our wounds.

Some of us have been in denial for a long time, using "They did the best they could" to keep from looking at our childhood wounds. We may be just beginning our child's journey.

Wherever we are is just fine. Wherever we are is just where we need to be. The best thing we can do is to continue our child's journey to its end faithfully.

Remember that in order for a wound to heal, we must first open it up, look at what's inside, pick the splinters out one by one, clean it and allow the natural process of healing to ensue. We would never expect a wound to heal if we closed it over with the splinters inside.

After we complete our child's journey, we may very well be able to see our parents as imperfect and as having loved us. We may be able to let in our parents' imperfect love at the same time that we have compassion for our inner child self who survived the hurts of that imperfection, and also at the same time we protect our inner child from wounding in the present. Reaching the place where we can see our parents as forgivable may, in fact, help us see ourselves as forgivable parents as well.

## Unrealistic Expectations

Our goal is to become willing to forgive ourselves so that we can heal. We want to be able to adopt a compassionate and caring attitude toward ourselves as imperfect human beings no matter what other people think. In order to forgive ourselves, we will need to begin confronting our children's, our culture's and our own unrealistic expectations of ourselves.

Our children, because they are our children, do not see us as the fallible human beings that we are. Because of their own needs, and because of our central importance in their lives, they feel wounded by our limitations and imperfections. Whether or not our children remain unrealistic, we can learn to adopt a more realistic, more compassionate attitude toward ourselves.

Even if the culture never becomes realistic, even if the climate of the culture continues to be one of parent-bashing, we can learn to accept ourselves as fallible and forgivable human beings.

## Special Status

We, too, suffer from unrealistic beliefs about ourselves. One of these unrealistic beliefs is what, in *Compassion & Self-Hate*, Theodore Isaac Rubin calls our "special status" belief. We believe that we should be treated differently from other human beings because we have special status.

For instance, we may feel that all other parents are forgivable for harm done but that we should have known better. Therefore, while we may be able to extend compassion to other parents, we cannot extend it to ourselves.

The special status we are assuming, by the way, is the special status of grandiosity. We believe we are somehow godlike and exempt from the human condition. It is not important whether or not we believe in God or a Higher Power. What is important is that we know we are not God. When we assume a position of special status or grandiosity or infallibility or unrealistic self-expectation, we are acting as if we were God.

We need to drop the rock. We need to accept the fact that we are as fallible as all other people. We have no special status. Since we are just like everyone else, we too are forgivable.

$$\boxed{\text{E X E R C I S E}}$$

In the first column below, list the unrealistic expectations you think that your children have, that your culture has and that you have about parenting and about how you should have been or should be now as a parent. Then next to each unrealistic statement, list the more realistic statement that should take its place. You will need another piece of paper to complete the list. I have filled in the first line as an example.

**Unrealistic**                    **Realistic**

**My Children Expect**

I should always listen atten-    I should listen attentively a
tively.                          reasonable amount of time
                                 and try to tell my children
                                 when I can't.

_____          _____

_____          _____

**My Culture Expects**

_____          _____

_____          _____

**I Expect**

_____          _____

_____          _____

## Reclaiming Our Selves

When we do not forgive ourselves, we sit in judgment on the parts of ourselves that we do not like. In order to forgive ourselves, we need to accept all of ourselves as fallible and as lovable exactly as we are.

Come with me on a journey to reclaim the disowned parts of ourselves. We will take this journey together by means of a meditation.

Get comfortable in a quiet place where you won't be disturbed for ten minutes. Uncross your legs, loosen your clothing and wiggle around until you feel comfortable. Then begin the process of paying attention to your breathing.

Breathe slowly in and out, in and out. As you breathe in, see in your mind's eye the vitality of the universe flowing into you. As you breathe out, breathe out your pain, your self-hate and your discomfort. Keep breathing rhythmically, in and out, in and out.

Visualize yourself in a bright, lovely meadow. The air is warm, the sky filled with puffy clouds. The meadow sits at the edge of a wood. Get up and walk toward the wood. As you enter, you are surrounded by tall sentinel pines and filtered sunlight. Birds abound, and beneath your feet is a carpet of wild flowers. You notice a path winding through the wood and you follow it with curiosity. The sun is warm, there is a breeze on your face. You are relaxed, at peace. You feel safe here.

As you round a bend, your path opens into a clearing. Opposite stands an inviting-looking log house — sturdy and well tended. You climb the steps to the porch and knock on the door. As you hear someone coming, you step slightly back. The door opens. The figure in the door looks familiar. As your eyes adjust to the light, you realize you are looking at a representation of yourself. Your host invites you in and beckons toward the table where two chairs sit opposite one another. You sit down, filled with curiosity and an eagerness to find out about this other self of yours whom you have found here in the woods.

As you and your host talk, you realize that you are speaking with all of the parts of yourself which you have disliked, sat in judgment of or attempted to discard. Here sits your shadow, your dark side — your regret, remorse, anger, greed, pettiness, emotional blindness, whatever about yourself you have failed to embrace and appreciate as part of the totality of you. As you sit and talk with your discarded self, you are filled with compassion for this other. You realize this is your wounded self that has already suffered so much. You acknowledge to yourself how much time and energy has been wasted hating this part of yourself — trying to push away and deny attributes and feelings that you did not know how to come to terms with or ask for help with. You have been one of the wounders of your wounded self. Suddenly you say to this other: "No more. No more. I will hurt you no more. You have never intended me harm. You have done the best that you have known how to do, given your own experiences. I will no longer attempt to banish you from my life. I will embrace you and try to learn from your experiences. Please forgive me. I am sorry for what I have done." This other replies, "I forgive you as I hope you will forgive yourself for your humanness. We both deserve mercy. Let us each allow the other back into our hearts. We are both forgiven and we are one — no longer divided against ourselves."

Slowly, you extend your hands across the table and clasp those of the other. As you each rise, you slowly step around the table and embrace this part of yourself. You are now one, no longer divided, no longer sitting in judgment of yourself. You embrace all of you, all of the parts of yourself. There is no badness or goodness here, only oneness. You are forgiven and forgiving. You have reowned this lost part of yourself.

You know that you can return to this place of oneness, reconciliation, and self-forgiveness whenever in the future you need to. You can come back to this place anytime that you forget that all of these parts make up the totality of you and you are tempted to discard or judge a part of yourself.

## EXERCISE

The meditation you just did will help you become more willing to embrace and reclaim the disowned parts of yourself. The process of actually reclaiming these parts, however, is again like cleaning splinters out of a wound. You need to search for each one and pull it out. You need to give each one your full attention. Once you see each disowned part of yourself clearly, you can work on reclaiming it.

Pull out two sheets of paper. On the first sheet, draw two large circles side by side. In one circle name some of the parts of yourself that you disown, condemn, judge or hate. In the other circle, name some parts of yourself that you own, like, accept or appreciate.

On the second sheet of paper, draw one large circle and put all the words you have just written on the first sheet in this circle. Notice how you feel.

Add to these sheets as you think of more parts of yourself you like or dislike, own or disown.

Which of these parts of yourself do you want to change? Is it realistic to expect yourself to be able to change these parts, or are they part of being human? Which parts do you simply need to accept?

This might be a good time to put a copy of "The Serenity Prayer" in a spot where you can refer to it often. Remember that you can address it to the Higher Power of your understanding:

> *God grant us the serenity to accept the things we cannot change, the courage to change the things we can and the wisdom to know the difference.*

---

## Developing Compassion

Are we willing to develop a sense of compassion for ourselves? Many of us have lived lives of self-hate and self-punishment. Although we are always responsible and accountable for our actions, many of us have meted out to ourselves punishments that don't fit our "crimes." We act as though our patron saint were Our Lady of Perpetual Punishment.

Even criminals are allowed an end to their punishment. At some point it is recognized that they have paid for their misdeeds, and they are released.

When we talked about the child's journey, we talked about developing compassion for our wounded inner child of the past. As we took an inventory of the tools in our parental toolbox and looked at the external events that had affected our parenting, we talked about developing compassion for the young parent we once were. Even though this book has been full of compassion, we may have fallen into our old patterns and used this book and these exercises to buttress our self-hate. We may have had so little experience with compassion for the self that we found this feeling unfamiliar when directed toward us.

Let's stop for a moment and think about our history with compassion. Did we grow up in a compassionate home where mistakes were just mistakes to be learned from, or were mistakes capital crimes to be ferociously punished? Were our parents able to say they were sorry? Did they acknowledge when they were wrong?

Did they forgive us for our misdeeds? Did they soothe and comfort us when we felt guilty and were being too hard on ourselves?

Our lack of compassion for ourselves as adults is often a reflection of lack of compassion in our childhood homes. We may need to make a special effort to learn what we didn't learn in our family of origin.

## Compassionate Role Models

A number of years ago, a friend was helping me move. She had parked her brand new Acura automobile outside my driveway.

Because of the height of my car, I didn't see her car when I backed out of the drive. As I made the turn out of my driveway into the street, I demolished her bumper and her left front fender.

I was aghast; I was chagrined. I went into the house to look for my friend, thinking that I should be drawn and quartered for what I had done. I fully expected her to go ballistic.

I was stunned by her response. She said, "It's just a car; a car can be fixed. Let's go and see what happened."

I assumed that when she really saw how badly the car was damaged, she would stop being so benign and start screaming at me. As we walked out to look at the fender, I told her that I, of course, would take time off from work to take the car to the shop. I, of course, would see to it that my insurance paid and that the insurance deductible came out of my pocket. I, of course, would pay for a rental car for her so that she would not be inconvenienced.

When she looked at the car, she said, "Well, it looks like the fender and the bumper need to be replaced. It's no big deal. We'll work out the details between the two of us."

Her behavior was an act of compassion. She acted as though I were a fallible human being and, therefore, like all human beings,

I make mistakes. I did not deserve to be drawn and quartered for having made a mistake. Her compassion helped me learn to have more compassion for myself.

In our quest to learn about compassion, we can consciously make an effort to look for role models. I'm not talking about people who are passive when things bother them, and who then harbor resentments and get us later. That is not compassion. I'm talking about people who are truly compassionate and forgiving.

Sometimes I suggest that my clients pretend they are anthropologists going out to visit a neighboring, but somewhat unfamiliar, tribe. As anthropologists, they are to take field notes on acts of compassion that they see.

For instance, a client might write down that when he was stuck in traffic, someone paused to allow him into a line of traffic and waved at him in a friendly way. Once we start noticing, we will find many examples of compassion to write down.

I also suggest that my clients watch children. Children can not only be very cruel, they can also be extraordinarily compassionate. A child can be very responsive to another child or to an animal or to us when we are sad, disappointed or hurt.

God, or a Higher Power, is the ultimate role model of compassion. As we attempt to learn about compassion, it will be helpful to look at our spiritual beliefs. Would the power of good in the universe, would God, would our Higher Power forgive someone else who had done what we feel we are guilty of? If that person is forgivable and worthy of God's compassion, why should we not also be worthy?

## EXERCISE

Write down the names of people in your life right now who are compassionate role models for you. Study them. Ask their advice when you have questions about compassion. Talk about the subject of compassion with them. Ask them how they developed compassion.

Keep a journal of compassionate acts you notice.

## Random Acts Of Kindness

A popular bumper sticker suggests, "Practice Random Acts of Kindness." One way to develop compassion for ourselves is to practice random acts of kindness toward ourselves.

For instance, if I notice that I am characterizing myself in a pejorative way, I can perform a random act of kindness toward myself by stopping and correcting myself. I can instead speak of myself with compassion.

Let's say I am describing myself as stupid and incompetent because I have difficulty programming my VCR. I can stop and say to myself, "I have never had any instruction on how to program a VCR. I am not particularly good with electronic devices, but there are many things I am good at. My lack of proficiency with my VCR does not mean I am stupid. I merely lack experience." That is a random act of kindness toward myself.

## EXERCISE

List some random acts of kindness you might perform toward yourself. Add to this list as you think of more. Ask your support people for suggestions.

## Becoming Our Own Best Friend

Our best friends are naturally compassionate toward us because they truly care about us. We, in turn, are compassionate toward our best friends. We can draw upon our experiences with our friends to learn about compassion.

## EXERCISE

Sit in a comfortable chair and put an empty chair across from you. Imagine for a moment that your best friend is sitting in that chair. It might be your current best friend; it might be a best friend from high school; it might even be your grandmother. Whoever it is, you know that person loves you and cares about you.

Picture in detail what your friend looks like. How is your friend sitting? What is the look on your friend's face?

Now go sit in that chair. Sit as your friend was sitting and picture yourself in the other chair. For just a few minutes, let yourself be your friend. Feel how your friend feels toward you. Feel the love, the caring, the concern.

Now speak to the chair you started out sitting in. Speak as your friend would speak to you if you had just told your friend how remorseful you feel. Start by saying, "I'm your best friend, and I love you a lot." Continue saying whatever you imagine your friend would say next.

After you do this exercise, you may realize that you do know how to be compassionate. You do have the words in your head and the feelings in your body. You simply have never focused those abilities on yourself. You can start now. You can use this exercise any time you are feeling hateful toward yourself.

## Looking Back

Another way to practice compassion is by using photographs. Sometimes when we have the distance of time between our present self and our past selves, we can be more compassionate.

## EXERCISE

This is a powerful exercise, so be prepared to do pieces of it on different days. You will need a chunk of uninterrupted time in a comfortable place each time you work on it.

Get out some photos of yourself at various ages from childhood through the present. As you look through them, notice which ages you have positive feelings toward and which ones you have negative feelings toward.

You will need to separate the pictures into groups with five years to a group. The first group will contain photos of you from ages one day of age to five years; the second group will include photos of you from six years of age through ten, etc.

Now spread out the photos of you from the first group. Looking at each picture as you speak, say out loud, "I'm sorry for the hurtful things that happened to you. I'm sorry for the hard things you had to live through." Notice how you feel as you look at the photos and talk. Don't be surprised if you cry or feel deeply tender feelings toward your younger self.

Then take the next group, ages six to ten, and start with the same two sentences. Then say anything else you would like to say to these photos. Continue this with each group of photos until you have talked to all the photos up to and including your present age.

When you began this book, you might have said to many of the photos, "I'm ashamed of you" or "I hate you" or even "I can't stand to look at you." Hopefully, by now, you will say that rarely.

When you do feel negatively toward a photo of yourself at a particular age, it means you have more healing to do on the issues you faced at that age before you can be compassionate toward yourself. You can talk about yourself at that age with your therapist or support group. You can look at your time line to see what you were dealing with around that age. Take some time to heal whatever self-hate you discover.

---

## Fake It

Initially, if we have had little experience with compassion, being compassionate toward ourselves will feel foreign and unfamiliar. One of the sayings in Alcoholics Anonymous is, "Fake it till you make it." We can fake compassion toward ourselves until we can finally feel compassion toward ourselves.

Most important, we need to remember that self-forgiveness is possible. We can make amends to ourselves; we can become realistic; we can stop our self-hate and own all the parts of ourselves. We can learn compassion and become our own best friends.

# CHAPTER

## 14

# Healing And Forgiveness

### by Chandra Smith

About a year and a half into my own recovery from alcoholism, I came home from work to find my teenage son, Jonathan, lounging in front of the TV. He had come home late from school and had not picked up his things.

I asked him to turn off the TV. Reluctantly he complied. From the expression on his face, I could tell my request did not please him.

I asked where he had been and why he had not put his things away. He crossed his arms and said nothing. His face was sullen.

"Jonathan," I persisted, "where have you been? What's going on?"

305

His face and tone of voice now challenging, Jonathan said, "You didn't always come home on time."

I could feel my face flush. I knew he was referring to my drinking days when I rarely got anywhere on time. I felt ashamed and caught. I was so flooded with my own feelings, I couldn't listen to him.

"Jonathan," I said tearfully, "I am really sorry about that. You are right. I wasn't always on time."

Before I could continue, Jonathan jumped up with his fists clenched, ready for a fight. This was more than a teenage challenge to my authority. He was angry about my previous neglect and poor parenting.

I tried again to make amends. Caught in his own anger, Jonathan could not hear. His feelings escalated, and he began to move toward me. He clearly wanted to fight.

I did not want to fight. I ordered him to his room. He argued with me and finally stormed off. This was not the way I wanted things to be between us.

Even though I had spent considerable time grieving about my disease and inadequate parenting before this fight with Jonathan, when confronted face-to-face so unexpectedly, I did not know how to respond. Clearly I needed to do more healing work myself before I could heal my relationship with Jonathan.

In his own way, Jonathan was asking me to acknowledge that he had not had a safe and protected childhood — the kind of childhood every child deserves. He was trying to express this in his anger and challenges. I, however, had not healed enough to respond appropriately or to sort out his childhood pain from his teenage challenge to authority.

Jonathan was not in a place to have a healing conversation either. He could not hear much of my amends because his anger was serving a purpose for him. It was protecting him from possible future hurts.

Since working with recovering parents, I have seen this stage of the process many times. A parent will try to make amends in the midst of a conflict. The child can't hear the amends because he is overwhelmed by his own grief or anger. The parent's wound is not sufficiently healed for the parent to be able to stay out of overwhelming emotion, and the situation gets worse instead of better.

## Healing Takes Time

I want to share a metaphor with you that has been meaningful to me in understanding the healing process. In some Native American traditions, they talk about grief and healing as being a time of going within, being self-reflective and letting go so that something new can be born or imagined.

The totem animal for this healing time is the bear. The choice of the bear is significant because when she gives birth, she does so in semiconsciousness. The cub then nurses in the cave for several months while the mother is still in her semiconscious state.

The cub has time to grow in the safety of the cave. If the mother were to take the cub out of the cave too soon, mature bears at the watering hole might attack the cub. Taking enough time to grow first inside the safety of the cave is essential for the cub's survival. In the interaction with Jonathan, I had not given my healing enough time to grow in the safety of my own cave before I tried to take it to the watering hole and share it with my son.

When we are in the semiconscious state of grief, we give birth to new ways of being. But our new life has to grow up a bit before we take it into the world. If we take it into the world too soon, we are in danger of losing it. We see this happen with celebrities from time to time. When their recovery is openly exposed to the world too soon, the pressures make them vulnerable to relapse. Their recovery needs more time to grow up.

Healing is a function of time. It becomes part of you, like breathing. Initially its birth may be almost imperceptible and small, like a newborn cub in a cave.

Through my personal experience and through my work as a therapist with recovering parents, both individually and in groups, I have discovered four essential steps to the healing process:

1. Learning to be "response able"
2. Learning to set boundaries
3. Learning to be accountable
4. Forgiving.

After we do the grief work, after we take stock of our past strengths and weaknesses as parents, we need to take these four steps in order to complete our healing.

Before we go on, let me caution you. We can do our work conscientiously, and we can make excellent plans about how we will heal our relationships with our children. Still, we must keep in mind that a good deal of the healing is simply not in our hands. Some of it is up to our children, and some of it, I believe, is in the hands of a greater power — call it Mystery, Higher Power or God.

## Response Ability

Ted Buffington, a colleague of mine who is an educator and consultant, wrote a book called *Mindset: Response Ability, A New Attitude For Managing Change.* In it, he maintains that the only thing we really have any power over in this life is our ability to respond.

Responding is different from reacting. When we react, we are acting only from our emotions without thought. When we engage our mind in a thoughtful way, we are "response able".

I have found as a recovering parent that my capacity to be response able with my children is directly related to how much healing I have done. In my exchange with Jonathan, I was *reacting* to feelings of shame and guilt I had not yet worked through in my healing process. Because my feelings were overwhelming me, I could not think clearly or *respond* appropriately. Because Jonathan's feelings of anger were overwhelming him, he could not hear my amends. We were both reacting. Before I could respond and not react, I had to reduce my feelings of shame and anger at my parental shortcomings.

Other recovering parents have shared similar experiences with me. They have learned that displays of feelings, especially of tears, may distance their adult children. These children report that such displays evoke in them the same feelings of helplessness and hopelessness they had as kids. As one adult child said, "Mom's feelings are just too big for me to deal with, so I go away."

When we are response able, we feel our feelings, but our feelings do not dominate or control our response. We still have spontaneous feelings, but we are in charge of how we respond to those feelings.

A year or so after my exchange with Jonathan, when my healing had grown up a bit, I had another chance to be response able with one of my children. Jonathan's brother, Stephen, was getting ready to graduate from high school and leave home.

I had noticed that Stephen was becoming increasingly downcast. He seemed angry or depressed.

One evening when it was fairly quiet, I knocked on his bedroom door and asked if we could talk. He was packing his personal things and getting ready to leave for the summer. I suspect that as he was putting away his most precious childhood possessions, he was reviewing his past and reliving old memories.

We sat on the edge of his bed. We were beginning something unusual for us. Stephen is a rather private person, and personal discussions involving feelings are not easy for him.

I asked him if something was bothering him. He responded with, "Sometimes it was so hard, Mom."

I asked, "What was hard?"

He responded with that familiar phrase, "You know."

I said, "I think I might know, but I'd like to hear exactly what you mean."

"Mom," he said, "it was so hard when you drank. Things were so crazy. I was so scared." As his large brown eyes filled with tears, so did mine.

Initially, the familiar feelings of guilt and shame washed over me. But almost immediately I was able to engage my mind and think clearly. My feelings subsided.

I could hear my son's pain and grief as he shared his anger and disappointments with me. He talked about the times I didn't show up at soccer games when I had said I would. He talked about the time there was no food in the house and about the time I just plain didn't come home. Since my recovery had grown up some, I was able to hear him without my guilt and pain presenting themselves in torrents.

Because I was able to engage my mind, I could remind myself that Stephen needed me to listen nondefensively, and I could have a real discussion with him. Indeed, discussions such as these became part of our healing process. I was becoming response able.

Timing can be critical. When I had finally got into consistent sobriety, Stephen had been in early adolescence. He had not and would not have been able to talk to me about his feelings. It had not been the right time for him and possibly not the right time for me.

---

## EXERCISE

To become response able, recovering parents have found that several old tools used a little differently have served them well. Your goal in this part of the healing process is to reduce the emotional intensity you feel so that you can be response able when confronted with painful past events.

1. *Use counseling* to release the intensity of your feelings in a safe place away from your children. Counselors and therapists are trained to help you find safe ways to release anger, pain, shame and guilt. You can make therapy a safe healing cave to grow up in.

One of my clients, for example, learned that pummeling a stuffed animal in private was a good way for her to release anger. She also found that holding mock court hearings with her stuffed critters was a wonderful way to identify her judgmentalness and thoughts of revenge so that she could release those as well.

2. *Tell your story.* Telling your story releases the emotions around the events you are recounting. It helps you own your life history — the good and the bad. It can also help you access pieces of information you did not know you had.

For example, I have often told the story of my difficulty getting holiday dinners together when I was drinking. My judgment, timing and coordination were impaired.

Because of my disability, I had to serve Thanksgiving dinner in courses. Potatoes were served as a single course while I tried to organize the other vegetables. The turkey had difficulty making it from the stove to the counter top without taking a side trip to the floor; it then had to be washed before being eaten.

This Thanksgiving story may sound funny, but it wasn't. Holiday meals were a nightmare for all involved.

It wasn't until I had told this story several times that I found myself saying, "You know, holidays have been a nightmare for me ever since I was a little kid, even though my childhood holidays did not include alcohol." Until I heard myself speak those words, I hadn't realized that I had passed on a holiday legacy of negativity.

There are many safe places to tell your story:

a. You can find a 12-Step or other supportive group where it is part of the group's process for you to tell your story and listen to other people tell theirs. It is important that this be a group of people whose focus is on examining their parental behavior and working toward healthy relationships with their adult children. This group should have a format that allows people to reflect back to you what they hear you saying without being shaming or blaming, and it should have an agreement regarding confidentiality. A side benefit of attending group meetings is that you can hear others share their stories and learn how they did or did not handle difficult situations.

b. Find out if your community has any groups for recovering parents. If it does, attend at least two meetings to see what they are about.

c. Identify at least one recovering parent you can share your story with.

Tell the same story more than once, and notice whether you learn anything new about the event or yourself. Notice whether your level of emotion changes as you tell it several times.

3. *Experiment with keeping different kinds of journals.* Keeping a journal is a way of telling your story to yourself. Different kinds of journals will help you reflect on different aspects of your story.

For instance, Sarah spent much time recording the experiences she had growing up in an alcoholic home and raising her children with her alcoholic husband. In group meetings, she shared some of those memories and the accompanying feelings. One day she said she was sick and tired of this process. She felt mired down by all the negative memories.

The group asked whether anything positive was happening to her. She could identify one or two things. The group suggested she balance the negative memories by writing down the positive things in her life. She decided to write down one or two things she was grateful for each day. This was the beginning of her Gratitude Journal. Here are some types of journals I have found helpful:

a. *The Gratitude journal.* Get a small notebook you can keep in your pocket or purse. Write down at least two things each day you are grateful for about yourself, your children or life in general. In order to be response able we must encourage our minds to remember the good as well as the bad. Remembering both is how we come into balance.

b. *The children's journal.* In a loose-leaf notebook, make a section for each of your children and one for your own inner child. Write down parental memories about each child. A good way to begin is to write your memories of each child's birth. Note how your parenting may have differed from child to child depending on their birth order and where you were in your disease. Ask yourself, How response able was I to each child? To my own inner child?

Here are some examples:

Stephen: Pregnancy was a joy. Birthing him was unexpectedly easy. I was thrilled and excited to have a beautiful baby boy. I never dreamed I would miss parts of his childhood because of my drinking.

Jonathan: Jonathan moved into our lives at 23 months of age like a tank. What a tough adjustment for a little guy to go from home to home. He clung so tightly to me when he thought I was going to leave that I had black and blue marks. He was so terrified of abandonment.

Inner Child: I remember the delight of my own inner child self at taking trips on the ferry with my dad and how scared I was that he would leave me.

c. *The What-if Journal.* In this journal write out any of your what-if scenarios to their ultimate conclusion. For example, in those dark days when I had awful moments of such regret I wished I were dead, I would write about what would happen if I did die. How would my children feel? What legacy would this leave? This process allowed me safely to release pessimistic feelings and self-pity that got in the way of being response able.

Some parents who do not like to write have found talking into a tape recorder just as effective. Save the tapes and journals for the next exercise.

4. *Reread your old journals or listen to your old journal tapes.* Reading journal entries we wrote weeks or years ago can often surprise us by revealing patterns we are unaware of.

For example, it wasn't until I reread my journals that I realized how defensive I was about my own parents' dysfunction. In entry after entry I excused them because of "their hard life." Rationalizing their behavior had kept me from seeing how I was carrying their legacy of workaholism and negativity into my own life and family. After seeing this pattern of rationalization, I was able to respond to their dysfunction differently and hold them accountable. This helped me in understanding the need my children have to hold me accountable.

Rereading journals can also stimulate thoughts about how you would like your life to be now, or where you would like to go in your relationships.

---

## Setting Boundaries

The mother bear puts a boundary between her cub and the outside world to protect it while it grows. The boundary might be a snow bank or her own body. We also need to set boundaries to protect our healing process and our new selves.

Many of us never learned to set limits as children. Others of us were punished when we tried to set limits, to say no. Instead of learning that setting boundaries was essential to our health, we learned it was dangerous. Learning to set boundaries now can be a major part of our healing process.

Pia Mellody, in her book, *Facing Co-dependency,* describes boundary systems as invisible and symbolic fences that have three purposes:

1. To keep people from coming into our space and abusing us
2. To keep us from going into the space of others and abusing them
3. To give each of us a way to embody our sense of "who we are."

The purpose of good boundaries is to protect both people. Boundaries are often violated when one party is in a reactive, rather than a response able, stance. In the emotional flood of reactivity, we often say things we later regret.

In order to maintain a boundary, we must monitor our emotional state. If we find our emotions getting out of hand, or if we observe our adult child's emotions escalating, we can set a boundary by taking time out — leaving the situation for a while. Before we leave, we tell our adult child when we will return. During the time out, we can experience and process our feelings; we can calm down; we can get support; we can decide rationally how we want to handle the situation.

One of the parents in my group, Thalia, reported having a difficult time with boundaries. While she was raising her young children, she had not been able to protect either herself or her children from her physically abusive husband. In other words, she had not been able to establish and maintain boundaries to keep herself and her children safe.

In the group meetings she expressed her grief. She realized that she had rationalized his behavior at the time to herself and to her children, thus allowing his behavior to continue.

When her adult daughter unexpectedly confronted her with her unprotectiveness, she first pleaded ignorance about the extent of the abuse. Then when her daughter asked why she hadn't left her husband and taken the kids with her, she became defensive. Overwhelmed by her own emotions about the abuse, Thalia became immobilized and started to cry. Her daughter, perceiving that her pain had not been acknowledged by Thalia, became verbally abusive, shouting at Thalia about her incompetence as a mother.

When Thalia brought this incident to group, the group helped her recognize that her own boundaries had just been violated by her daughter's abusive attack. Just as she should have stopped her husband's abuse, she needed to stop her daughter's abuse.

She learned to stop a conversation when she felt overwhelmed — and how to schedule it for another time. She learned to ask in advance what the topic of conversation was going to be, and to assess whether or not she was up it. She learned to call her daughter to accountability for violating her boundaries.

Maintaining good boundaries is a common difficulty for recovering parents. We so identify with our children's pain that we fail to hold up our boundaries and find ourselves being abused in the process.

The Native American community has given me another metaphor for understanding and respecting boundaries. In some tribes the women carried a basket known as a burden basket. They carried this basket on their backs for gathering wood, grasses or other small items. When it was not in use, it hung on a pole outside their lodge or tipi. Then it served to remind guests to leave their burdens outside before entering.

I have often thought of this image when exchanging visits with my adult children. Each of their homes is their sacred space, as the lodge or tipi was in tribal communities. Before entering, I check to see that my personal burdens, and any excess emotionality or reactivity, are left outside and do not intrude into their space. We do not dump our personal burdens uninvited into each other's spaces. These small acts of respect support healing.

There is another kind of boundary we need to learn to set as well as we heal with our children — the boundary of detachment. It is difficult to watch our children begin to live out the same destructive behavior patterns we engaged in. We want to go back and reparent them. We want to save them from repeating our mistakes. Part of our healing process is to detach — to let them make their own mistakes and be in charge of their own lives.

Mary, another member of my group, struggled with this issue. Her son, who had two children of his own, was a cocaine addict. Seeing her grandchildren unkempt and often without proper clothes reminded Mary of her own childhood in poverty. She consistently found herself spending her limited income buying them food and clothes, taking them to school or caring for them in some other way. She also lent her son money or bailed him out of his difficulties.

In raising her son, Mary had done the best she could. Still she grieved that it hadn't been good enough. She had not protected her son from his father's violent outbursts. Even though she had had good intentions for working outside her home — so her son would not have to grow up in the poverty she had experienced as a child — she still felt guilty that she had not given him enough time and attention.

As her work in the group progressed, she learned to grieve for herself — for her lost opportunities and her own wounded child. She inventoried her parental strengths and liabilities. She came to see that her son's father also had some responsibility for her son's pain. With the group's help, she learned to see the irrationality of berating herself for not giving her children skills she hadn't had at the time herself. Finally the group confronted her gently when she reported engaging in behaviors she wished to change — like trying to rescue her son and grandchildren.

Mary needed to learn how to keep clear boundaries between her life and her son's life. She needed to allow him to have his own journey. With the group's support and encouragement, she learned to allow him the consequences of his behavior even though she knew her grandchildren might suffer.

For Mary, this meant no longer rescuing her son with money. It meant watching her grandchildren be placed in protective custody instead of trying to take them into her own home, something her ill health and limited resources would have made very difficult. Rescuing her son might have temporarily assuaged her guilt, but it would not have let him feel the consequences of his actions, nor would it have let him take responsibility for recovering from his disease.

With the group continually reminding her, she could see that she was not solely responsible for her son's deteriorating life. She could also see how rescuing her son supported his addictive behavior. With support from her allies, she learned to set firm boundaries and keep herself safe from her son's addictive, abusive and manipulative behavior.

---
**EXERCISE**
---

1. Imagine a boundary you would like to set with your adult child. Write it down.

2. What do you fear about setting this boundary? What makes you uncomfortable about setting this boundary?

3. If you set this boundary and get a negative response, will you survive?

4. If the answer to 3 is yes, write out an imaginary situation in which you set this boundary with your adult child.

5. Write out some realistic supportive statements to remind yourself it is okay to set boundaries. Mary's supportive statements looked like this:

---

I have the right to say no to my son when he asks me for money which he uses for his drug abuse habit. I do love him and my grandchildren. If I am financially able, I will buy the children clothes or toys. If he threatens me with not being allowed to see the children, I will be sad; but I will survive.

---

6. Write the names of people who can support you in setting boundaries. If you don't have much experience in setting boundaries, you will need a friend, a sponsor or a therapist as backup. Write a plan for how you will contact that person to discuss this issue.

---

## Negotiating Boundaries

Often boundaries can be defined by negotiating them before the next situation arises. Here is a four-step process for negotiating boundaries adapted from *Lifeskills For Adult Children* by Janet Woititz and Alan Garner.

1. *Define* your boundaries as specifically as possible. Identify what is acceptable and what is not.

2. *Express* to your adult child what your concerns are and what your absolute boundary is.

3. *Listen.* Once you have stated your limits, listen to your adult child's considerations and feelings. Determine what boundary is best.

4. *Act.* Develop and agree on a plan of action. This will undoubtedly involve some compromises for both of you.

---

## EXERCISE

1. Ask a partner to do this exercise with you.

2. Pick a boundary you would like to set with your adult child. If you have several boundaries you need to set, start with the easiest one on your list.

3. First, play your role and ask your partner to play your child's. Practice setting the boundary in various ways.

4. Then switch roles. Notice what it feels like to be in each role.

5. Finally, repeat the exercise with you once again playing your own role. Ask yourself how response able you are in this negotiation.

---

## Maintaining Boundaries

Once you have clearly communicated your boundaries, you can use "the broken record technique" if the boundary is challenged. Using this technique, you repeat your boundary over and over again like a broken record. For example, "If I have enough money, I will buy the kids shoes, but I will not give you cash. If I have enough money, I will buy the kids shoes, but I will not give you cash."

Pay attention to your tone of voice and body language. If you speak too softly or are too hesitant, you may not be taken seriously.

It is important to decide what you will do if a boundary is not honored. What is your contingency plan? What consequences will you set in motion? Make sure the plan is something you can really follow through on when the time comes.

You need to tell your adult child the consequences in a non-threatening, matter-of-fact way. Mary told her son, for example, "If you continue to call me only to ask for cash, I will need to hang up on you."

---

## EXERCISE

1. With a friend or sponsor, role-play using the broken record technique with your adult child. Remember to switch roles.

2. Write out all the possible ways the boundary you have set, or plan to set, can be broken.

3. Write out your contingency plan or consequences.

4. Role-play telling your adult child about the consequences.

5. Role-play carrying out the consequences.

---

## Accountability

As a parent I am accountable for my parenting. I am not excused because I have a disease or because I was ignorant.

Every child has the right to a nurturing and protected childhood. Even when I was a parent in recovery, I was not always able to provide that.

My adult children have feelings about not having received what was rightfully theirs. They have the right to call me to account for that.

## Forgiveness

When we forgive someone, we acknowledge the real and perceived hurts that person caused us. We acknowledge the person's imperfections. We release our resentments and our desire to punish that person.

When we forgive ourselves, we acknowledge the real and perceived hurts we caused other people and ourselves. We acknowledge our own imperfections. We release our anger and our desire to punish ourselves.

Forgiving does not mean we forget the hurts or the imperfections. We will always have scars to remind us. But when we forgive, we release the pain around the memory. The wound is allowed to heal. We regain our balance. People who have experienced forgiving themselves, or someone else, sometimes call forgiveness grace.

Forgiveness most benefits the one doing it. Being forgiven may assuage guilt, but forgiving moves us into serenity, tolerance and openness. Both forgiving and being forgiven allow healing and the bridging of broken relationships.

## Not Forgiving

When we have not yet forgiven ourselves, our parents or our children, those relationships are broken. In extreme cases, there may be a physical break. We may have no contact at all with people we have not forgiven. But even if we do have contact with them, being unforgiving — holding resentments, guilt, fear or anger — makes us feel out of balance. We become extremely cautious. We rarely feel joyful or spontaneous or relaxed around them. The relationship is fragile.

Miriam, for example, had never forgiven herself for her imperfect parenting. As a result, she had mixed feelings about spending time with her adult children.

On the one hand, she was excited to see them and to see her grandchildren. On the other hand, she always felt she was walking on eggshells when she was with them, worrying she might do or say something to offend them.

Both her son and daughter had openly expressed anger to her about their childhoods. Discussions about the past, however, had ended in stalemates.

Finally Miriam's daughter wrote her a letter stating she would no longer be in contact. She said she needed a time out to heal. She felt their conversations were hurtful.

Miriam was devastated by this complete break in their relationship. It was further proof of her failure. "Besides," Miriam said to herself, "if I don't forgive myself for my own imperfections, why should I expect my daughter to forgive me?"

## Forgiving Ourselves

Most recovering parents have a difficult time with self-forgiveness because we struggle with our own imperfections. I have agonized over the effect I had on my adopted son, for example. What a shame that he was given up by one mother only to be adopted by me, an alcoholic mom. How could I have done that to him? To me?

For many of us, self-forgiveness is a long, slow process. It comes over time as we are able to place our lives in the context of life events. We are accountable for any harmful or hurtful behavior we have engaged in, but we cannot go through life being our own ongoing judge, jury and executioner.

For example, to continue to punish myself for my alcoholism does not allow my life to move forward in a healthy relationship with my children or with myself. Forward movement is supported by heartfelt amends and behavioral changes that move us toward self-forgiveness.

When I adopted Jonathan, I did not know I had the disease of alcoholism. In order to move toward self-forgiveness, I needed to make amends to him for my actions. However, before making amends to Jonathan, I had to make amends to myself. I found that over time this was possible as I understood my alcoholism was my path to spirituality and I had a purpose in my life. My recovery from alcoholism taught me how to have a deeper and more honest relationship with myself, with others and with my Higher Power.

Jonathan's acceptance of my amends allowed the relationship between us to continue. Making amends and changing my behavior — becoming sober — in turn allowed me to forgive myself and supported me in that undertaking.

## Receiving Forgiveness

Sometimes receiving forgiveness from an adult child can allow us to forgive ourselves. Sometimes our children can give us a new perspective on the failings and struggles we feel so guilty about.

At the beginning of this chapter, I described a very emotional exchange between my son Jonathan and myself during my early recovery. Our exchanges during that time were less than satisfactory. Little did I know then that a precious healing was slowly taking place in him.

A few years after that exchange, Jonathan elected to go into the Army instead of working or going to college. While he was in the service, the Persian Gulf war broke out. On the eve of the war, he wrote each of his family members a good-bye letter. Here is part of the letter he wrote to me:

---

Dear Mom,

I am really scared. I don't know if I will ever see you again. . . . There are some things I want to tell you. I am very proud of you for the way you have changed. That takes courage! I admire you, Mom, and hope when the time comes for me to face my own stuff that I can be like you. You have been a tremendous role model for me. . . . I love you!

Your son,
Jonathan

---

Although I had long since surrendered to knowing I had a disease that is in part genetic, I had not forgiven myself for the hurts I had caused while drinking. Deep inside I still believed that I should have been perfect — I should have been able not to drink — and therefore not to cause harm. Like Miriam, I believed I was unforgivable.

The reality was, of course, that aside from my alcoholism, I had many other imperfections. Knowing that Jonathan not only forgave me but also had received something valuable from me helped me forgive myself and helped our relationship grow stronger.

## EXERCISE

1. Turn back to Chapter 12, "Taking Stock". Look at the attitudes or behaviors or events you feel guilty about. Are there any positive lessons your children might have learned from them? Are there any positive lessons your children might have learned from your recovery or from changes you have made in your attitudes or behaviors?

2. Remind yourself that if you were perfect, you would be God.

## Forgiving Others

Sometimes it is we parents who have trouble forgiving others: our spouse or partner, our parents or even our adult children. If we come from a long line of alcoholics, we may feel unforgiving rage about having inherited alcoholism from our family. Or we may not be able to forgive our dysfunctional family for the legacy of destructive behaviors they passed on to us.

If we are not addicted and there is no substance abuse in our family, we may feel furious that our adult children are addicted and irresponsible in their parenting. I have worked with several grandparents who have had the painful ordeal of witnessing their adult children surrender to addictive disease. In the process their grandchildren were taken from their adult children by Children's Protective Services and placed in less-than-adequate foster care. Their grief has been enormous, and their effort to forgive, heroic.

As I said earlier, forgiveness most benefits the one doing it. We increase our own serenity, tolerance and openness when we forgive. A side benefit is that we also show our children that it is possible to forgive. We model forgiving for them — a skill that will come in handy for them when they run into things they need to forgive us for.

## EXERCISE

1. Write down the names of people you need to forgive.

2. For each one, write the answer to these questions:

a. How is holding on to the anger or resentment toward this person serving me? (For instance, sometimes I have found we hold on to guilt or anger so that we don't have to confront the offense or the offender.)

b. If I were to let the anger and resentment toward this person go, what would my life be like?

c. Is there something I need before I can do this?

3. Make a plan to get what you need in order to forgive.

4. Imagine yourself being able to forgive each person.

---

## What Allows Forgiveness?

*Being willing.* Be open and vulnerable to forgiving.

*Understanding.* Place the event in its correct historical context. As a parent, it may have taken you time to get the strength, skills and resources to move your children and yourself from an abusive situation. Domestic shelters and treatment centers were not readily available 20 years ago.

*Acknowledging.* Without judgment, acknowledge your imperfections or the imperfections of others.

*Letting yourself feel your loneliness.* Notice that the absence of the other person is more painful than his presence.

When Miriam's daughter cut her off, Miriam's loneliness gave her the impetus she needed to work on her own self-forgiveness. Adult children who take space from their parents often miss them. A time of complete absence allows the children to heal, as well as to reconsider all that their parents mean to them — the positives as well as the liabilities.

Miriam's daughter did eventually reconnect with Miriam and express her appreciation for what Miriam had done in the way of positive parenting. This supported Miriam's self-forgiveness.

*Letting yourself feel your commitment.* Feel the depth of your commitment to the relationship, for then you are often more willing to release the resentments and no longer assign blame. I have frequently witnessed this happen in Al-Anon.

*Letting yourself feel your pain.* Consider, as my colleague Constance Huey says, "It may just be less painful to forgive and let go than to keep a wound open by hanging on to resentments."

## What Disallows Forgiveness?

*Continuing the behavior* that caused pain initially. For instance, if you say you are sorry but then continue to violate your adult children's boundaries with abusive behavior, they won't be able to forgive you for abusing them.

*Repeatedly calling attention to past hurts and scars.* For example, when Miriam visited her son, he always asked her sarcastically how she was doing with her recovery "this time."

*Talking as though the past were the present.* Miriam's son also made remarks about how Miriam was a "late person," even though Miriam had not been late in meeting with him for the past year.

*Not believing an event or behavior is forgivable.*

## Chronic Unforgiveness

When we are chronically unforgiving, we are constricted or tightly bound. We can't let go of past hurts and resentments. We stay stuck in a static place.

For example, if I can't forgive my past, I am stuck in it. Because it is not resolved, it holds my present attention and I focus on it. Being stuck feels like being a victim. I feel trapped. I can't go back and I can't move forward.

Because I can't resolve the past, the best I can do is try to forget it. Addictions that numb feelings and anesthetize assist this process. They support a victim stance of immobilization and non-resolution.

I have observed that many recovering parents suffer from a belief that they, as human beings, were unworthy to begin with. They see their alcoholism as evidence that supports this belief. They feel in some way irreparably damaged.

Their feeling of unworthiness may stem from having been born a girl when Mom or Dad wanted a boy. Subsequently it has been made worse by the self-inflicted wound of addiction.

Because they cannot forgive themselves either for a mistaken belief, such as being born the wrong sex, or for having a disease, they perceive the world as not being good or safe, and they want to get out or go away. The getting out or going away is done through self-destructive behavior, such as addiction. Their internal sense of personal unworthiness and the world's being unsafe is passed unwittingly on to their children.

For some parents, the unpardonable sin is that they were born feeling unworthy. If they are in a stance of chronic unforgiveness about this, they have difficulty receiving or giving love. Because they don't feel worthy of receiving love, they don't take it in when it is given, and they have difficulty giving love because they haven't received it.

---

## EXERCISE

Take some time to ask yourself the following questions:

- Am I suffering from a wound of unworthiness?
- Is this my unpardonable sin?
- Is it possible that my belief about myself is incorrect and that I am and always have been adequate?
- Am I keeping myself a victim with my unforgiveness?

---

## The Unpardonable Sin

What if you believe you have committed the unpardonable sin? What if you are the parent who has to own that your child's learning disorder may well be the result of your drinking during pregnancy? Or what if you were under the influence of drugs when you drove your car into a telephone pole, leaving your child permanently damaged or even dead? What if you are the parent who introduced your child to drugs or molested him or her? For many parents, coming to terms with these events is like dealing with unpardonable sins.

A woman at one of our seminars for recovering parents tearfully talked about how she felt responsible and unpardonable for the death of her child. The room became totally silent. I am not sure any of us knew exactly how to respond to the enormity of her loss. We felt, and indeed we were, powerless.

In the back of the room, another woman moved closer to a staff member and whispered, "I have had a similar experience." At the break we brought these two women together.

Sharing with someone who has had a similar experience is the beginning of the healing and forgiveness process in such circumstances. Each woman thought she alone had committed the unpardonable sin. Finding someone who was dealing with the same issue released the tension of guilt and allowed the possibility of other feelings and outcomes.

When we are responsible for something as significant as the death of a child, we may carry grief about that at some level for the rest of our lives. The fact that we always carry some grief, however, does not mean we must also carry unforgiveness toward ourselves.

## When Is Forgiveness Appropriate?

It is appropriate to forgive someone when we have boundaries to protect us from further wounding by that person. It is also appropriate to forgive when we feel complete with an issue, that is to say, when we have examined it, released our emotions and made peace with imperfection.

Jonathan had worked through much of his anger with me in the years preceding the letter he wrote. He took the time to examine the effect of my behavior on him, and he was able to complete the issue by accepting my alcoholism, seeing that it held some meaning for him and forgiving my parental imperfections.

## Phases Of Forgiveness

In a presentation on forgiveness, Martin Rossman, M.D., and Roxanne Whitelight, M.A., shared these thoughts about the process or phases of forgiveness:

1. Recognize the wound is there.
2. Feel the feelings.
3. Express the feelings in a nondestructive way.
4. Find a frame of reference, a way of understanding or a context for feelings and experience: How have I been hurt? In what way have I been hurt?

5. Look for benefits or gains from the experience.

6. Let go of any grievances or resentments toward self and others.

7. Use imagery, meditation or rituals to formalize the letting go.

## Forgiveness Tools

In my work with recovering parents I have found that imagery, meditation and rituals are effective tools for forgiveness.

To use *imagery,* find a quiet place where you can close your eyes and relax. Take some deep breaths. Find in the quietness of your mind a safe or peaceful place. It might be a real place or a place you imagine. When you have located your safe place, find somewhere inside it to sit down.

Invite a wisdom figure, an inner advisor or someone you respect to come and be with you. Talk to that person about your concerns with forgiveness. Ask that person to share related thoughts and feelings. And express your thanks.

Imagery is a good way to access your own inner wisdom. All the answers are not outside you. I believe, in fact, that you already have the answers. You only need to find a way to access them.

*Meditation* is an excellent way to de-escalate from overwhelming feelings. It is a way to clear or quiet the mind so your inner self can speak.

Your conscious mind does not have all the answers. You also have an unconscious self whose wisdom can be accessed if you are willing to sit in silence. You have wisdom and healing energy that can be tapped into by quieting your mind.

Some people do this by focusing on their breath or by chanting. To focus on your breath, sit in a relaxed position and pay attention only to the feeling of your breath as it passes by the tip of your nose each time you inhale and exhale.

If you want to try chanting, an easy chant to clear your mind is the Eastern chant of *om.* As you exhale, say in your mind, "Ooooooooommmmmmm," until you run out of breath. Then inhale and begin again.

*Rituals* make our internal beliefs external. Some parents who were participating in a 12-Step program were encouraged to make a God box. This was a cardboard box with a slit on top.

After working through an issue for which they needed forgiveness — after they had examined it, grieved over it — they named the issue on a piece of paper. As a symbol of releasing it, or of giving it to God, they placed the paper in the box.

One recovering parent created a ritual that could remind her of having been forgiven and of her strengths. She made herself a tape stating what she was forgiven for and what she perceived to be her strengths. These were affirmations.

Then she brought the tape to a group meeting, and other parents added their affirmations to the tape. She found that other people's affirmations made her statements more real because these were people who knew her and her story. She plays the tape during her morning meditation as part of her personal ritual.

## How Do We Know We Are Healed?

We know we are healed when we can name and claim all the parts of ourselves — when we know and accept our strengths as well as our weaknesses. We know we are healed when we can accept both the strengths and weaknesses of the people who have hurt us as well.

We know we are healed when all our emotions are accessible. When we were out of balance, we felt or acted only in limited ways.

For example, when I was working through my grief about the impact of my alcoholism on my sons' lives, my emotions were largely negative — regret for what I had done, sadness at what it must have been like for them and anger at the genetics and legacy I had inherited and passed on. I did not feel joy, curiosity about life, exhilaration or peace. Once we have done some healing, positive feelings are again part of our lives.

We know we are healed when our stories include not only the pathos we have experienced in the past but also the serenity and hope we feel in the present.

We find that, as we are able to forgive ourselves, we become more able to forgive others for their imperfections and hurtful behaviors.

I found that when I couldn't forgive myself, I was disconnected from myself; I didn't trust myself. My negative judgments and dislike of myself kept me from being me.

In early recovery, for example, I was always watching myself for any slips or inappropriate behavior. I was stiff and controlled. As healing and forgiveness inched their way into my life, I became lighter and more spontaneous and smiled more easily. Moments of joy began to balance torrents of grief.

We know we are healed when we can maintain our serenity and be compassionate even in the midst of chaos, disappointment and ambiguity. We are aware of the self-knowledge and wisdom we have gained.

We know we are healed when we can let our adult children live their lives as they will. They may repeat our mistakes because they carry our legacy, but if we are truly healed, our lives will not be dominated by guilt or sadness about what they are doing or by plans to rescue them.

There is a 12-Step saying: "The more you recover, the more you remember." For a while, the more I recovered, the more memories I accessed that called for grieving, healing and forgiveness. But it became easier as I learned how the healing worked and saw that it yielded wonderful gifts. Now the process is mine to keep and use whenever I need it.

As we heal, we often claim a spiritual dimension to our experience. Even though we may still struggle with the most difficult situations — like having a child who is alcohol fetal affected or being cut off by our angry adult children — we find ourselves sustained by a belief: even though we don't always know why such terrible things have happened, somewhere it is known. This belief, that somewhere it is known, has been enough to bring our lives back into balance.

The gift that healing and forgiveness bring is the gift of relationship. We can have a whole, healthy relationship with ourselves instead of being distant or disconnected from parts of ourselves. We can own who we are, totally, without denigration, shame or guilt. We can build loving relationships with our adult children, recognizing who they are in their own right. And we can have a relationship with a Mystery, Higher Self or God who reassures us that out of painful experiences can come new life and unexpected gifts.

# SECTION

## IV

# INTER-GENERATIONAL HEALING

# CHAPTER

# 15

# Before We Talk
# With Our Children

In this chapter we are going to look at the nuts and bolts of preparing ourselves to talk with our children. We will assess our own readiness and our children's readiness. We will determine what we should do if our children confront us.

Before we focus on the specifics, however, it's important to put this conversation with our children into a context. Just as we looked at our time lines to see how external events were affecting us as we parented our children, we need to look at what's going on in our lives right now.

## Midlife

We are at midlife. It may sting when I say that, but for most of us, that is a reality.

We can divide life into three fairly large segments: ages 0 to 30, 31 to 60 and 61 to 90. During the first segment, the morning of our life, we move from childhood into young adulthood; we leave home, stand on our own two feet and begin taking on the commitments of intimacy, children and work.

In the middle time period, the afternoon of life, we begin reckoning for the first time with our own mortality. As this time period starts, we begin realizing that the amount of sand in our life's hourglass is one-third in the bottom and two-thirds in the top. When this time period ends, two-thirds of the sand will be in the bottom and one-third will be in the top, depending upon how long we live.

Facing the issues between ourselves and our children is only a small part of what we need to do during this time in our life. It's important to look at all the tasks of midlife for a moment so that we can identify the feelings we may be flooded with that arise from our relationship with our children, and those that arise from the natural challenges of midlife.

As we face our own mortality, and the aging and mortality of our parents, we realize we have limited time to sweep the debris of unfinished business off our life path and limited time to realize our dreams. We also realize we have limited financial, emotional and health resources. We must set priorities.

## Self

Some of the business we will be cleaning up in the next decades will have to do with our own self-development — midlife is second only to adolescence in terms of presenting an opportunity to develop our own unique sense of self more fully. That is to say, it is our next major, and in all likelihood our last, opportunity to become fully ourselves, owned by no one but ourselves, governed and directed by our own values and beliefs.

Up to this point, we have often been governed by the unconscious beliefs of our childhood and by our unfinished business with our family of origin. Much of what we have done has been done either to please or displease our parents, the parents of our partner, the culture or our partner. Someone else has been piping the tune for our behavior. Midlife is an opportunity for us genuinely to throw off the shackles of other people's expectations and to write a blueprint for our lives that really fits us.

Some of this life evaluation is set in motion by the onset of what I call the "nevers." When we get to midlife we begin realizing that certain things are never going to happen. We're never going to be an Olympic gold medalist; we're never going to be a ballet dancer.

At this time in life, we are confronted with our own limitations, with the likelihood that certain things we thought we would achieve will, in fact, go undone. We begin to recognize that there is only so much time left to accomplish what we most want to accomplish.

For example, as men, were we taught that our role in adulthood should be to support our family financially and to commit ourselves to our work life? At midlife we may begin questioning whether we want work to have such primacy.

Maybe we're tired of being so responsible. Maybe long ago we ceased to find our job exciting. We may suddenly find that there are a million things that intrigue us, some of which we have not thought about for 20 years because we were committed to the work harness and didn't have the luxury of even looking beyond our blinders.

Maybe we no longer want to be so competitive and so aggressive. Maybe we find ourselves becoming more interested in things that are philosophical and spiritual. Maybe we find ourselves more tender, more feeling and more gentle.

As women, we may have been taught that our worth and value was predicated on our youth, our attractiveness, our willingness to provide for our children and our ability to nurture and take care of the needs of others. Perhaps we, too, are beginning to feel tired and to wonder when it will be our turn.

With the gradual onset of menopausal symptoms, we have to confront the loss of our capacity to bear children, as well as the loss of our youth and a change in our attractiveness. If we do not reorder our priorities and redefine our identity to establish a new sense of personal and social value, we will go into the next decade of our lives in a state of despair.

Now that our children are grown, we may decide to go into the work world for the first time or to quit the job we've had and go back to school. It becomes increasingly acceptable for us to be competent. We assume a sense of personal authority that men had conferred upon them by the social order far earlier.

## Couple

Midlife may also be the first time in 20 or 30 years that we can focus on our couple relationship unencumbered by children. We may have grown distant from our spouse or partner over the years of family life. We may have become so busy with work and income, with succeeding and with raising children, that we lost one another along the way. We may not even have noticed the vacuum in our intimate life.

Midlife brings with it the often frightening and risky opportunity to stop and look at our spouse or partner and say, "Who is this person? What kind of relationship do I want with this person now?"

We may find that the compromises we made with our partner no longer meet our individual needs — the compromises about who was to lead and who was to follow, the compromises about who had the power and how much, and over what and when. We need to renegotiate, and this renegotiation can be terrifying.

If we take the risk of changing our relationship and of upsetting the balance we have created, we fear the relationship will shatter. This is not an unrealistic fear; the forties are the decade of unnecessary divorces and separations. We sometimes fail to realize that the source of our unhappiness is not our partner, nor is it the discord we are having with our children. The source of our unhappiness is the set of assumptions by which we have lived our lives and which no longer suit us.

During midlife we can end up feeling tremendously disoriented, confused and in a crisis. We may feel that the only difference between a rut and a grave is one of dimension.

Maybe everything we have been doing up to this time has fit just fine, but suddenly it doesn't seem to fit any longer. It's taken us half a lifetime to feel we have become good at certain things, and all of a sudden the value of those things is thrown into question.

We may think we are going crazy. We may feel burned out. Although we may be in a crisis, it is really the crisis of growth, opportunity and transition. And it's important to know that it is normal.

## Losses

A tremendous number of losses are scheduled to occur during midlife as part of our natural life cycle. Some of us may have lost a parent in childhood because of death, desertion or divorce, or we may have lost a parent in our twenties or thirties to substance abuse or mental illness. It was probably difficult for us to mourn the loss at that time because we were out of sync with what was happening with other children or other young adults. They could still maintain the illusion that their parents would always be there, but we could not. If we haven't lost a parent yet, as we come into our late thirties, forties and fifties, we and our peers have to confront the loss of our parents through aging as part of the natural life cycle.

During our forties, probably more than any other decade, life can feel as though all hell has broken loose. We may have a parent who is seriously ill, a spouse with a major crisis such as infidelity or a layoff at work and a child who can't emancipate or who is having serious emotional problems. We may also be confronting the feeling that if we had known we were going to live so long, we would have taken better care of ourselves because our own health may be starting to falter. During midlife, women face hysterectomies and mastectomies, and men face prostate cancer and heart trouble.

We cannot stay the hand of time for ourselves or for our parents, and we begin anticipatory mourning. We mourn the growing up and launching of our children, the anticipatory or real loss of our parents and the "I'll-live-forever" feeling of our youthfulness. We may no longer experience ourselves as having limitless vitality and zest. Our bones may creak, our knees may not work like they used to, and we may get tired more easily than we used to. We are not only being confronted with our parents' illness, aging and death; when we look in the mirror, we are beginning to see our parents looking back.

Because we no longer live with the childhood illusion that our parents will live forever, we begin the process of finishing unfinished emotional business with them. If they are still living, we have the opportunity to resolve more issues with them. Potentially we can come to forgive them, and they can come to forgive us. They can be freer to go, and we can be left behind less burdened by our own anger, disappointment and hurt.

We also begin finishing unfinished emotional business with our siblings. We realize that we had best reopen cutoffs and reestablish our relationships because they will be our family 20 and 30 years after our parents have died.

## Finances

As all hell seems to break loose in our lives, we may begin to have serious questions about whether we will have enough money for our own retirement. Will we be able to realize the dream we have dreamed of the postchildren era of our lives?

It costs so much more for our children to go to college than we had ever anticipated. Our daughter's husband has left her with a small child and no education.

We find we cannot allocate our resources only to ourselves. We feel that it is incumbent upon us to help each of our children who is in trouble, each of our siblings who is in trouble and each of our parents who is in trouble. We wonder what will happen to us. We had never anticipated these demands on our financial resources.

We had never anticipated how expensive it would be to live when we arrived at this time in our lives. Nor had we anticipated that the companies for which we have worked would not take good care of us in retirement. Suddenly we are expensive objects in a volatile global economy that they cannot afford to keep. We may be approaching an expensive retirement and thus be "let go" before we are fully vested in our company's pension plan.

## Spirituality

It's no wonder that many of us begin pursuing a spiritual path for the first time in many years. We turn to God or a Higher Power in the hope that faith will be a buffer against the vicissitudes of midlife.

I think of a woman I know who is in midlife. During the past ten years a sibling has committed suicide; both of her parents had been ill with long, painful illnesses and finally died slow deaths; she has lost property to a fire; her husband of many years has hit his own midlife crisis complete with multiple affairs; she and her husband have divorced and gone through a very painful property settlement. On top of this, one of her grown children has developed multiple sclerosis, and she herself has become preoccupied by a fear that these ten difficult years will result in an illness in her fifties, as happened with her parents, who also had difficult lives. All of these events totally altered her vision of what her future would be like.

When I asked her how she had stayed vertical with her nose holes above the water line during these ten years, she said that she had turned to God for solace. That had it not been for turning to God, she would have succumbed.

At this time in our lives, we may find ourselves preoccupied with our own mortality, and we may, for the first time since we were children, renew our interest in spirituality. We may rework our beliefs about the meaning of life and the meaning of death. We may ask ourselves upon whom we will rely when our partner and our parents are either no longer here or here but no longer sources of solace? We may, in fact, decide to rely on a power greater than ourselves in order to get through these difficult times.

## Grandchildren

During midlife, some of us take on, either willingly or grudgingly, the responsibility of raising our grandchildren. Large numbers of adult children are disabled by drugs or alcohol or by lifestyles that do not allow them to generate enough income or to have sufficient responsibility to commit themselves to child-rearing.

If we have taken legal or custodial responsibility for our grandchildren because our children are dysfunctional, at some level we probably feel it is our fault that our grandchildren are deprived of capable parents. We have the midlife task not only of figuring out what is best for our grandchildren, but also of sorting through our own guilt so we can give appropriate weight to the adult choices our children are making that contribute to their parental dysfunctions.

## Children

Finally, we have the midlife task of dealing with our children. If our children leave home, we will have to mourn their leaving. Even if we have been saying for years that we'll be glad when they're gone, we will grieve when they actually go.

We may have to confront our children who don't leave, who don't emancipate. Some of our children may see home as comfortable and the world out there as scary. Or we may have given our children a covert message that we needed them at home with the result that they didn't leave home and are still with us through midlife.

We may have to deal with our children's "boomeranging." In their thirties and forties, some adult children boomerang and come back home to live, not so much because they can't make it economically in the world as because they have been socialized to a standard of living they cannot create for themselves. At this time in history our children have to confront the expectation that they and their children will, in all likelihood, never achieve the standard of living that we were able to provide for them.

This poses a dilemma for us. Do we allow them to stay for a while, hoping we can help them relaunch, or are they digging in like chiggers under our skin to stay forever?

Even if our children have successfully and permanently emancipated, our relationships with them will most likely be more complicated during midlife. All children, particularly in their late twenties and early thirties, need to repudiate us at some level as part of their process of separating.

It is very difficult for us as parents when our children need to have distance from us. It's difficult for us to remember that this is a normal part of the growth process. Our children take ownership of their own lives partly by remembering, with a distorted retrospective lens that leans toward the negative, how we reared them and what we did to them.

Sometimes their perspective isn't distorted by their having incorrect facts; all children take in their experiences in idiosyncratic ways. Because they were small or immature, they didn't have the capacity to check out with us the conclusions they came to and the assumptions they made about what was happening to them or why.

The reality is that in order for our children to fully emancipate from us, they need to remember everything they feel we did wrong and all of the experiences they absorbed in a wounding way. We may have had a close relationship with our children until they hit their middle or late twenties, when suddenly we became the bad guys. It's important to remember, through the pain, that this part of their child's journey is natural and temporary, even though *temporary* can mean years in duration.

## Parenting

Finally, we must deal with our own remorse and regret about our parenting, which is what this book is about. During midlife, we see our children as the fully grown adults they have become, and perhaps as the young parents they now are, and we can see some imprints of the past in their present lives.

Perhaps we see them making the same mistakes with their partners or children that we made. We view our children with the wisdom and experience of the present, and we wish we could have been more mature, more adequate parents when they were small. We begin mourning our past inadequacies.

Each of us will respond differently to this time of looking at our children and our parenting from a new perspective. Some of us were raised in families where our parents said, "Look, we did the best we could; don't cry over spilled milk; don't look back; just move on." We may have the same style ourselves as we pause and look at our children. We may not realize that we feel defensive or anxious. If our children confront or rebuke us, we may give them either a silent or a verbalized "Don't talk" message: "The past is the past; I did the best I could; you didn't turn out so bad; don't complain now."

Some of us will be at the other end of the continuum of parental-reactions. We will view every nuance of our adult children's behavior as a living indictment of our inadequacy as parents and as human beings. We will be parentally co-dependent to the nth degree. We will meddle in our children's lives. We will confess and *mea culpa* until they want to kill us. We will offer them therapy and buy them self-help books, constantly telling them how dysfunctional they are and how much it is our fault.

The fact is that they may experience themselves as being fine. They may not reproach or rebuke us. What they do experience is our neuroticism, meddling, anxiety and guilt.

Somewhere between these two extremes lies a more useful middle position where we are willing to look at what we feel remorse about, sort out what parts of our remorse are realistic, mourn what we regret and take our own healing journey.

When we reach midlife, there is a whole series of tasks to complete and a whole list of unfinished business that needs to be finished, including healing in our parental role. As we go about that job, we must keep in mind the other stresses and challenges we are facing in midlife. We must give ourselves credit for the work we are doing on these tasks and acknowledge the time and energy we are spending. We need to give each task its due.

How we resolve the tasks of midlife will determine the quality of the evening of our life. If we do not deal with our own psychological tasks at this time in life, we will go into the evening of our life with a sense of stagnation and despair. It is essential to our own future that we resolve our multitude of issues.

It is also essential to our children and our grandchildren that we complete our midlife tasks. What we do with this time period will determine the kind of person they will relate to in the future.

## EXERCISE

How much time and energy is each of the midlife tasks taking up in your life right now? Is each issue difficult, or are some of them easy? Is each one mostly resolved, or are some of them still waiting to be addressed?

For instance, your finances may be fine right now, but when you look ahead, you may see expenses coming that may surpass your budget. Or even though you have done some financial planning, you may know you have a lot more financial planning to do. In this case, you might say that finances are not an issue right now, but pretty unresolved. If you used an *M* to represent Myself, and plotted yourself on two scales — they might look like this:

## FINANCES

```
_____ M _____
Easy                                    Difficult
```

```
_____ M _____
Resolved                              Unresolved
```

Putting yourself on the scales can give you a picture of how much energy you need now, and how much energy you can expect to need, for the issue of finance.

Now it's your turn. Place an *M* for Myself on the scales below. You can't know for sure, of course, how much each issue is resolved, but make your best guess.

## SELF/NEW BLUEPRINT

```
_____
Easy                                    Difficult
```

```
_____
Resolved                              Unresolved
```

## COUPLE

```
_____
Easy                                    Difficult
```

```
_____
Resolved                              Unresolved
```

## LOSSES

```
_____
Easy                                    Difficult
```

```
_____
Resolved                              Unresolved
```

## FINANCES

```
_____
Easy                                    Difficult
```

| Resolved | Unresolved |
|---|---|
| **SPIRITUALITY** | |

| Easy | Difficult |
|---|---|

| Resolved | Unresolved |
|---|---|
| **GRANDCHILDREN** | |

| Easy | Difficult |
|---|---|

| Resolved | Unresolved |
|---|---|
| **CHILDREN** | |

| Easy | Difficult |
|---|---|

| Resolved | Unresolved |
|---|---|
| **PARENTING** | |

| Easy | Difficult |
|---|---|

| Resolved | Unresolved |
|---|---|

When you look at all the scales together, you have a snap-shot of how much energy your midlife tasks are consuming right now. Although no one can predict these things perfect-ly, you have some idea how much of your midlife journey may be behind you and how much may be still ahead.

## Preparing Ourselves

Now that we have put our unfinished business with our chil-dren into its proper perspective as only one of the midlife tasks, let's move on to look at how we might prepare ourselves to talk with our children or to make ourselves available to them when they are ready to talk with us. We will go through a number of questions and checklists in order to get a sense of how ready we are to deal directly with our children.

First and foremost, keep in mind that healing is a time-dependent process. Healing takes time, and there is no way to speed it up.

## For Whom?

One of the first questions we need to ask ourselves is, "For whom are we taking this journey?" That is to say, Why do we want to talk to our children? Is it for someone other than ourselves?

Are we feeling compelled, pressured or shamed by our partner, by one of our siblings, by one of our children, by a friend, by our therapist, by our church or by other members of a self-help group to which we belong? Have we recently watched a talk show on television and felt shame because other people on the show have been able to talk with their children and we have not yet talked with ours? It's particularly important that we look at our motives, because talking to our children for inappropriate reasons will generate more harm than simply saying nothing.

## Why Now?

When our children give us a self-help book that details how we ruined their lives, we do not say, "Thank you for sharing."

In a similar manner, when we have been exposed to a talk show, read a book or heard recovering parents in a co-dependency group talk about making amends to their children, we may feel a sense of urgency and excitement about correcting harm done with our children. If our children are not yet ready to hear from us, we cannot expect that our children will say, "Thank you for sharing." Our children, as a matter of fact, may react to our premature disclosure of regret and remorse in a number of ways.

Some of our children will look at us with blank stares, as if to ask, "What are you talking about?"

Others will anxiously reassure us that we were wonderful parents. Their inner loyal child will be compelled to jump in to quell our anxiety, to quell their own anxiety.

Others may respond as though we were being controlling, meddling and manipulative. They may feel we are again being overprotective and giving them the message that they are not capable of running their own lives.

If we try to talk with our children before they are ready, and before we are ready, we may inadvertently give our children a "Don't talk" message. The degree of our discomfort and anxiety may be sufficient for them to deduce that this is to be a one-time conversation. Surely we will never want to have this conversation again. And certainly they will never want to have this conversation again. Although our intention is to open the door and dialogue with our children, the effect is to shut down communication rather than open it up.

---

## EXERCISE

Take a moment to write your answer to each of the following questions.

Why are you doing this? _____

For whom are you doing this? _____

Whose needs are you meeting in doing this? _____

Why are you doing this now? _____

Are you and your children ready for this conversation now?

_____

---

## Boundaries

Before we begin our conversation, we may want to think about boundaries and boundary-setting procedures discussed in the previous chapter. We may want to agree upon specific boundaries with our children.

If our children are at the beginning of their child's journey, feeling that horrible mixture of love and hate toward us, establishing boundaries may protect our children from abusing us. This is both to our advantage and to our children's advantage. On the one hand, our children may be very angry and want to beat us up psychologically, but on the other hand, they will also feel guilty and find it intolerable if they actually do so.

In order to establish boundaries that will protect both us and our children, we may want to arrange to have our therapist, or one of our children's therapists, or both therapists, present. We may want a therapist present who has no established therapeutic relationship with any of us. A third person, who is trained to aid clear communication and to stop abusive behavior, can make all the difference.

## Our Worst Fantasy

What is our worst scenario of what will happen when we talk with our children? If we analyze our worst fears and share them with our support people, we may find they are truly unlikely; or we may be able to take steps to prevent them from occurring.

Perhaps in our worst fantasy we would be confronted by all of our children at once and be terrorized by this "lynch mob." Perhaps in our worst-case scenario we would accompany our children to a treatment facility or therapist and then be shamed and judged for our inadequacies by a stranger.

We need to remember that we have something to say about where we meet and with whom we meet. We can bring a support person into a meeting with our children, or we can ask to meet with each of our children individually before meeting as a group. We can talk to our friends about their experiences in therapy and get referrals to therapists they trust. We can try meeting with a therapist and stop the session if it doesn't feel right.

Many of us imagine that a conversation with our children will be like a nuclear blast that will strip the meat from our bones. While I advocate setting boundaries so that the exchange between us and our children will be respectful, the reality may be that only a nuclear blast will get our attention and get us to take our children's pain seriously. Although I am not recommending that we foster a screaming confrontation, I am recommending that even if our children blow up, we take some time to look for the grains of truth in what they are saying. If we have practiced boundary-setting, we know we can stop the conversation or take a time out whenever we choose.

Even when ideal conditions are met, we may still have terrifying fears about what our children wish to hold us accountable for. These fears are usually based on the things about which we feel the most guilt, the most remorse and the most regret.

After years of working with families as a therapist, I can say that our children's complaints will most likely be about things very different from what we feel bad about. Often we will discover that they don't even remember the things we feel most remorseful about. At the same time, we may be surprised at the slights and hurts our children have harbored and have never talked to us about.

One of our fears may be that we will be abandoned by our children. Or we may fear that, in the face of too much stridency from our children, we will abandon them.

If these are our worst nightmares, it's useful to think about what we know about our ability to tolerate a range of feelings. How well do we tolerate being on the receiving end of someone else's blame, anger, sadness, fear, hurt, rage or distortion of the facts as we understand them? How well do we tolerate our own feelings of helplessness, hopelessness and despair? During our conversation with our children, we may feel some or all of these feelings if it seems as though our children are rebuking us and discrediting the job we did as a parents.

Go back to Chapter 4, "Our Family Emotional Process," to look again at the range of emotions allowed in our family of origin and the communication skills modeled by our family or origin. If there are skills we would like to learn before we talk to our children, we can take some time to learn them first. We are less likely to abandon or be abandoned if we have strong communication skills and can handle a wide range of emotions.

It will also be useful to think about which feelings our children handle well and which feelings they don't handle well. What are the communication strengths and weaknesses of each child? Making a realistic assessment of ourselves and our children can calm some of our worst fears and encourage us to prepare ourselves with better skills and firm boundaries.

| EXERCISE |

Write your worst fantasies about talking with your children. Share each fear with at least one support person to check out how realistic or unrealistic it is. With your support person, list some ways you might (a) prevent the occurence of each fantasy and (b) stop the conversation if this worst-case scenario begins to happen.

Complete the following sentences:

I am most uncomfortable when my children express feelings of _____

_____

My best communication skills are _____

My weakest communication skills are _____

(You may have more skills to add to these two lists after you read the next chapter.)

I could improve my skills by _____

My children are most uncomfortable when I express feelings of _____

_____

My children's best communication skills are _____

My children's weakest communication skills are _____

I can maximize their strengths and prepare myself for their weaknesses by _____

## Where Are Our Children?

Several years ago in a seminar I was conducting, the mother of a 25-year-old daughter spoke with relief about how well her child had turned out. Her daughter was "over the hump." The mother no longer feared her daughter would someday rebuke her with a litany of her shortcomings as a parent.

A father in the group responded, "She hasn't done it yet!" He went on to tell how the warm, loving relationship between his daughter and himself had become strained and acrimonious, in her middle twenties, to the point of a complete breakdown in communication, which had continued for a number of years.

I can only speculate that the father's daughter had begun her child's journey. Although this process is a normal part of growing up and leaving home, it can be more than normally painful to the degree that the child's needs went unmet or were inappropriately met. It is also more painful to the degree that the child's pain and adamancy about harm done may be fueled by fervor in the ACoA movement or by an irresponsible therapist who has not completed his or her family-of-origin work and hence is acting out unfinished business through a client.

As a side note, for all the wonderful healing that has come out of the ACoA movement, it has had a down side, too, which is the parent-bashing atmosphere. Some of us have had the misfortune of being confronted by our children with "abuse" which we do not remember and/or did not commit. When we have been less than forthcoming with an admission of guilt, we may have been told we were very sick or in denial. Our children may have terminated their relationship with us until we sought treatment as prescribed and approved by them.

If such has been the case, first and foremost, we need to search our heart for any evidence that may confirm what our children have accused us of. Second, we need to consult other adults who have seen our behavior over the years to see if any of them can lend any credence to our children's accusations.

As parents, if we are not in touch with our own wounded inner child of the past, we will have little empathy for our children's wounds and we will not understand their need to take the child's journey. The greatest gift we can give our children is what we are doing right now — looking into the toolbox with which we started our parental journey, confronting the wounds of our own childhood and the remorse we feel about our parenting.

## Time Line For The Child's Journey

Although it is not unusual for our children's lenses on childhood to begin to change when they reach their late twenties or early thirties, their emotional emancipation can begin at any time after the early twenties. In the process, our children will confront both their internalized, distorted perceptions and their actual recollections of childhood experiences that were hurtful for them as children.

The child's journey is composed of a number of stages that may take from two to three years or longer for our adult children to complete. It's important to remember that not all of our adult children will feel compelled to take this journey, and those who don't are not necessarily in denial.

It's also important to remember that our incompetence or dysfunction were not the only adverse influences on our children. A host of variables determine how family life affects children, including gender, birth order, inborn temperament, what we projected onto them, etc. Some of our children were enmeshed with us and were more affected by our unfinished emotional business than others. In any case, the environment around them only accounts for 50 percent of their personality; their inborn qualities account for the other 50 percent.

At stage one in the child's journey, our children confront the problems in their lives — addictions, depression, etc. — and acknowledge that some of this pain is a result of early childhood experiences with us. At this stage, many of their realizations are on an intellectual level. They think about their past; they figure out the patterns in their lives.

Alice Miller writes, in *The Drama Of The Gifted Child*, that developmental loss is to be mourned, not blamed. Nevertheless, the first stage in the child's journey, appropriately, is blame. Our children move out of their loyal child position, where they were protecting us by blaming themselves for their problems, and shift the blame from themselves to us.

Blame serves an important function, whether it is our children who are blaming us or we who are blaming ourselves. It is intolerable for us, as humans, to feel powerless and helpless. If someone is to blame, we have a defense against feeling the capriciousness of life and feel that someone can do something about what is wrong.

As our children begin to blame us, they want what David Freeman calls "change by cooperation." According to his experience, reported in *Multigenerational Family Therapy*, they make their wellbeing and healing contingent upon our agreement with their list of believed harm done and with reality as they perceive it.

When our children reach stage two, they begin to feel the feelings associated with their childhood losses and wounds. When they were little, like all children, they repressed many of their negative feelings because their loyal inner child required that they feel neither too angry at us nor too hurt by us. They may have had letter-perfect recall of their childhood but been totally divorced from any feelings associated with it. At stage two, many of these disavowed feelings begin to emerge. Often most disconcertingly for our children, they don't have letter-perfect recall, and some of their feelings emerge disconnected from specific memories.

As our children start to feel their anger, sadness and fear, they realize they will need more support for this journey than they had expected. During stage three, they construct an emotional net of support people to provide them safety as they change their lenses on the past. Within stage three, they may choose to disengage from us temporarily as they construct new internal and external boundaries.

*Temporarily* is different for each adult child. For some adult children, it may encompass weeks or months, and for others, years.

Hopefully our children are creating a timeout rather than a cutoff of their relationship with us. Hopefully our children aspire to a different, better and more healed relationship with us.

It is necessary, both for us and for our children, that they have a safety net of people to support them.

Stage four in the child's journey is the stage wherein our children mourn what was that should not have been and what was not that should have been. As parents, we will be experiencing a parallel mourning process. We will grieve over our lost opportunities; we will grieve over our inability to go back and apply then what we know now.

When our children are in stage four, they will often be quite emotionally reactive. They may confront us in person or by letter with the "abuse" they experienced at our hands.

For them to heal, they must stand up for their wounded inner child. For them to heal, they must stand in their truth. The most difficult part of this stage for us, as parents, is to remember that their truth is not *the* truth. It is only *their* truth, and it must be witnessed and honored as such.

At stage four, it is helpful to remember that much of our children's emotional adamancy and volatility is not just a reaction to the list of hurts they feel we're guilty of. It is also a reaction to the terror their inner child of five or seven or eleven feels when confronting the all-powerful, 25-foot, 600-pound giant we were experienced as being when our children were small.

Understanding the reasons behind their intense emotions does not mean we have to stand and be stripped bare by their nuclear blasts. We still need to set boundaries and expect them to do their intense emotional work elsewhere. In fact, up to this point, most of our children's work should have been done with surrogate parents: friends, siblings, therapists.

When they reach stage five, they will be ready to deal with us directly as separate adults. They will have beliefs, values and lives of their own. They will feel their power as adults. They will have moved from being reactive to being response able, and they will confront us more from the position of being equal adults than from the position of being frightened children.

They will set new limits with us about how they will or won't relate to us and how they will or won't allow us to relate to them. For instance, if our children feel we have used them in an emotionally inappropriate way by telling them our troubles and by inadvertently making them feel responsible for our lives, they may set a limit with us. They may say they won't listen to our troubles any more, and they may ask us to take our feelings to an adult of our own generation. If they have a no-smoking rule in their house, they may ask us to smoke outside just as all their other visitors do. A new relationship emerges between us with different rules.

## EXERCISE

Where do you think your children are in their child's journeys? Using their initials, plot them on the following scale.

## STAGES OF THE CHILD'S JOURNEY

| 1 | 2 | 3 | 4 | 5 |
|---|---|---|---|---|

## Letting Go

One of the most important things I can say to you in this entire book is that the child's journey our children must take has its own time line and can only be determined by our children and what their emotional, psychological and spiritual needs are. It is their prerogative to establish the time line for their own healing and to heal in their own way.

For instance, when we began our own inner child's journey and found that our siblings did not view the family in the same way we did, it may not have occurred to us that our siblings may have had an experience in our family completely different from ours. Instead, we may have decided that they were in denial; we were in recovery, and we were right.

The same may happen when we, in our parental co-dependency, offer our children self-help books, therapy and self-help conferences, and our children refuse. We can make the error of assuming that our children are so badly wounded that they are in denial, and we may redouble our efforts to heal them.

In fact, one of two things may be true: First, they simply may not be ready to take their own journey.

Second, since not all children are equally affected by a dysfunctional family, no matter how dysfunctional it is, they may have been less adversely affected than we may have expected. Those children who were less enmeshed with the pain in the family may not take the child's journey at all, or they may take a version of the child's journey that is relatively watered down compared to what we think it should be. Their journey may be unrecognizable to us. They may make their journey through surrogate parents or through sources of which we are unaware.

The point is that the child's journey belongs to the child, not to us. All we genuinely have control over is our own healing. We can take our own parental journey, and then we can do what may seem like the hardest part — get on with our lives and wait for our children until they are ready for us. We can wait with other parents and share support with other parents.

One of the realities here, by the way, is that if we have made our own journey, our children may see the changes. If we are facing the challenges of midlife and creating our own identity, our children may see that we are getting on with our life, not simply waiting for them.

In getting on with our own life, we are no longer hovering, we are no longer hypervigilant about how our children are or are not doing. That is to say, we are no longer pursuing them for relationship.

One of the ironies of life is that whenever one person pursues another, the person who is being pursued has little choice but to distance himself. The more he does so, the more the other person pursues.

Parental co-dependency occurs when we pursue our children for their recovery and for ours. The minute we get on with our own life, not excluding or banishing or punishing our children but simply recognizing that ours is the only life we can pursue fruitfully, our children will look up at some point and say, "Where's Mom? Where's Dad? They are no longer hovering; they are no longer orchestrating; they are no longer gnashing their teeth or wringing their hands or looking anguished or guilty or angry."

At that point, our children may get curious and come looking for us. They wonder what we are up to, and a new kind of relationship between us can begin.

Some of our children may have felt that they had to help us sustain our life. We may, in fact, have asked them to be our cuddly teddy bears or to take care of us, or we may have asked them to share the mouthpiece of their oxygen tank with us so that we could buddy breathe.

If we have done enough of our own work at this point, we will have acquired our own oxygen tank and our own mouthpiece. We will also have acquired sufficient lateral support from our own generation to give up depending on our children to keep us alive, keep us happy, keep us sane, keep us out of the hospital or keep us from killing ourselves. This will free up our children to be curious about us without fearing their life energy will be usurped again.

Some of our children may feel as though they have been the pursuer in their relationship with us and that we have always been distant. We need to pause for a moment and ask ourselves, have we been distant? Have we been so withdrawn, self-involved, distracted or preoccupied with our own life and our own problems that our children's experience of us is one of unavailability and lack of interest?

If the answer is yes, then getting on with our own lives in the way just mentioned is going to look to our children like an acceleration of more of the same. We may, in fact, need to be the parent who begins to pursue.

By *pursuing*, I mean we need to touch base with our children periodically and express an interest in what they are doing. We need to be genuinely interested in being involved in what our children are involved in to the extent that our children want us to be. In so doing, we signal our availability and our interest, while at the same time we are respecting where they are in their journey.

## Are We Ready Enough?

We will never be "perfectly" ready to talk with our children. We will probably never have a flawless conversation with them or have totally contained reactions and godlike empathy. We are human; we will make mistakes. We will apologize and try again.

The question is, *Are we ready enough*? Have we taken enough of the parental journey to talk productively with our children?

First, have we taken the time to go back and inventory what we had in our parental tool box as we began this journey as a young parent? Do we know what helpful tools and what hurtful tools we brought to parenting? Do we know what tools we were missing? Have we developed some compassion for the young adult we were who attempted to parent with that set of tools?

Second, have we been able to put our parenting in its appropriate context setting up our time lines? Since each of us has a tendency to oscillate wildly between denial and profound, crushing self-blame, it is important to get more balanced by remembering what lateral supports we had available as young parents, what the cultural context was and what events in our extended family we were responding to.

Third, have we been able to do our grief work? Have we been able to acknowledge the reality of our losses and feel the feelings associated with those losses? Have we been able to mourn the things we regret doing or not doing so that our own feelings of grief will not overwhelm us or our children when we talk?

Fourth, have we taken stock both of what we feel remorse about and of what we feel proud of? We need to be clear about what we want to make amends for before we talk with our children, and we need to be balanced in our self-assessment.

It may be helpful at this point to get some reality checks from people who saw us parent. We may want to talk with our parents, our siblings, our aunts and uncles, our grandparents, our best friends or our next-door neighbors. We can ask people who were in some way intimately involved with us what they remember about us as a parent.

In asking for their input, we need to remember that there is sometimes a fine line between asking people to whitewash our past and asking people to tell us how they experienced us in our interactions with our children. We want to be wary of people who feel so protective toward us that they are willing to lie to us.

We are looking for people who love us, who are honest with us and who will neither magnify nor minimize the harm done. We are looking for people who have a sense of our strengths and our weaknesses.

Fifth, how much compassion have we acquired for the young parent we were? It is easy to blame and hate ourselves. It is much more difficult to forgive ourselves for harm done. Forgiving ourselves when we talk to our children gives them a role model that says, "You, too, can forgive both yourselves and other people."

Sixth, we need to take our temperature with regard to our reactiveness. Are we emotionally reactive to things that are still so painful and so unprocessed that we cannot move into our rational self, that we respond only out of our emotional, reactive self?

## Reactivity

If we forfeited our childhood by taking care of our parents, then forfeited our adulthood by taking care of our children in a co-dependent way, we may have two sets of underlying feelings.

First, we may feel defective, inadequate and unlovable. Our child self may reason that had we been lovable enough, our parents surely would have loved us without requiring that we take care of them.

Second, we may feel there should be some bonus paid to us for having given up our childhood and our adulthood for other people. We should get gratitude or recognition or appreciation.

When what we have wanted in exchange for our sacrifice is not forthcoming, our primitive childhood rage will be restimulated, and the defense that we have built against our underlying feelings of worthlessness and unlovability will no longer work. We will be reactive.

We may also become reactive because we compare our relationship with our parents when we were young adults to our adult children's relationship with us. If our parents would have seen us as impudent and ungrateful to have held them accountable for harm done, even though we had the same wounds our children have and the same longing for accountability that our children have, we may feel outrage that our children are doing with us what was forbidden for us to do with our own parents.

To take our reactiveness temperature, we can listen to our tone of voice. Do we sound defensive when we talk about certain issues? We can notice the tension level in our body. Do we get knots or butterflies in our stomach when certain issues come up?

We need to know which issues we feel reactive/defensive about and which ones we can discuss calmly. We can draw appropriate boundaries around the issues we are not ready to talk about and do more work on them. In so doing, we will protect both ourselves and our children from our reactivity.

Do we have a life? Have we confronted enough of our midlife tasks so that our children do not have to be concerned about our well-being. Do we have enough adults from our own generation who can fund our sense of "okayness" so that we don't have to use our children?

Finally, what lateral supports do we have available for this parent's journey? As we inventory our lateral supports, it is important to look at what function these individuals have in our life. It is possible for us to form collusive alliances with parents who are stuck in their own guilt and to use these alliances to white-wash the reality of our past with our children.

Do the people who are available to us collude with us in our denial? Do they play the game of "Aren't they awful" when we talk about our children? Or are they willing to stand shoulder to shoulder with us, willing to stand in their grief and shame as we stand in our grief and shame? Are they willing to help us inventory and look fearlessly at both the harm we've done and the good we've done?

It is helpful for us to have several kinds of supports. It is helpful to have a therapist, a support group, other parents who are healing the wounds between themselves and their children and any other adults who can be present for us and not get in our way while we feel and talk. We must be sure we have enough support before we talk with our children.

---

## EXERCISE

Mark an *M* for Myself on the following lines to show how much work you think you have completed on each task of the parent's journey listed below. Again, remember that these are just your best guesses.

**TOOLBOX ASSESSMENT**

---

Completely done                              Not at all done

**CONTEXT/TIME LINES**

---

Completely done                              Not at all done

**GRIEF WORK**

---

Completely done                              Not at all done

**TAKING STOCK**

---

Completely done                              Not at all done

## SELF-FORGIVENESS

| Completely done | Not at all done |
|---|---|

## EMOTIONAL READINESS

| Response able | Reactive |
|---|---|

## MIDLIFE TASKS

| Completely done | Not at all done |
|---|---|

## LATERAL SUPPORTS

| Enough | Not enough |
|---|---|

## Healing Our Wounds

Our unfinished business with our parents and siblings may be affecting our relationships with our children. To the extent that we can heal the wounds from our own past, we are less likely to act out our neediness, emotional unfinished business and shame-bound defenses against our sense of unlovability with our children.

For instance, maybe we have not spoken to our brother for years, but our children have maintained contact with him. The strain between ourselves and our children may, in part, be a function of our feeling that they have been disloyal for maintaining a relationship with someone we were angry with.

Would it now be possible to reopen the cutoff with our brother? We may be able to resolve some of the unfinished business with him so that the pressure of this generational problem does not affect our relationship with our children.

In a similar way, there may be work we could do with our parents that would help us in this work with our children. Let's say we have never been able to deal with our parents about our underlying feeling that no matter what we do, they never think it's the right thing to do. We may be willing now to deal with this issue with our parents to see if we can either come to some resolution or at least feel the relief of having acknowledged it.

If we can resolve this piece of unfinished business with our own parents, then when our children hold us accountable for harm done, our inner child will hear their complaints and be less likely to say, "I never do anything right. No matter how hard I try, I never do anything right." We will be less reactive.

---

## EXERCISE

Let me suggest another brief inventory here. Take three minutes to list what you feel is unfinished between yourself and your parents. Then take three more minutes to list what is unfinished between yourself and your siblings.

### UNFINISHED WITH PARENTS

_____     _____

_____     _____

_____     _____

### UNFINISHED WITH SIBLINGS

_____     _____

_____     _____

_____     _____

Now look at both lists. Put a star next to anything on either list that makes it more difficult for you to deal with your children. Circle the star by any item you are willing to try to resolve.

---

## Expectations

If we do our work and let our children know that we are ready to talk when they are ready, what do we expect will happen? Do we expect that they will immediately respond? What if we make an overture and it is never accepted? What if our children carry on their lives as if we had said nothing? Are we prepared to deal with this?

What can we expect if we do our work? Ideally, whether our children ever talk to us about the past or not, we can expect to go forward into the rest of our life with less remorse and regret. Even if our children never dialogue with us, we will be more at peace. We will carry into our own future less emotional unfinished business and therefore, we will be less likely to act out our emotional unfinished business through our children, our grandchildren or our partner.

---

## EXERCISE

Let's pause for a moment and do an honest appraisal. What did we hope for when we began this journey? If our hopes come true, what will the outcome be? If our hopes don't come true, what will the outcome be? How can we make this process useful whether or not anyone else cooperates with us?

---

## What We All Want

If we could talk successfully with our parents about our childhood wounds, what would we want from them? How would we like them to respond?

I suspect we would want what all human beings want. We would want to be seen and heard and witnessed by our parents. We would not want to be invalidated or shamed or told we were wrong. We would like them to validate whatever they could — we would like them to say, "Yes, I agree with you about this." And we would want them to say they were sorry.

I think of a woman who took her child to a doctor. The doctor said that a certain procedure would not be painful. However, when he performed the procedure, it was extremely painful for her child. She was enraged with the doctor for misleading her, but she didn't say a word about it.

Many months later, after having worked through her anger at herself for not having made the doctor stop, she confronted him. He immediately said, "You are absolutely right. I was wrong. My judgment was not good. I am sorry."

Her rage with this man vanished on the spot. It did not take away the hurt her child had experienced. It did not make her feel she could trust this doctor completely again. It did not take away her awareness that she had not protected her child appropriately. It did, however, take away her rage and her sense of having been wounded without acknowledgment. It also reinforced her sense of reality. It gave her a renewed commitment to trust her own judgment and to question authorities.

Our children want the same things from us that we would want from our parents. Our children want the same things from us that we would want from any other adult who had caused us harm, either consciously or unconsciously, deliberately or without intent. Our children want us to be respectful and to listen, to be accountable and to get our reactivity and our shame out of the way.

---
## EXERCISE
---

This exercise may give you some surprising insights into what your children may want from you. You can do this with your eyes closed as a meditation, or you can write out your answers.

Let yourself fantasize the perfect conversation with your parents about your childhood. This is just a fantasy, so you can let yourself imagine perfection you would not expect in real life.

Visualize where you are sitting; imagine what you might say. After you have spoken, see in your mind's eye the looks you would like to see on your parents' faces. Hear each phrase you would like to hear in just the tone of voice you would most like them to use. Watch them do exactly what you would like them to do. Receive the amends you most desire.

Take at least five minutes for this fantasy. Let yourself feel whatever feelings come up. You may find that there is healing in this exercise for your inner child, as well as information you can take to your conversation with your adult children.

## Being Confronted

There are many ways in which our children may confront us. They may confront us indirectly or directly, calmly or emotionally. They may confront us one-on-one or with siblings and extended family present.

Our children may confront us indirectly by using sarcasm or sniping to indicate they are angry and unhappy with us. In such instances, we may attempt to discern what the problem is and be told that nothing is wrong or that they are not ready yet to discuss what's wrong. At some level we may feel that we are being asked to read our children's minds.

We may be confronted by our children's taking a timeout or cutting off their relationship with us for a while. Particularly if our children are in therapy, this should be a planned disengagement rather than an impulsive cutoff.

Sometimes a cutoff will not occur in a dramatic way. Our relationship with our children will drift into what I have called a fixed-distance, perfunctory relationship. Our children may put more physical or emotional distance between us without saying why. They may slowly reduce the amount of telephone or letter contact they have with us.

Our children may confront us indirectly by letting us know that they talk about us in therapy. They may even report to us what their therapists allegedly think of us and our behavior.

Sometimes we don't understand the language that our children use, particularly if they are involved in the ACoA movement. They may speak a language out of 12-Step groups that sounds to us like psychobabble. Not knowing what their words mean may make us less prepared to meet with them.

Lastly, our children may not confront us directly, but may stay in therapy for what seems like forever. We experience their being in therapy as a rebuke for our inadequacy, but we can also experience it as an indirect message that they will need to talk to us at some point.

Some of our children will confront us in a direct and blaming way, holding us responsible for all of their life problems.

When we feel blamed, it's important to remember that blame is often a defense against realizing the capriciousness of the world and against feeling hopelessness and despair.

## The Letter

Here's a hypothetical letter one of our adult children might send to us when wanting to confront us directly. I've purposely made it a letter that would be difficult to respond to without being reactive.

---

Dear Dad,

I've been in treatment for three years dealing with your sexual abuse of me. My therapist says that I come from an incestuous family and that you made me your wife. Although I have no specific memories of your having touched me inappropriately, I have all of the symptoms of a sexual abuse survivor, and at the least I am an emotional incest survivor.

Since your behavior has been toxic and damaging to me, I am severing contact with you until you can demonstrate to me that you are in an approved sexual abuse treatment program, that your counselor feels you are no longer in denial about your illness and your behavior and that you are dealing with how profoundly you damaged my life.

Do not contact me until you verify your successful participation in sexual abuse treatment.

Your daughter,
Sue

---

We might have a whole host of reactions were we to receive such a letter from one of our children. Before we should even think of responding to our child, however, we should first ask ourselves, "What is my reaction? Do I feel shame, shock, hurt, dismay, rage, confusion, fear, puzzlement?" It is important to let ourselves feel the full range of our emotions rather than to suppress the negative parts of our reaction.

What do we want to do with our feelings? Do we want to lash out, punish, retaliate, deny, cringe, crawl, beg, bargain, confess, cry, scream, withdraw, become mute or go numb?

Whatever our immediate response is, it's important to *do nothing* directly with our child for a while. We need to wait, hold our tongue and digest what's been said.

I would even recommend that initially we not confirm any information with which we are confronted unless we are absolutely sure it's true and are relieved that it is out in the open. I suggest this for a number of reasons.

First, some of us, out of our feelings of guilt, will confess to things that we are not guilty of. For some of us it's simply a habit to accept whatever blame is laid on our doorstep. We may have a poor self-concept or a history that taught us to accept all blame. We may have difficulty with boundaries — knowing where we begin and end and where someone else begins and ends — so that our children's perceptions automatically become our own.

Second, even if what our child has written is true, we will need to take some time to work through our feelings. We will need time to consider thoughtfully what's been said before we will know fully how we want to respond.

During this time we can talk to another adult, preferably someone who is a parent, to help us process and clarify our own feelings. We can talk to our therapist, to our sponsor or to other support group members.

## Two Responses

If we fail to process our feelings before we respond, we may write a letter we later regret. Here's an example of a blaming, reactive response we might write if we feel our daughter's accusations are wrong:

---

Dear Sue,

You always were too sensitive. You always had your own unique, distorted way of processing reality. Your recent letter is a beautiful example.

I can see that you are still in therapy rather than growing up and taking responsibility for your life.

Your mother and I were good parents to you kids. You are the only one of our children who makes complaining about us a full-time job. Needless to say, we evidently no longer have a relationship.

No, I won't be going to "treatment." In the years to come, I want you to remember that you severed our relationship, not me.

Signed,
Your Dad

---

We may need to write many letters like this one to process our feelings. However, letters like this are called "not-to-send" letters. We can use them to get all of our feelings out in a safe manner. Then we can either throw the letters away or keep them in a private journal when we have finished. It is not helpful to send such letters.

A more helpful response to our daughter's letter might be the following:

---

Dear Sue,

I was stunned and dismayed by your recent letter, although I was grateful to know why our relationship has been strained and difficult for so long.

I don't understand exactly what it is that you are accusing me of having done that has been so harmful to you. You were not specific in your letter in a way that would be helpful to me in understanding what the charges against me are.

I am willing to discuss this with you when we are both ready, but your letter has basically cut off communication between us. You have given me an ultimatum and only one method by which I can respond if I am to have further contact with you.

I would like an opportunity to hear you out in a setting and under circumstances that provide each of us with appropriate safety and support. My hope is that at some point you will become willing to meet me halfway.

In the meantime, you can be assured that I will seek professional help in attempting to understand what I may have done that could be construed as "emotional incest."

I hope to hear from you again. I also hope to meet with you when you are ready to be more specific in your grievances against me, so we can see if there is some way I/we can heal this painful breach between us.

Lovingly,
Your father

---

In this letter we are expressing our feelings without being reactive. We don't label her or call her names; we stick with statements about how we feel.

We also state our needs: We need more information and an appropriate way to discuss the issues. We show our caring and respect by saying we intend to look into the accusations and to leave communication lines open.

## We're Ready

We have done our work. We've decided to talk with our children when they are ready. We don't expect ourselves to do it perfectly, but we are pretty confident we can do it in a responsive way rather than a reactive way.

# CHAPTER

# 16

# Listen Up — How To Talk With Our Children

I have said many times that healing is a process, not an event. Talking with our children about the past is also a process, not an event.

We may have several in-depth conversations with them in a month's time. We may have a series of short dialogues with them spread over years. We may exchange letters for years on the subject and have only one face-to-face conversation.

What's most important is that we should not convey to our children, either verbally or nonverbally, "I want to talk to you about the past once and once only." When we talk with our children, we want to open a door. We want them to know that when issues from the past surface for them, they can bring those issues to us for discussion.

369

## Beginning

Sometimes our children will initiate the first conversation about the past; sometimes we will. If we decide to initiate the conversation, we might do so in several ways.

We can tell our children that when they are ready to talk to us, we are ready to hear them. We can tell our children we would like to make some amends to them, and we would like to know when they are ready to hear them.

We may be able to use a misunderstanding or an argument between us and our children as an opportunity to open up the issue of what's wrong between us. We may say, "Let's talk about what's not being said in this argument. There seems to be more here than meets the eye."

We can point out our children's avoidant behavior — whatever they are doing to maintain a fixed-distance, perfunctory relationship with us. We can then tell them that when they are ready, we would like to repair the damage between us so that we can be closer.

When we are the one to initiate the first conversation, we need to recognize two things. First, although at some level our children will want such an overture from us, at another level they will feel threatened. Second, our children will have their own timetables for taking up our invitation and acting on it.

If our wish is to repair our relationship with them and to make amends, we must leave it to our children to decide when the conversation begins. Once we are ready, it is their readiness that needs to pipe the tune for this conversation.

## Listening

Once the conversation is initiated, the most important thing we can do is listen to our children. We need to hear them out without interrupting or justifying ourselves.

In order to listen well, we need to pay particular attention to the "stoppers" we have developed over the years that have served to intimidate our children or to throttle their feelings of pain and anger with us. We are using stoppers when we burst into tears or when we glare, look bored or impatient, or when we say something like, "You think *you* had it bad."

It is incumbent upon us, first, to be aware of our stoppers; second, not to engage in them; third, to stay present; and fourth, to listen to our children respectfully.

If we need to stop our children's confrontation because we feel unsafe, abused or provoked beyond our ability to maintain good emotional control, we need to ask for a timeout. We can resume later, preferably with a therapist, a minister, a sponsor or a trusted family friend present who can cool the situation down and keep it safe.

It's so important to remember that we are still powerful figures to our children, even if our power now is only the memory of us as the giants of their childhood. When our children confront us, they are at cross purposes with their loyal inner child, and they are taking the side, sometimes for the first time, of their wounded inner child. The level of their anger and adamancy is a manifestation of the degree of hurt they feel, the degree to which they long for repair and connection with us and the degree of terror they feel in confronting us, the giant whose love they feel they will lose or whose love they feel they have never been assured of.

## Not Defending

Our children need to be seen, heard and witnessed by us. They need to tell us their story.

As I said before, their story is *their* truth, it is not *the* truth. We do not need to defend ourselves against our children's accusations or give our side of the story to make sure they have the truth.

There is no absolute right or wrong. If we do not remember the situation the same way, it is not because our children are wrong or right. All experience is subjective. Someone's saying that something is so does not make it ultimately so. It is only a reporting of that person's subjective experience of the situation.

If we can, we need to treat our children's story as a gift. It is information that allows us to have access to our children's inner world of perception and emotional experience. Our children are giving us the gift of knowing how they took in a particular experience. It allows us to know in some measure why they feel as they do and why they view the world as they do.

## Abuse

What about children who are abusive? If our children seem to have endless rage and complaints, if they endlessly pass off responsibility for their present lives onto us and others, we will need to set some clear boundaries when we deal with their confrontation. If we, in fact, deeply harmed these children, allowing ourselves to be abused by them now will neither solve their problems nor repair the past.

When we feel guilty, it's easy to unconsciously encourage or allow others to savage us. It will be important for us to draw a line between hearing our children's grievances and setting ourselves up to be beaten up because of our own guilt.

Our highly dysfunctional children may feel like living indictments of us as a parent. And our self-indictment may be fueled by unrealistic cultural expectations of parenting that result in an inaccurate cultural assessment of parental responsibility.

However, even if we are totally responsible for a particular child's dysfunction, which is highly unlikely, the most we can do is come to terms with what we feel responsible for, forgive ourselves, make amends and create the most compassionate, loving and respectful relationship with our child that is possible under the circumstances. Our children's lives, for better or worse, now belong to them.

This, by the way, would be a good time for us to do some reality checks with lateral support people who not only knew us when we were parenting our children years ago but also know us as parents now. They can help us sort through what is happening between ourselves and our children.

If we have a particularly dysfunctional child we feel terribly responsible for having damaged and whom we have allowed to abuse us, we may be surprised when we ask our family for feedback. The entire family may say, "Oh, that's just Joyce. Everybody knows how Joyce is. She came out of the womb difficult/easily angered/spaced out/self-absorbed/pushy. We expect she will always be that way. There's never been anything anyone could do to get her to change." Even if we can't always see it, sometimes other people can see and acknowledge the 50 percent of our child's personality that comes from genes.

## Responding

After we listen, the next step is to *thank* our children for sharing — to thank them for being willing to trust us enough to tell us their truth.

Next we need to *validate* their reality. That is, we need to acknowledge the parts of their story that are also true for us. For instance, if we placed too much responsibility on our daughter and she says she feels her childhood was forfeited because of our demand for hyperresponsibility and pseudomaturity, it is important for us to tell her that we agree with her perceptions. It is our job to look for every grain of truth we can agree with.

Even if we don't remember something in precisely the same way, even if we interpret a situation differently, we need to see if we can step into our daughter's shoes and say, "I can understand how it would have seemed that way to you. I can see how you would have felt you needed to take care of me."

Next we *express our regret* for what we did, for how our behavior affected them, for the pain they experienced. It's essential here to stay out of justifying, explaining or rationalizing our behavior. We need to be aware of our stoppers especially. If we move into maudlin self-pity or self-justification, we will be placing our need for emotional comfort before our children's need to be seen, heard and validated.

The hardest thing that we do here as parents is to *contain* — not stuff, but contain — our own feelings while we listen, validate and express our regret. We need to promise ourselves that we will process this experience with at least one of our adult support people later in order to release and work through our feelings about it. It is inappropriate for us to process our feelings about this experience with our children.

It is essential that we *be authentic*. We must not own what does not ring true for us or express regret unless it is genuine.

Our children are not the only ones who are feeling terror in this exchange. We are, too. In order to relieve our fear, we may be tempted simply to confess and get it over with.

We may be in shock or in a dissociative state. If our own childhood history was replete with trauma, we may have unconsciously learned to protect ourselves by "dissociating," that is, by "going away" emotionally and psychologically in the face of what feels threatening.

If such is the case, we can tell our children what is going on with us. We might say, "I might be in denial. Little or none of this rings true for me, but I believe it may be my problem rather than the validity of what you are saying. I will need to do some work on this and get back to you."

It is important that we be sure we are not stonewalling our children. Stonewalling happens when we don't want to deal with what they are saying, so we avoid the issue by being nonresponsive. We might need to say, "I would like to stay present, but my defense, in my own fear, is to go numb, and mute or to emotionally leave the room. I want to hear you, and I want to repair the hurt between us, but I need some time to process this and take it in. Can we talk again soon? In the meantime, I will get some help so that I can be more fully present for you in what you need me to understand."

As part of expressing our sorrow and our regret to our children, we need to *make amends* for what we feel bad about. It is important that we follow our children's lead on this. We can ask them whether they are ready to hear our amends. If they are ready, we can tell them that there are things we deeply regret for which we wish to stand accountable and for which we would like to make amends. We can say the words, "I'm sorry."

*I'm sorry* does not mean "I am a heinous, bad, awful person." *I'm sorry* means "I am sad. I wish it were possible to rewrite the past, but I can't. I am responsible. I am accountable to you, to myself and to God."

We make direct amends to our children when we are ready to make the amends, and when our children are willing and capable of receiving the amends. We do not make an amend when to do so would harm our children or some third party.

For instance, let's say that one of our children is the product of an affair but doesn't know it. To disclose to our child the secret that he or she is not our spouse's child does not involve only our child; it also involves our spouse and the biological father of our child.

Before we can disclose this information to our child, we will need to disclose and discuss it with both the biological father and with the man our child believes to be his or her father.

After that, the information should be disclosed to our child only if our child wants this information. We may prepare our child by saying, "There is a piece of information that I have withheld from you that is important and has an impact on your life, but I am hesitant to disclose this information because it may have a negative effect on you. Do you have sufficient lateral support in your life? Are you far enough along on your own child's journey to be ready for what may be disquieting information? If you are not, please tell me when and if you ever want this information made available to you."

The point is that it is our children's prerogative to decide whether or not to receive the information, and when to receive the information. Our own need to disclose, to relieve our conscience or to come clean is not sufficient reason to provide our children with information or amends. Our children's needs and situation determine what is to be shared, not our needs.

## Recompense

Our children wish for reunion with us. They may wish for a connection they have never had. Our children yearn for us to care about them — to see them, to hear them and to honor them for the unique beings they are. They also want recompense from us. Making recompense is part of making amends.

At this point in the healing process between us, it is important to find out from them what would help. What would make a difference in healing the relationship between us? What would serve as recompense?

A child whom we physically abused might ask us to pay for his or her therapy. Another child might want us to set aside time to talk about the past as it comes up.

In my experience as a therapist, the recompense most children want is for us to be genuinely remorseful about harm done, to be willing to hear them on an ongoing basis and to be willing to establish new footing for a relationship. Children who live with the terrible consequences of having been been sexually and physically abused are most likely to want us to pay for their treatment.

It is my belief that if we are able, and if we truly feel that our children are living daily with serious consequences of the harm we did, it is incumbent upon us to pay for this treatment. Although our children's lives now belong to them, our children are burdened by the experiences of the past engendered by us.

There are all kinds of less direct ways to offer recompense to our children as well. One way is to get ongoing help for ourselves. Again, remember that this reconciliation between ourselves and our children is a process, not an event. If we continue to heal and grow, we will be better prepared for each successive conversation.

We can offer recompense by being a better parent now. We can help our children with their children by baby-sitting, by giving them time off as a couple. We can do the considerate, supportive things for them as young parents that we longed for but didn't get when we were a young parent. We can be a truly superb lateral support person for them.

If we have grandchildren, we can also be a wonderful grandparent. Here we can use the 20/20 hindsight that we have gained from life experience and from our own recovery; we can be more loving to our grandchildren in the present than we were able to be to our own children in the past.

I must issue a warning here. We must follow our adult children's lead about what they feel is appropriate and inappropriate with their children. It is important that we do not undercut them or compete with them.

We will need to watch for our children's reactions to our grandparenting. Our children may feel anger or jealousy when they see their children get from us what they longed for and didn't get from us as children. If we notice negative reactions, we may be able to create some healing by saying, "I wish I had been able to do this for you" or "I wonder if it's hard for you to watch me play with Johnnie since I let my workaholism keep me from playing with you as a child."

Sometimes we will not be able to offer direct or indirect recompense to our children because they are not available to us. Sometimes they will not allow us to repair our relationship with them, or they are inaccessible because of death or mental impairment. In this case, we can make symbolic recompense. Symbolic recompense is a way of saying, "I'm sorry and I am making recompense, but I am doing it in the larger society rather than directly."

We might become involved in civic affairs that improve the quality of life for families, for parents and for children in the community. For instance, we might join a chapter of MADD (Mothers Against Drunk Driving), run for the school board, become a guardian *ad litem* and be a protective person to a child in a custody dispute. We might contribute money or food to the local fund for hungry families, volunteer at a mission for homeless families, take care of crack babies at a local hospital.

One father I know made monthly donations to a local rape crisis center. Another went back to school to become an expert on parenting skills so that he could offer classes to new parents.

In making symbolic recompense, we become one of what former President Bush called the "thousand points of light." We can make a difference in the world even if we feel we cannot make a difference with our own children.

When we offer recompense, we are not just healing our relationship with our children; we are healing ourselves. It is important for us to restore our own sense of self-respect, personal dignity and integrity. Our symbolic recompense can move us from a state of regret, remorse and despair to what Erik Erikson calls a state of ego integrity.

If we have ego integrity, we feel that our life has meaning. We can go into the late afternoon and the evening of our life with a sense that the positive in our life outbalances the negative.

We may ask, "Is there any end to this, or is this a life sentence of making recompense?" Each of us must decide what is a reasonable attempt to repair the past with our children. We can ask our lateral supports for advice, but in the end we alone must decide what is enough.

## Forgiveness

Forgiveness is the last step in the process. Depending upon our children's history with us, they may or may not be willing to forgive us or to take further steps in repairing their relationship with us.

Remember, this is a process not an event. Healing takes time. Our initial dialogue is just a beginning. Our children may not be ready to forgive us after the first, second or third conversation, but as we continue working on our own healing and on our relationship with them, forgiveness may come.

If they forgive us, if the bond between us is repaired or strengthened, this forgiveness is a gift. We cannot demand it. Whether or not they forgive us, it is essential that we forgive ourselves. We did, in fact, do the best we could at the world's hardest job.

If we were inadequate or damaging to our children, it is not inconsequential. We have been reading this book in an attempt to work through the regret and remorse that we feel. However, our remorse cannot be a life sentence. We are not to be sentenced to eternal damnation or prison, either for having been less than perfect or for having been terribly imperfect.

In some branches of the military, when a person is dishonorably discharged, he is stripped of his insignia. Then he marches between a double line of drummers who literally drum him out of the corps. It is a way of stating, "You are excluded, dishonored and no longer part of the group."

Society has a multitude of ways of drumming people out of the corps of humanity and very few ways of drumming people back in. It is essential that we find ways to drum ourselves back into the corps.

This has not been an era of forgiveness. Once upon a time society believed that if people went to prison, they had paid for their crimes. If people held themselves accountable and said they were sorry, they had paid for their errors.

The current climate of our society is much more focused on punishment than it is on forgiveness. Lack of forgiveness in the culture is one of the gaps that 12-Step groups try to fill. Twelve-Step groups not only attempt to help people recover and be accountable for harm done to themselves and others, but also offer avenues for forgiveness and a means to drum people back into the corps.

Some of the ideas behind 12-Step groups originated in the Protestant congregations in Europe. John Wesley, the founder of Methodism, would meet with small groups of people who would confess their sins to the group in strict confidentiality. They would be forgiven, and they would be brought back into the fold.

One root for the word religion is *ligare*, which means to bind with one's fellows and one's community. So *re-ligare*, or religion, therefore, acknowledges that humans will sin, will violate the precepts of their community and in so doing become alienated from themselves, from God and from their community.

If a religion or a society does not provide a way back, people will continue to be alienated and will continue to sin. So *ligare* is one way in which we can confess having fallen away, can re-embrace the precepts of our community, can repent, can be forgiven and can be taken back into the community.

## EXERCISE

You will need all the communication skills you can get when you talk to your children. I suggest you read books, take communication-skills classes and practice all the exercises you are given until you are comfortable with them. Write out conversations you imagine with your children, and have a support person look them over. Role-play conversations with your support people.

Practice in the mirror to see what your face is conveying as you talk. Tape record your practice sessions so you can hear what your tone of voice is conveying.

It may seem as though I am suggesting a lot of preparation for what may be only one conversation. The fact is, the communication skills you develop will be valuable in a wide range of situations. You will be amazed at how handy your new skills will be with your boss, your employees, your partner, even with your friends. After you have lived with these skills for a few years, you will wonder how you ever got along without them.

I have found two books to be particularly good at teaching communication skills: *Parent Effectiveness Training* by Thomas

Gordon and *Straight Talk* by Sherod Miller and others. They are listed among the references at the end of this book.

# CHAPTER

---

# 17

# Intergenerational Healing

N one of us stands alone in time. We are all held and shaped by a magnetic force field created by the generations before us. We add our pattern to the force field and pass it on to hold and shape the next generations. Usually we are oblivious to the effects of this intergenerational force field.

When Molly took her time lines back two more generations, for instance, she saw that the patterns of alcoholism and fundamentalist response to alcoholism in her family went back at least to the generation of her great-grandparents. With her own recovery through AA and therapy, she had faced much more than her own personal "bad habit" or a pattern modeled by her mom.

She had changed a powerful intergenerational rule that said, "This is how we deal with loss and pain and trauma."

Perhaps we have become curious about our grandparents and great-grandparents. The further back we can trace our family patterns, the clearer those patterns will become — the clearer it will become that in taking our parent's journey we are cleaning up pain and changing patterns that have traveled down generations.

At this point, it's time to congratulate ourselves for whatever amount of healing or change we have been able to bring to our intergenerational family system. It has taken all of us enormous courage simply to pick up this book. It has taken even more courage to do the work that this book has entailed.

During our journey together we have carried healing both up and down the generations. It's time to celebrate.

## Our Generation

The most important healing to celebrate is the healing in our own generation, within ourselves. Many of us were governed by guilt, remorse and regret. Hopefully, in reviewing our own history, we have been able to develop some self-forgiveness.

In the process of forgiving ourselves, we may have found ourselves feeling compassion for other members of our generation. Perhaps we have developed compassion for our siblings. Perhaps we have healed wounds in our relationships with other people who parented our children: our partner, spouse or ex-partners. Perhaps we have forgiven teachers or counselors who should have helped us, or our children. Certainly, if we have been members of a parents' support group, we have felt compassion for other parents of our generation who have had to face their own fears and their own children.

Every bit of compassion we have felt for other people has increased our ability to forgive ourselves. Every time we have forgiven someone, we have given our children a role model, and permission, for forgiving.

## The Future Generations: Our Children

If we have taken our parental journey, and if our children have taken their own child's journeys, we may now be able to celebrate the beginning of healing in our relationships with our children. We and our children have the possibility of becoming three-dimensional people to each other.

They can see us as real, live adult human beings who have interesting generational histories that formed us in the same way that they have interesting generational histories that formed them. We can see them as separate, emancipated adults who belong to themselves. All of us can let go of the expectations and demands that we make on each other as "parents" and as "children," and instead see each other for the unique human beings that we are.

Some of our children will continue to maintain distance in their relationships with us. They will continue to cling to their story of how it was, rather than to take the journey back in time to confront their pain, heal their wounds and move from an emotionally cut off position with us to a more potentially conflictual, but a more alive, relationship with us. For our children who cannot, for whatever reason, take the child's journey, we will continue to be one-dimensional figures called parents.

Whether or not our children take their own child's journey, we can heal our own side of the relationship. If we are allowed any contact with them at all, we can become better parents in the present than we were when they were small. We can be wiser and more mature lateral supports and consultants. We can be role models.

I think of the woman who came to see me in anguish about the lives of her adult children. She berated herself unmercifully for having been a horrible parent. She was sure her horrible parenting had caused the misery in her adult children's lives.

I asked her, "How many times did your own mother notice when you were having a difficult time as a young adult? How many times did she come by and offer to take the children for an afternoon or for a weekend? How many times did your mother notice when you and your husband needed couple time alone and offer to take the children so that you and your husband could work on some of the difficulties in your intimate relationship? How many times did your mother notice, let alone care, when your children were hungry or without appropriate clothing?"

384 • WE DID THE BEST WE COULD

The answer she gave to each question was, "Never." I suggested
to her that she was already being a better parent to her adult
children than her mother had been to her as an adult. Although
she couldn't go back and undo the harm she had done to her
children in their childhood, she had already changed the family
legacy for her daughters as adult women.

This woman's legacy from her family of origin had included
drug addiction, alcoholism, neglect, sexual abuse and physical
abuse. She herself had been an addicted and alcoholic parent and
had been neglectful; also, she felt that she had been emotionally
abusive, although not physically abusive.

There was no way she go could back in time and change the
past. The past was like a football game that had been played. The
score was in; the game was over. No matter how much regret she
had about the score, she could not go back and replay that game
and change that score. All she could do was take what she had
learned from that game and apply it in any subsequent game in
her life.

Over time she did, in fact, apply what she had learned in the
multiple recovery journeys she accomplished. She recovered from
alcoholism and drug addiction. She went back and did her child's
journey, dealing with the tremendous wounding she had experienced as a child. She completed the parent's journey — mourning and taking stock, forgiving herself and standing accountable
for the inadequacy of her own parenting. She stopped the transmission down the generations of substance abuse, neglectful behavior and emotionally abusive behavior. She stopped the transmission of the unconscious behaviors her ancestors had used to
cope with losses, anxiety and a lack of lateral supports.

Although she couldn't change her children's pasts, as an adult
woman she provided her grown daughters with a different kind
of role model. They could see that it was possible for a parent to
change. They could see that it was possible to recover from
addictions.

She could now give her children the most important ingredient
for their own healing: the reassurance that their mother's ne-
glectfulness and abusiveness had been about her and her own
unhealed history rather than about them.

## Future Generations: Our Grandchildren

Some of us have grandchildren but have been denied access to them. I have seen many clients over the years who have come to therapy specifically because of the deep anguish they feel over having been denied access to their grandchildren.

Our adult children may deny us access because they are taking their inner child's journey. They may be identifying themselves as abused and temporarily cutting off contact while their feelings and memories surface. From a therapist's point of view, I know that this is often a planned disengagement rather than a cutoff. It is sometimes in our children's best interests to sever or limit contact during the time they are in the greatest pain and are most reactive over their history.

Many of these adult children will reopen the cutoffs with us once their own wounds are healed. They will, hopefully, hold us accountable and then forge a new relationship with us.

Other adult children will not complete their child's journey. They will use our grandchildren as chess pieces in a game of retribution with us.

Sometimes the cutoff is motivated by a fear for their children's wellbeing. This would certainly be the case if we were still actively alcoholic, drug-addicted, emotionally or physically abusive, actively mentally ill, bitter, hateful, negative, critical or behaved in a sexually inappropriate or abusive manner.

If our children have terminated contact between us and our grandchildren, we have an opportunity to stop and ask ourselves, "What is it that I am being accused of? Am I guilty as charged? Am I an unsafe person for my grandchildren to be around? Do I need to seek extensive specialized help to heal my own wounds in order that I not wound my grandchildren as I have, in fact, wounded my children?"

Even if we are clearly "safe", our children may choose never to heal their relationship with us. They will decide that their "enemy" is also to be their children's "enemy." Our letters to our grandchildren may be intercepted. Our presents may be unwelcome. Our presence may be unwelcome or rejected.

If we have done our own work in the parent's journey, if we have done everything in our power to heal our relationship with our adult children and are quite sure that our relationship with our grandchildren is appropriate, the only option we may have available to us is to wait. Someday our adult children may complete their own healing and become willing to reopen the cutoff and provide us some access to our grandchildren.

We may not be able to have a relationship with our grandchildren until they themselves are adults and have the freedom and courage to be disloyal to their parents and open up a relationship with us. If such is the case, we may be able to give them some perspective on their family issues and their intergenerational inheritance when they are ready.

If we do have access to our grandchildren, we may be able to celebrate some changes in our relationship with them. We may be able to be better grandparents than we were parents.

I've mentioned before that when children have at least one person present for them who can truly see them and hear them and love them unconditionally, they are more resilient in the face of difficult life circumstances. We may have an adult child who is severely dysfunctional and who is not capable of being appropriately present to his or her children. We may be the one safe person in our grandchildren's lives. We may be the teddy-bear person who can make a difference in the lives of our grandchildren even if we cannot make a difference in the life of our child.

I cannot tell you how many times in therapy clients have said to me that the saving grace of their childhood was a grandparent who loved them unconditionally. Even though the grandparent could not completely rescue them from the situation or save their severely dysfunctional parent, that grandparent had made them, as children, feel loved and, to some degree, protected.

When clients are doing frightening work in therapy, I often ask them to evoke the memory of safe people or guardian angels of their past. The times a grandmother or grandfather has been called upon have been legion. These grandparents have been internalized as part of the safety net for children who have felt a paucity of safety with their own biological parents.

When we are grandparenting, it's particularly important that we ask ourselves these questions again and again: Are we meeting our own needs rather than our grandchildren's needs? Are we triangulating with our grandchildren and our children in a way that is potentially hostile and competitive?

When we have clearly examined our motivations, when we are sure we see our grandchildren for the unique little beings whom they are, when we are willing to be confronted by our own children with the grief or anger they feel as they see their children receive what they longed for as children and when we use that confrontation as an opportunity for healing, we are ready to be healing grandparents. We are ready to move the legacy of healing on to the next generation.

## The Past Generations

We have come to the time in our life that when the face looking back at us from the mirror is the face of our mother or our father. The older we become, the more we identify with our parents as parents, as people and as older adults.

Perhaps, at this point, we can take a moment to celebrate the changes that have occurred in our relationship with our own parents. Taking the parent's journey has most likely changed our relationship with our parents whether they are living or dead.

We may have had a few conversations about the past with our parents in the course of this healing journey. Maybe we have only imagined a conversation with them.

Perhaps the fact that our children's perceptions and ours have sometimes been different during this journey has made us curious about the memories of our own childhood. It may be that some of our "stories" are just stories — ways our unconscious explained certain feelings or events to us — just as sometimes our children's stories are just stories. Perhaps we have surmised, or discovered, that our parents have different, and equally valid, stories. Perhaps we have been able to hear from them the larger context of their lives and their parenting.

I will never forget something my mother once told me. We were talking about what it had been like for her to have children, and she said, "You know, no one ever tells you that when you have a baby, you're having a *baby*."

I looked at her with curiosity. She said again, "You know, you think you're just having a baby, but what you're really having is a *baby*."

I was still looking puzzled, so she went on. "My fantasies, at the age of twenty, were about having a baby doll, completely different from the reality of what it was like to be responsible for a child, to raise a child and to have a lifelong relationship with a child."

Hopefully, we have become curious in the course of this book to find out what it meant to our parents to have the *baby* that happened to be us. Perhaps we have become more curious about their hopes, fears and dreams for our family of origin. We may be curious about where those dreams came from and whether they were realized.

Many of our parents' dreams came down through the generations without our parents being consciously aware of them. In "Next Steps," which follows this chapter, I finish Molly's story by taking some parts of her time lines back to the era of her great-grandparents so that I can show the impact these earlier generations had on her and her family. I suggest, as a future exercise, that we do the same for our own families. These time lines can be invaluable for our own healing. They can also be invaluable visual aids when our children ask about the larger context of our lives.

## Anything Is Possible

At this point, our celebrations may be celebrations of beginnings. Perhaps we are *beginning* to learn self-forgiveness and to heal our relationship with ourselves. Perhaps we are beginning to heal our relationships with our parents and our children.

If we feel stalled at any point, either by the time it is taking our children to complete their own child's journey or by the time it is taking us to grieve or to complete any part of this process, let me remind us again that healing takes time. With time, anything is possible. No matter what kind of cutoff we are in with our parents or our children, there is always the possibility that eventually the situation will change.

Recently I was invited to conduct a workshop 35 miles away from the town where my stepfather lives, and I invited him to come see me work. Over the years, though my mother has attended many talks and workshops I have given, my stepfather has never had the opportunity.

He accepted my invitation and said he would arrive about midday. We had a delightful lunch together. When it was time for my part of the workshop, he said he would probably stay for only a few minutes and then have to leave for home. His wife has a terminal degenerative illness, and his having taken a half a day away from her bedside was a big deal for both of us.

As I began to give my talk, I glanced over at my stepfather and I immediately became choked up. The look on his face was one of pride. For whatever reason, I had not expected him to be proud of me.

I was delighted, surprised and emotionally very moved. I was feeling so intensely, in fact, that I began to wonder whether I would be able to complete my talk.

My topic was adult children of alcoholics as parents. When I came to the last ten minutes of the talk, I began telling the story of a young woman who had been at a workshop I had conducted recently on intergenerational healing.

The woman said her parents had divorced when she was in her mid twenties. She had blamed her father for the divorce and had felt very angry with him. He had tried to contact her every three or four months, asking her out to lunch, and each time she had rebuffed him. This had gone on for several years.

She began crying and said that she was so relieved that her father had neither attacked her nor withdrawn from her. He had just lovingly stayed present and kept asking her to lunch every now and then.

I looked down into the audience and saw that my stepdad was sobbing. Tears welled up in my eyes and I said to him, "I didn't realize it, Dad, but I'm telling our story."

I then looked at the audience and said, "I was very angry at my stepfather for leaving my mother because of her alcoholism. As a result, I did not speak to him or respond to any of his correspondence for ten years."

I turned back to my stepfather and said, "Thank you for not abandoning me. Thank you for sending me cards at Christmas and on birthdays, and for dropping me a note every now and then."

I told the audience the rest of the story. About five years ago my mother was so ill that she asked me and my brothers to come home because she thought she was dying. It became apparent to me that she needed several things.

First, she needed to know before she died that the three of us were getting along with one another. She had invited us home to finish our business with one another. Second, she needed us to tell her good-bye, and she needed to tell us good-bye.

Third, she needed me to know how much grief she carried about the rupture between me and my stepfather. She and my stepfather had made peace with one another long ago. I was the one who was still carrying anger toward him.

I looked down at my stepdad in the audience and continued: "As a result, I initiated contact with him, and we have built a better and better relationship with each passing year. Not until today did I realize that he did not abandon me or intrude on my life in a way that would push me further away. I am ever grateful that he did not go away."

At that point I invited my dad to come up and give the audience his perspective. The woman with whom I was co-leading held her breath. She wondered if there would be some revelation that I was not privy to that I would be aghast at having disclosed in front of an audience of more than 200 people. I was relatively sure I knew the whole story, so I was probably the least anxious person in the room.

My stepdad is 86 years old, wears double hearing aids, works out at the gym three times a week and still does sit-ups and push-ups every day. Although he is elderly and a little bitty peanut, he is still very vital and mentally and physically intact. He has always had tremendous presence in front of audiences.

He came up and took the microphone. He turned to me and said, "Lorie, can I tell them the story?"

With my consent, he told the audience, "My daughter was very, very angry at me for a long, long time. But she didn't know the whole story. There was a great deal that she did not know." He then went on to relate some of the factors involved in my parents' separation of which I had not been aware until he and I had healed the breach between us years later.

He encouraged people to not give up on trying to heal their relationships with their parents and their children. He said he wanted people to know that it is possible to reconcile.

There was probably not one dry eye in the room by the time he finished talking. He cried; I cried; the audience cried. At the end of his speech, the workshop was over and people lined up to give him a hug and to thank him.

I knew as I watched the workshop participants that they were hugging him as a role model and as a surrogate parent. They all hoped they could end up with the same kind of relationship with their parents and with their children some day.

He is a wonderful example of someone who did not give up. It takes incredible persistence, and a willingness to contain our own pain, to stay in contact for ten years with any human being who is consistently rejecting us, let alone one of our children.

I don't want to give the impression that a healing with our parents or with our children means that we all immediately go to heaven. About a week after this experience, I received a letter from my dad. I was excited as I opened the letter, thinking it would say something warm and affirming about this wonderful experience we had had together.

All it said was that he had enjoyed speaking to an audience with a microphone — and he asked whether I could possibly help him, at the age of 86, to develop a public speaking career. Thank God, I no longer need him to be perfect.

## Congratulations

We are the *last* generation of children who were raised under the rule that required us not to cry over spilt milk, not to hold our parents accountable. We are the *first* generation of parents with access to enough information and support to stop, in large numbers, passing down the pain and dysfunctional patterns of previous generations. No other generation on a worldwide scale has been given the chance, or the imperative, to heal our relationships with our children and our parents.

When we do the exercises in this book, when we talk with our children and our parents about our past, when we talk with other parents and start support groups, we do so as part of a worldwide movement. We are a piece of worldwide healing, as well as a piece of personal healing. Congratulations to us!

# NEXT STEPS

**For More Information**

Lorie Dwinell offers workshops, training and consultation both nationally and internationally on the following topics:

Parents of Adult Children/Parents in Recovery
Adult Child/Inner Child
Individual/Family Addiction Recovery
Sibling/Only-Child Issues
Grief Work/Trauma/Loss Resolution
Midlife Transitions/Adult Development Issues
Surviving the Effects of Abrupt Relationship Abandonment

She can be contacted in Seattle, Washington, at (206) 448-8832; or in Santa Fe, New Mexico, at the Enchanted Mesa Training Institute: (505) 299-2266, 856-1717.

## Support

Some of you may have read this book straight through without doing the exercises, either in order to get an overview or because you knew you didn't have enough support to do the exercises. If the latter is the case for you, your next step is to find or create the support you need.

You can ask friends if they would like to form a group that meets weekly to work on the exercises in the book. You can call counseling agencies or the local AA chapter in your area to see if there are groups you can join. You can invite a speaker to your area and ask all the participants, or specific people you meet there, if they would like to form a support group that continues to meet once the workshop is over.

You can call counseling agencies or ministers to find out which therapists in your area have the training and experience necessary to lead a group for parents. You can then ask those therapists to start a group or contract one of them to lead a group for yourself and your friends.

Once you commit yourself to finding or creating support, you will think of countless ways to do it. The first step, as always, is commitment. Commit yourself to a small step, perhaps making one call a day or one call a week. You can do almost anything, one step at a time.

## Completing The Picture

I mentioned in the last chapter that it will be helpful to extend your time lines to the generation of your great-grandparents. I'll show you why.

Let's look at Molly's life one last time. When Molly made time lines for her grandparents and her great-grandparents, she discovered part of the four-generational emotional force field within which she grew up.

Molly's great-grandfather was a chronic alcoholic in a dry, fundamentalist midwestern town. In those days the legitimate treater for alcohol addiction was the church. Someone who was alcohol-addicted was seen as a derelict and a person who had fallen away from God. The appropriate treatment for that individual was to "get right with God."

There was, of course, no Al-Anon for family members of actively addicted alcoholics in Molly's great-grandmother's day. Molly's great-grandmother used the only resource available to her at the time: the church. Molly's great-grandmother, feeling powerless, hopeless and ashamed of her husband's wayward behavior, would sit in the back room of the church and cry and pray and read the Bible. She became a fundamentalist.

Molly's grandmother, growing up in this pain-filled home, was not only a fundamentalist but also an alcohol-abstainer. She lived during the heyday of the Women's Christian Temperance Union, when Carry Nation, the great saloon buster, was active. Molly's grandmother was in her glory in such an environment. Her motto might have been, "Lips that touch liquor will never touch mine."

Since Molly's mother grew up in a fundamentalist, dry, alcohol-eschewing home and had a genetic disposition toward alcoholism, one could speculate what her response to such an environment might be. We know that individuals who develop alcoholism come disproportionately either from actively alcoholic homes or from homes in which there is a strong anti-alcohol bias, particularly when that bias is part of a religious prohibition.

Molly's mother, as we know, did not become alcoholic. In order to be loyal to her family belief system, she developed a pharmaceutical addiction instead. She was a modern woman.

During the time periods when she abstained from pharmaceuticals, her abstinence was a "fundamentalist sobriety." She returned to her fundamentalist beliefs; "Anyone who uses alcohol or any drug in any form is not welcome in this home" she conveyed.

Molly followed the family tradition of becoming a fundamentalist in her teens, but in spite of her conversion, she began drinking in late adolescence and developed alcoholism relatively quickly. A crisis in her faith, wherein she no longer believed that the church and religion were the answers to all her problems, occurred at the same time that her alcoholism worsened.

As the pendulum in Molly's family continued to swing between fundamentalism and alcoholism, one of Molly's brothers not only developed an active alcohol problem; he remained an active alcoholic while active in a fundamentalist church. When Molly looks down the four generations from her great-grandparents to her brother, she can see two for the price of one in her brother. Both fundamentalism and active alcoholism lived side by side within one generation in the same person until her brother recovered.

I'd like to make something clear here. In no way do I represent an antifundamentalist bias. In talking about the fundamentalism in Molly's family, I am being descriptive, not judgmental. Both the alcohol addiction and the fundamentalism were extremely important issues that traveled down the generations in tandem. Both exerted tremendous unconscious effects on each member of Molly's family system.

After Molly completed these extended time lines, she could see the tremendous impact the culture had had on her family through the decades. It is significant that Molly's grandmother came to young adulthood during prohibition, during the heyday of the Women's Christian Temperance Union and during the time when the church and psychodynamic psychological beliefs were wrestling for the souls of individuals in America. The historical time period gave a twist to what happened in Molly's family of origin around religion and alcohol addiction that is different from the twist today's historical period would give Molly's daughter were she to develop an alcohol problem.

Molly could also see that her ancestors were doing the best they could with what they had available to them at the time. They were struggling with addictions that were still a mystery to the culture and reaching for the only cures the culture could offer. She could feel not only her anger at the legacy she had had to overcome but also compassion and respect for her predecessors who had tried and failed to stop the transmission of alcoholism because of lack of support.

With her four-generation time line in her hand, Molly is ready to talk with her daughter when her daughter is ready. She can show her daughter the generational patterns she herself has tried to change, to which her daughter will be susceptible.

For instance, the rigidity of the fundamentalism in Molly's family and the destructiveness of the alcoholism in Molly's family were not gifts in any generation. When Molly talks with her daughter, she can talk about alcohol addiction as both a genetically mediated disorder to which her daughter may be disposed, and as an attempted solution to the unconscious pain that has come down through the generations from unmourned losses. Although alcohol was intended to relieve the pain, it has, instead, been one of the two major generators of pain throughout the history of the family.

Looking at the time lines together, Molly's daughter will be able to see that she has more choice about what she does with her pain than Molly, Molly's mother, Molly's grandmother or Molly's great-grandmother did. Psychological counseling, support groups, self-help books and a variety of spiritual approaches to her emotional problems are more refined and more available to her than they were to her predecessors.

## EXERCISE

At this point, I would like to encourage you to take out several sheets of paper and extend your original time lines back beyond your parents' generation. Gather together any information you can find about your grandparents and great-grandparents.

You may discover, as you may have discovered when you did your parents' time lines, that you have very little information about your grandparents and your great-grandparents. This may be the time to begin eliciting information from your parents, your aunts, uncles and any grandparents that are still living. You may even want to do some formal genealogical research through the library or through classes on genealogy, or through the extensive records maintained by the Mormon Church.

Were your ancestors native to this country or did they immigrate? If they immigrated, what was the impact immigration had on the generation that accomplished it and the generations that followed?

What patterns did each of your ancestors bring to your family from their cultural roots and from their attempts to blend their cultures within their marriages?

Remember to take into account what was going on in the culture. Notice what resources were available at the time to help your ancestors deal with addictions, unwanted pregnancies, disabilities. What were the norms of the time in relation to wife abuse, child abuse, child labor?

We do all this work, by the way, to discover the invisible four-generational force field within which we grew up and within which we still live. We have a better chance than our forebears did of healing, because we can scrutinize and process patterns that are conscious.

# NOTES

## Introduction

The 12 steps which Alcoholics Anonymous recommends to the alcoholic seeking to recover are as follows:

1. We admitted we were powerless over alcohol — that our lives had become unmanageable.
2. Came to believe that a Power greater than ourselves could restore us to sanity.
3. Made a decision to turn our will and our lives over to the care of God *as we understood Him.*
4. Made a searching and fearless inventory of ourselves.
5. Admitted to God, to ourselves and to another human being the exact nature of our wrongs.
6. Were entirely ready to have God remove all these defects of character.
7. Humbly asked Him to remove our shortcomings.
8. Made a list of all persons we had harmed, and became willing to make amends to them all.
9. Made direct amends to such people wherever possible, except when to do so would injure them or others.
10. Continued to take personal inventory and when we were wrong promptly admitted it.

11. Sought through prayer and meditation to improve our conscious contact with God *as we understood Him*, praying only for knowledge of His will for us and the power to carry that out.

12. Having had a spiritual awakening as the result of these steps, we tried to carry this message to alcoholics, and to practice these principles in all our affairs.

xviii     Milkman and Sunderwirth, p. 165.

xxi     The quote is from Stephanie Brown's presentation, "A Developmental Framework For Understanding The Adult Children of Alcoholics," at the Children of Alcoholics Conference, Los Angeles, California, 1983.

xxi     See Middelton-Moz and Dwinell, *After The Tears: Reclaiming The Personal Losses Of Childhood*, for the child's journey and the elements of grief resolution which are integral to this journey. Many of the ideas about the child's journey and recovery as a process are derived from *After the Tears.*

## Chapter 1

1     "Please don't shoot the piano player" is a paraphrase of a quote by Oscar Wilde: "Over the piano was printed a notice: Please don't shoot the pianist. He is doing his best." Wilde's quote is in John-Roger and Peter McWilliams, p. 354.

3     Campbell, pp. 8-9.

4     The description of the three child selves is from Nancy Whitaker-Emrich's presentation, "Healing The Lingering Resentments: Self-Forgiveness And Spiritual Principles In Family Of Origin Work With ACoA's," at the Seventh Annual Conference on Adult Children of Alcoholics and Others Who Identify, Bellevue, Washington, 1990.

## Chapter 2

16     "The Little Match Girl" allusion is taken from the story of the same name by Hans Christian Andersen.

## Chapter 3

22　"Family emotional process" is used here to refer to "what we do" rather than "what we say" and is different from Murray Bowen's concept of "nuclear family emotional process." Bowen's concept deals with how families handle levels of individual differentiation and anxiety levels by emotional distance, marital conflict, dysfunction in a spouse or the transmission of the problem to a child. For further elaboration on Bowen's point of view, see Murray Bowen, pp. 475-477.

23　Schutz, pp. 13-33. This entire chapter draws heavily on Schutz's work as elaborated in *The Interpersonal Underworld*.

24　Research cited by Carl and Sharon Leman Hollander during psychodrama training workshops, 1973-1977, Colorado Center for Psychodrama, Sociometry and Sociatry. See Sharon L. Leman, "Action Learning." See also Carl E. Hollander.

50　Throughout the book, several concepts related to the presence or absence of health in a family are derived from the work of Alan J. Hovestadt, William T. Anderson, Fred P. Piercy and Samuel W. Cochran, "A Family-of-Origin Scale."

## Chapter 4

54　For further discussion of triangulation, see Papero, pp. 49-51.

57　The quotation, "There's nothing wrong here; don't talk about it," comes from Stephanie Brown's presentation in 1983, op. cit.

65　For a perspective on light and heavy "control" talk and on direct versus indirect communication, see Miller, et al., pp. 29-37.

69　The concept of "relational nomads" comes from Bowen, p. 536.

73　The concept of "imperfect people in an imperfect world" is derived from Shauna Smith, p. 57.

76　The entire quote from Ecclesiastes 3:1-8 in the Bible is as follows:

*To every thing there is a season, and a time to every purpose under the heaven.*

*A time to be born, and a time to die; a time to plant, and a time to pluck up that which is planted;*

*A time to kill and a time to heal; a time to break down, and a time to build up;*

*A time to weep, and a time to laugh; a time to mourn, and a time to dance.*

*A time to cast away stones, and a time to gather stones together; a time to embrace, and a time to refrain from embracing;*

*A time to get, and a time to lose; a time to keep, and a time to cast away;*

*A time to rend, and a time to sow; a time to keep silent, and a time to speak;*

*A time to love, and a time to hate; a time of war, and a time of peace.*

77      The concept of "multigenerational shock waves" comes from Bowen, p. 506.

86      "Are we allowed to prioritize ourselves before our family of origin?" is derived from the work of James Framo, "The Integration Of Marital Therapy With Sessions With Family Of Origin" in Alan S. Gurman and David P. Kniskern, editors, p. 139.

## Chapter 5

92      For an elaboration on the concept of role and division of labor, especially in dysfunctional families, see the books by Claudia Black, Virginia Satir and Sharon Wegscheider-Cruse.

93      Rosalie Cruise Jesse "Children Of Alcoholics: Their Sibling World," in Michael D. Kahn and Karen Gail Lewis, editors, cites on p. 247 that all children in an alcoholic home need help, but that youngest and middle latency-age children are most likely to be referred for professional help. Kevin Leman, pp. 77-78, cites that adult middle children are the last to seek help from counselors. Firstborn

professionals and last borns are more likely to seek help, although Leman does not factor in alcoholic homes as a variable, as does Jesse.

94      "Squeezed from the bottom and squeezed from the top" is a concept developed by Leman, p. 74.

96      For an explication of gender and role compatibility in marital/partnered relationships, see Walter Toman, "Basics of Family Structure And Sibling Position," in Michael D. Kahn and Karen Gail Lewis, editors, pp. 45-65.

100     For more information about resiliency, see Summar, pp. 10-13.

102     For a discussion of sibling sexuality and incest, see Stephen P. Bank and Michael D. Kahn, p. 170.

## Chapter 6

105     The title for this chapter and the one that follows is taken from the song "O Little Town Of Bethlehem" written by Lewis Henry Redner and Phillips Brooks.

105     I am indebted to David Freeman for increasing our understanding of individual behavior by putting it into the perspective of a three-generational emotional field. Dr. Freeman's work has helped me clarify the presentation of my concepts in both this chapter and the chapter which follows.

106     For more information on Resonance, see William Bridges, pp. 66-68.

107     For more information on identical twin studies, see Loehlin, pp. 1285-1292.

113     For more about the unconscious pull of birth order position as manifested by teachers with students, see Toman, "Basics Of Family Structure And Sibling Position," in Michael D. Kahn and Karen Gail Lewis, pp. 57-58.

114     "Crown prince" is a term used by Kevin Leman to describe the pressure felt especially by firstborn males.

## Chapter 7

119     "Unfinished business" and the concept "You can't give what you didn't get" are both elaborated on by David Freeman, pp. 30-55.

120     The role of major generational losses which can't be processed and have a reverberating effect throughout the family system are themes elaborated on by David Freeman, p. 53, and Murray Bowen, p. 506.

120     The "Life is difficult" quote comes from M. Scott Peck, p. 15.

134     For more on sibling de-identification, see Bank and Kahn, pp. 224-227.

145     For an especially helpful discussion of empathic attunement, see the works by Rosalie Cruise Jesse, especially *Healing The Hurt: Rebuilding Relationships With Children*, p. 126.

146     For an elaboration of childhood developmental needs for merging, mirroring, idealizing, an alter ego and a benignly adversarial attachment figure, see Wolf, pp. 124-135.

## Chapter 8

156     The concept of horizontal and vertical vectors was developed by Elizabeth A. Carter and Monica McGoldrick, p. 10.

158     I am indebted to the *Chronicle of America*, Chronicle Publications, Mt. Kisco, New York, NY, for the "cultural timeline."

170     The concept that the most pronounced effects occur with the first events comes from Kenneth G. Terkelson, in Carter and McGoldrick, p. 41.

179     The concept that life cycle events are more traumatic if they occur off-cycle is from Bernice Neugarten in *The Counseling Psychologist*, 1976, Vol. I, p. 6.

180     The reference comes from the workshop by Claudia Black, Ph.D., "Healthy Families: Healing The Legacies Of Shame," sponsored by Solutions, Inc., Temecula, California, October 3, 1992.

180     I am indebted to Rosalie Cruise Jesse for the concept of restimulation of the child self and the wounded child as a result of the unfinished emotional business reverberating from childhood into adulthood and parenting. See the works of Rosalie Cruise Jesse, especially *Children In Recovery: Healing The Parent-Child Relationship In Alcohol/Addicted Families*.

## Chapter 9

183    For an updated presentation of the stages of the family life-cycle, see Joy K. Rice and David G. Rice, pp. 80-91.

185    For an explication of adult stages of development and the tasks of each stage, see Roger Gould.

188    See Jesse, *Children In Recovery*, p. 10, for a discussion of the restimulation of the child self and the wounded inner child.

190    "Thank God And Greyhound" words and music by Larry Kingston and Ed Nix, © 1970, Careers-BMG Music Publishing, Inc.

194    For a more complete understanding of the unconscious elements in coupling, see Harvil Hendrix.

209    For a more complete review of what Alcoholics Anonymous suggests see *Alcoholics Anonymous*, "Chapter 5, How It Works," pp. 58-71.

## Chapter 10

213    I dedicate my chapter to my exquisite daughter Jennifer and to her deceased father, in memoriam, who was the best father a child could ever have.

225    The concept of moving in the direction of the least pain comes from a series of support groups given by Elly Lindborg called, "Stepping Stones To Spiritual And Emotional Recovery," Seattle, Washington, 1987-88.

## Chapter 11

235    I express here my heartfelt thanks to the many great teachers of our time who influence my thinking. They are the pioneers of work in crisis intervention who recognized that grief in loss or in acknowledgement of long-felt loss is a crisis of the human spirit deserving attention and assistance.

    Norman L. Farberow, Elisabeth Kubler-Ross, Erich Lindemann, Karl A. Menninger, Edwin S. Shneidman — to name only a few — are men and women who have so influenced our thinking that their uses of crisis intervention in grief resolution have become simply common sense and standards of quality clinical training. As my own interests have moved over 25 years through issues of substance abuse, psychosocial responses to medical emergency, suicide prevention, and the processes of human mortality, their early work remains my solid foundation.

237    The Crisis Time Line was developed by Patsy Burnett Carter.

254    The Steps in Recovery graph was presented by Sydney and Suzanne Simon at a workshop called "The Dynamics of Forgiveness," April 26, 1991, Portland, Oregon. The same information, in a slightly different form, is in their book, *Forgiveness: How To Make Peace With Your Past And Get On With Your Life.*

## Chapter 12

257    The idea of digesting this a little at a time and sharing it with at least one other person is the essence of the grief resolution process.

258    The concept of having a vision for one's self and one's family infuses the work of David Freeman.

287    "Twelve Steps to Healing the Hurt", see Jesse, *Healing The Hurt: Rebuilding Relationships With Your Children,* pp.181-184.

## Chapter 13

289    The concept of our dilemma that we are our own worst judge and jury is derived from Tatelbaum, p. 159. The books by Rubin, Caplan, the Fourteenth Dalai Lama, Borysenko and Simon and Simon, which I have listed in the references, discuss forgiveness and self-forgiveness in depth.

289    I am particularly indebted to Theodore Isaac Rubin for many of the ideas in this chapter. To quote Rubin, "Despair is directly proportional to energy and substance used in service of self-hate. Emotional well-being and relational freedom from destructive inner turmoil are directly proportional to energy and substance used in the service of compassion," p. 5.

290     In my own life, I have been particularly grateful to Jack Fahey for his loving reminders that I need to "drop the rock."

290     Whitaker-Emrich, op. cit.

290     The stages of grief resolution include: (a) acknowledging the reality of the loss, (b) feeling our feelings, (c) acknowledging that that which is lost is gone for good and will never be again, (d) letting go, and (e) moving on. Step 3 in Whitaker-Emrich's Steps to Self-Forgiveness acknowledges that since grief is a socially facilitated process, we not only need to feel our feelings, we need to share them with and be witnessed by one other human being in order to resolve them.

291     Step 5, "We make amends to ourselves," follows the precepts of the 12 Steps of Alcoholics Anonymous and is part of the accountability/forgiveness/healing process.

294     The concept "fallible human being" was developed by Albert Ellis.

294     A "special status" belief is a belief which feeds our false self. It imbues us with the sense that our position is privileged and therefore not that of a fallible human being. It leads away from humility and toward grandiosity and false pride. See Rubin, pp. 138-141.

294     In June 1989, I was part of a plenary panel with Claudia Bepko, Claudia Black and JoAnn Krestan at the American Family Therapy Association Conference, Colorado Springs, Colorado. Our topic was "Adult Children Of Dysfunctional Families: A Social Movement." During the discussion period at the end of our presentation, an audience member wanted to know how we handled the issue of God and spirituality in our clinical work with adult children. JoAnn Krestan, in her superbly articulate way, stated that it was less important that our clients did or did not believe in God, and more important that they know that they were not God. For an elaboration of these ideas, see Bepko and Krestan.

298     There are several versions of the "Serenity Prayer." This version comes from *As Bill Sees It*, p. 20.

298     Rubin, p. 121, states: "Compassion is, ultimately, a state

of mind in which benevolence reigns supreme and in which a state of grace is established with ourselves. This state of grace is antithetical to the promotion of self-hate. In this state of grace loyalty to self, in all circumstances whatsoever, is a prime importance in the human hierarchy of values. Being responsible for ourselves and taking good care of ourselves without guilt or other forms of self-hate take precedence over all other activities." For an additional discussion of developing compassion for ourselves, see also Gerald G. May.

298    The concepts of "compassionate home" and "learning compassion toward the self" are central to the work of Whitaker-Emrich, op. cit.

## Chapter 14

308    For a further discussion of response ability, see Buffington.

314    See Mellody for more information on boundaries and co-dependency in general.

317    For further information on boundaries, see Woititz and Garner.

327    The information on forgiveness from the workshop is also presented on a tape by Rossman and Whitelight.

## Chapter 15

333    Thanks to Constance B. Huey who brainstormed ideas for this chapter with me.

334    See Bridges, pp. 28-56, for an elaboration of the change process within the context of life stages.

334    See Rhodes, pp. 301-311, for an explication of the tasks of each segment of adult life.

334    For a discussion of mid-life as both crisis and opportunity, and for an elaboration of the concept that unconscious childhood beliefs and unfinished business with our family of origin need to be addressed as part of growing up and becoming a separate self, see Gould, p. 307.

335    Bridges writes that existential psychologist James Bugental also refers to "the nevers," p. 44.

335      For a further discussion of being confronted with our limitations and with the reality of what is so, see Rice and Rice, p. 80.

335      See Bridges quoting Carl Jung on the issue of male substance/female substance in men and female substance/male substance in women at mid-life, p. 49.

336      See Gould for a further explication of the tasks of mid-life, including the opportunity/risk of reworking intimate relationships once children are launched, pp. 217-307.

336      For more discussion on divorce within the context of mid-life and the life cycle, see Gould, pp. 217-307, and Rice and Rice, pp. 70-104.

336      See Bridges for a model which explains and normalizes the disorientation felt at change points in our lives, pp. 90-110.

337      One of my favorite sayings is that mid-life feels like a balloon payment on a karmic debt.

338      For an elaboration of sibling-related issues at mid-life, see Bank and Kahn, and also Kahn and Lewis.

340      See Okimoto, *Boomerang Kids.*

342      See Erik H. Erikson's *"Eight Ages Of Man."* Stage seven is "generativity versus stagnation," and stage eight is "ego integrity versus despair," pp. 247-274.

350      For further explication of the concept that we will have little empathy for our children's wounds if we are not in touch with our own wounded inner child of the past, see Jesse, *Children in Recovery*, p. 214.

351      The "stages" model of the child's journey is an amalgam of several people's work: Bob Aylmer of Life Cycle in Newton, Massachusetts; Claudia Bepko and JoAnn Kreston, as presented in their workshop with Lorie Dwinell, "Adult Children: Two Treatment Approaches," at the Sixty-Fifth Annual Meeting of The American Orthopsychiatric Association, San Francisco, California, 1988; and Middelton-Moz and Dwinell, *After The Tears.*

351      See Alice Miller, pp. 56-57.

351      See Freeman, p. 274.

352    For a discussion of the defense of disavowal, see Jesse, *Children in Recovery*, pp. 208-209.

352    The concept of "planned disengagement" versus cutoff is a concept to which I was initially introduced by Claudia Bepko and JoAnn Krestan at a one-day institute that we co-taught called, "Adult Children of Alcoholics: Two Treatment Approaches," at the Sixty-Fifth Annual Meeting of The American Orthopsychiatric Association, San Francisco, California, 1988.

353    In family therapy, this limit-setting behavior is called "taking an 'I' position." It is the appropriate assertion of self in the emancipation/self-care process.

354    See Beattie for a more detailed discussion of the many manifestations of co-dependency.

360    For an excellent discussion of "shame-bound defenses" and respectful versus shame-bound family systems, see Fossum and Mason.

## Chapter 16

370    For the concept of "stoppers," I am indebted to Carol Allen and Pat Dunn, a gifted addictionologist/family therapy team who run workshops called Intensives. I heard them speak about stoppers at an Intensive they gave in Reno, Nevada, in January 1992.

371    As Gould points out, even if there has been no parental shortfall, i.e., even if we have loved our children with perfect parental empathy and understanding, the nature of being a child is such that our children ". . . will feel let down in some way and bear scars to prove it." p. 22.

372    Setting ourselves up to be beaten up because of our own guilt can take many forms. We can attract people who are harmful to us in some way; we can ask for "feedback" when the other person is likely to be abusive. Setting up these situations is a manifestation of our guilt and self-hate. It is particularly important that we not seek expiation of our guilt by inviting abuse rather than dialogue from our children. See Rubin, pp. 47-53, for examples of "dangerous situations" with a potential for self-hate.

374   See *Alcoholics Anonymous* for a model for making amends.

377   Erik Erikson discusses ego integrity, pp. 268-269.

379   See Nathan Hurvitz for a further discussion of *ligare*. To quote Hurvitz, "Re-ligion literally means a reconnection that can be achieved by confession and restitution. Through reconnection with his community one learns appropriate behavior and is encouraged to live it," p. 97.

## Chapter 17

386   "Safe people or guardian angels" are what I called "cookie people" in *After The Tears*. For those of you with eating disorders, this name can be changed to "teddy-bear people."

# REFERENCES

*Alcoholics Anonymous.* 1976. New York: Alcoholics Anonymous World Services.

Andersen, Hans Christian. 1987. *The Little Match Girl.* New York: G.P. Putnam's Sons.

Angel, Marc D. 1987. *The Orphaned Adult: Confronting The Death Of A Parent.* New York: Insight Books.

*As Bill Sees It: The AA Way Of Life . . . Selected Writings Of AA's Co-founder.* 1967. New York: Alcoholics Anonymous World Services.

Bank, Stephen P. and Michael D. Kahn. 1982. *The Sibling Bond.* New York: Basic Books.

Beattie, Melody. 1987. *Co-dependent No More: How To Stop Controlling Others And Start Caring For Yourself.* New York: Harper/Hazelden.

Beattie, Melody, ed. 1991. *A Reason To Live.* Wheaton, Illinois: Tyndale House Publishers.

Bepko, Claudia and JoAnn Krestan. 1985. *The Responsibility Trap: A Blueprint For Treating The Alcoholic Family.* New York: The Free Press.

Black, Claudia. 1982. *It Will Never Happen To Me.* Denver: M.A.C. Printing.

Borysenko, Joan. 1990. *Guilt Is The Teacher, Love Is The Solution.* New York: Warner Books.

Boszormenyi-Nagy, Ivan and Geraldine Spark. 1973. *Invisible Loyalties: Reciprocity In Intergeneration Family Therapy.* New York: Harper & Row.

Bowen, Murray. 1978. *Family Therapy In Clinical Practice*. Northvale, New Jersey: Jason Aronson.

Bridges, William. 1980. *Transitions: Making Sense Of Life's Changes*. Reading, Massachusetts: Addison-Wesley.

Buffington, Ted C. 1991. *Mindset: Response Ability, A New Attitude For Managing Change*. Carlsbad, California: Performance Press.

Campbell, Joseph. 1988. *The Power Of Myth*. New York: Doubleday.

Caplan, Paula J. 1989. *Don't Blame Mother: Mending The Mother-Daughter Relationship*. New York: Harper & Row.

Carter, Elizabeth A. and Monica McGoldrick. 1980. "The Family Life Cycle And Family Therapy: An Overview." In *The Family Life Cycle: A Framework For Family Therapy*. New York: Gardner Press.

*Chronicle of America*, Mt. Kisco, NY: Chronicle Publications, Inc.

Ellis, Albert. 1975. *A New Guide To Rational Living In An Irrational World*. Englewood Cliffs, New Jersey: Prentice Hall.

Erikson, Erik H. 1963. *Childhood And Society*. New York: W. W. Norton.

Forward, Susan. 1989. *Toxic Parents: Overcoming Their Hurtful Legacy And Reclaiming Your Life*. New York: Bantam Books.

Fossum, Merle A. and Marilyn J. Mason. 1986. *Facing Shame: Families In Recovery*. New York: W. W. Norton.

The Fourteenth Dalai Lama. 1988. *Kindness, Clarity & Insight*. Ithaca, New York: Snow Lion Publications.

Framo, James L. 1992. *Family Of Origin Therapy: An Intergenerational Approach*. New York: Brunner/Mazel.

Framo, James L. 1981. "The Integration Of Marital Therapy With Sessions With Family Of Origin." In *Handbook Of Family Therapy*, edited by Alan S. Gurman and David P. Kniskern. New York: Brunner/Mazel.

Freeman, David S. 1992. *Multigenerational Family Therapy*. New York: Haworth Press.

Gordon, Thomas. 1975. *Parent Effectiveness Training*. New York: New American Library.

Gould, Roger. 1978. *Transformations: Growth And Changes In Adult Life*. New York: Simon & Schuster.

Gurman, Alan S. and David P. Kniskern. 1981. *Handbook Of Family Therapy.* New York: Brunner/Mazel.

Hendrix, Harville. 1988. *Getting The Love You Want: A Guide For Couples.* New York: Henry Holt & Co.

Hollander, Carl E. 1978. "Psychodrama, Role Playing And Sociometry: Living And Learning Processes." In *Learning: Making Learning Environments More Effective,* edited by Dewayne Kurpius. Muncie, Indiana: Accelerated Development.

Hovestadt, Alan J.; William T. Anderson; Fred P. Piercy; and Samuel W. Cochran. 1985. "A Family-of-Origin Scale." *Journal Of Marital And Family Therapy.* 11:. 287-297.

Hurvitz, Nathan. 1974. "Peer Self-Help Psychotherapy Groups: Psychotherapy Without Psychotherapists." In *The Sociology Of Psychotherapy,* edited by Paul M. Rowan and Harrison M. Trice. New York: Jason Aronson.

Jesse, Rosalie Cruise. 1989. *Children In Recovery: Healing the Parent-Child Relationship In Alcohol/Addictive Families.* New York: W. W. Norton.

Jesse, Rosalie Cruise. 1990. *Healing The Hurt: Rebuilding Relationships With Your Children.* Minneapolis: Johnson Institute.

McWilliams, John-Roger and Peter. 1990. *You Can't Afford The Luxury Of A Negative Thought: A Book For People With Any Life-Threatening Illness — Including Life.* Los Angeles: Prelude Press.

Kahn, Michael D. and Karen Gail Lewis. 1988. *Siblings In Therapy: Life Span and Clinical Issues.* New York: W. W. Norton.

Kubler-Ross, Elisabeth. 1969. *On Death And Dying.* New York: Macmillan.

Leman, Kevin. 1985. *The Birth Order Book: Why You Are The Way You Are.* Old Tappan, New Jersey: Fleming H. Revell.

Leman, Sharon L. 1973. "Action Learning": *Sensorsheet.* A co-publication conceived by the Environmental Studies Project & Earthscience Teacher Preparation Project, funded via National Science Foundation; Boulder, Colorado: Newsletter No. 10. Revised by Sharon L. Hollander, 1976, for Colorado Center for Psychodrama, Sociometry and Sociatry; Englewood, Colorado.

Lerner, Harriet Goldhor. 1985. *The Dance Of Anger: A Woman's Guide To Changing The Patterns Of Intimate Relationships.* New York: Harper & Row.

Loehlin, John C. 1989. "Partitioning Environmental And Genetic Contributions To Behavioral Development." *The American Psychologist*, 44:, 1285.

May, Gerald G. 1988. *Addiction & Grace*. San Francisco: Harper & Row.

John, Roger and Peter McWilliams. 1990. *You Can't Afford The Luxury Of A Negative Thought: A Book For People With Any Life-Threatening Illness — Including Life*. Los Angeles: Prelude Press.

Mellody, Pia, with Andrea Wells Miller and Keith Miller. 1989. *Facing Co-dependency*. San Francisco: Harper & Row.

Middelton-Moz, Jane and Lorie Dwinell. 1986. *After The Tears: Reclaiming The Personal Losses Of Childhood*. Pompano Beach, Florida: Health Communications.

Milkman, Harvey and Stanley Sunderwirth. 1987. *Craving For Ecstacy: The Consciousness And Chemistry Of Escape*. New York: Lexington Books.

Miller, Alice. 1981. *The Drama Of The Gifted Child: How Narcissistic Parents Form And Deform The Emotional Lives Of Their Talented Children*. New York: Basic Books.

Miller, Sherod; Daniel Wackman; Elam Nunnally; Carol Saline. 1982. *Straight Talk*. New York: A Signet Book.

Neugarten, Bernice. 1976. "Adaptation And The Life Cycle." *Counseling Psychologist*. I:6.

Okimoto, Jean Davies. 1987. *Boomerang Kids*. Boston: Little, Brown.

Papero, Daniel V. 1990. *Bowen Family Systems Theory*. Boston: Allyn & Bacon.

Peck, M. Scott. 1978. *The Road Less Traveled: A New Psychology Of Love, Traditional Values And Spiritual Growth*. New York: A Touchstone Book.

Rhodes, S. L. 1977. "A Developmental Approach To The Life Cycle Of The Family." *Social Casework*. 58, 301-11.

Rice, Joy K. and David G. Rice. 1986. *Living Through Divorce: A Developmental Approach To Divorce Therapy*. New York: Guilford Press.

Rossman, Martin and Roxanne Whitelight. 1992. *Forgiveness And Healing*. Mill Valley, California: Academy for Guided Imagery. Audiotape.

Rubin, Theodore Isaac. 1975. *Compassion & Self-Hate: An Alternative To*

*Despair.* New York: Ballentine Books.

Satir, Virginia. 1972. *Peoplemaking.* Palo Alto, California: Science & Behavior Books.

Schutz, W. C. 1966. *The Interpersonal Underworld.* Palo Alto, California: Science & Behavior Books.

Simon, Sidney B. and Suzanne Simon. 1990. *Forgiveness: How To Make Peace With Your Past And Get On With Your Life.* New York: Warner Books.

Smith, Shauna L. 1991. *Making Peace With Your Adult Children.* New York: Plenum Press.

Summar, Polly. 1992. "The Resilient Ones: Rising Above Hard Times Isn't Easy, But It Can Be Done." Sage, *Albuquerque Journal Monthly Magazine For Women,* 4:, 10-13.

Tatelbaum, Judy. 1989. *You Don't Have To Suffer: A Handbook For Moving Beyond Life's Crises.* New York: Harper & Row.

Terkelsen, Kenneth G. 1980. "Toward A Theory Of The Family Life Cycle." *The Family Life Cycle: A Framework For Family Therapy,* edited by Elizabeth A. Carter and Monica McGoldrick. New York: Gardner Press.

Wegscheider-Cruse, Sharon. 1981. *Another Chance.* Palo Alto, California: Science & Behavior Books.

Woititz, Janet and Alan Garner. 1990. *Lifeskills For Adult Children.* Deerfield Beach, Florida: Health Communications.

Wolf, Ernest S. 1988. *Treating The Self: Elements Of Clinical Self-Psychology.* New York: Guildford Press.

# ABOUT THE AUTHORS

**Lorie Dwinell,** ACSW, is a psychiatric social worker, an addictionologist and an international trainer in the fields of Adult Children, grief and trauma, addictions, family recovery and women's issues. She divides her time between her private practice in Seattle, and her position as co-director of the Enchanted Mesa Training Institute in Santa Fe, New Mexico. She has been a specialist in the treatment of addictions for 26 years and involved in the Adult Child arena since 1977. She is co-author, with Jane Middelton-Moz, of *After The Tears: Reclaiming The Personal Losses Of Childhood.*

**Ruth Baetz,** MSW, is a psychotherapist in private practice in Seattle, and has specialized in therapy for women since 1978. She is also a ghostwriter, a writer and an editor.

**Patsy Burnett Carter,** ACSW, has had a private psychotherapy practice in Seattle since 1977, with a special emphasis on grief work and recovery from trauma and loss. Since 1968 she has studied and worked with people in crisis in the context of emergency medical care as well as with outreach trauma teams. She has taught crisis intervention at the University of Washington School of Social Work and now regularly teaches emergency personnel, in Medic I programs, how to help people suffering in acute grief.

**Constance B. Huey,** M.Ed., a psychotherapist has been in private practice for the past 13 years, specializing in inner child exploration, issues among siblings and reconciliation between parents and their adult children. She has also taught at the University of Washington and in the Addictions Program at Seattle University.

**Chandra Smith,** MSW, has been a director of alcohol and drug treatment programs in both Oregon and Washington. She is a writer, consultant and therapist on recovery and women's quality of life choices. She is the author of *Healing The Feminine.*